NEUROANATOMY
Text and Atlas

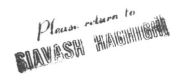

NEUROANATOMY
Text and Atlas

John H. Martin, Ph.D.

Center for Neurobiology & Behavior
Department of Psychiatry
College of Physicians & Surgeons
of Columbia University
New York

Medical photography by
Howard J. Radzyner, R.B.P., A.I.M.B.I., F.R.M.S.

Illustrated by
Michael E. Leonard, M.A., A.M.I.

Assisted by
Terese Winslow, M.A., A.M.I.

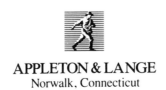

APPLETON & LANGE
Norwalk, Connecticut

93 94 95 96 97 / 10 9 8 7 6 5 4 3 2 1

Prentice Hall International (UK) Limited, *London*
Prentice Hall of Australia Pty. Limited, *Sydney*
Prentice Hall Canada, Inc., *Toronto*
Prentice Hall Hispanoamericana, S.A., *Mexico*
Prentice Hall of India Private Limited, *New Delhi*
Prentice Hall of Japan, Inc., *Tokyo*
Simon & Schuster Asia Pte. Ltd., *Singapore*
Editora Prentice Hall do Brasil Ltda., *Rio de Janeiro*
Prentice Hall, *Englewood Cliffs, New Jersey*

ISBN 0-8385-6691-X

Library of Congress Catalog Card Number: 92-055059

The magnetic resonance image used on the cover courtesy of Dr. Neal Rutledge, Department of Psychology, University of Texas at Austin.

Photographs © 1988 Howard J. Radzyner (unless otherwise credited)

PRINTED IN THE UNITED STATES OF AMERICA

To Carol
and our triumph of daughters,
Caitlin, Rachel, and Emma

Contents

12 General Organization of the Cranial Nerve Nuclei and the Trigeminal System 291

13 The Somatic and Visceral Motor Functions of the Cranial Nerves 321

Preface

Neuroanatomy has always played an important role in the health science curriculum, particularly as a means of preparing students for understanding the anatomical basis of clinical neurology. Recently, the development of high-resolution brain imaging techniques, magnetic resonance imaging, and positron emission tomography has created a new relevance for the study of human neuroanatomy. These techniques provide detailed information about the structure, chemistry, and function of the living brain. The physician can use these techniques to localize brain trauma with remarkable clarity. Even the particular brain regions where some neuroactive and psychoactive drugs may be acting to produce their effects can now be mapped. New brain imaging techniques equip the neuroscientist and clinician with an armamentarium for elucidating the localization of function in the human brain and for studying the biological substrates of disordered thought and behavior. Yet, even with these powerful tools in hand, to interpret the information obtained requires a high level of neuroanatomical competence.

An important goal of *Neuroanatomy: Text and Atlas* is to prepare the reader for interpreting this new wealth of images through the development of a fundamental understanding of the *anatomical basis of brain function*. To provide a workable focus, I have restricted this book to a treatment of the central nervous system, its gross structure, and component parts and their interconnections. I utilize a traditional approach to gaining neuroanatomical competence: the locations of brain structures are examined on two-dimensional *myelin-stained sections through the human central nervous system*. This approach is particularly pertinent because the basic imaging picture is also a two-dimensional section through the brain. In addition to myelin-stained sections, the three-dimensional configuration of brain structures is considered in order to increase the depth of neuroanatomical knowledge. Moreover, there is a greater consolidation of neuroanatomical information when the three-dimensional shape of brain structures is correlated with their locations on two-dimensional sections. Combined with this morphological approach, structure and function are also correlated to obtain an overall view of the spatial organization of functional neural systems.

Neuroanatomy: Text and Atlas is written as a companion to *Principles of Neural Science*, edited by Eric R. Kandel and James H. Schwartz (Elsevier). It is aimed at the graduate level, in particular at medical, dental, physical therapy, and other allied health science students. Designed as a self-study guide and resource for information on the structure and function of the human central nervous system, this book could serve as the text and atlas for an introductory laboratory course on human neuroanatomy.

Acknowledgments

I take this opportunity to acknowledge the help of many friends and colleagues. I am indebted to Susan Billings-Gagliardi, Bob McMasters, Jane Sargent, Jerome Sutin, and David Ruggiero for critically reading the manuscript. Their helpful suggestions proved to be invaluable in the preparation of the final manuscript. I would like to extend a special note of thanks to Claude Ghez and Eric Kandel for their support and encouragement during preparation of this book.

I am grateful to the Center for Neurobiology & Behavior of the College of Physicians & Surgeons for use of many of their excellent teaching materials. I also thank the Departments of Anatomy and Cell Biology, Neurology, and Pathology for use of histological materials. I thank my friends on the neuroanatomy teaching faculty at the College of Physicians & Surgeons for many helpful discussions. I was particularly fortunate to have had the opportunity to discuss many aspects of the teaching of neuroanatomy with Dr. Robert Payette, a gifted teacher and researcher, whose untimely death is felt by all who have had the occasion to work with him. I am grateful to Dr. Neal Rutledge for providing a wealth of superb neuroradiological material. In addition, the following friends and colleagues have kindly read portions of the manuscript or provided histological or radiological materials: David Amaral, Brian Boycott, Vincent Castelucci, Becky Craik, Michael Crutcher, Richard Defendini, Mahlon Delong, John Dowling, Ronald Dubner, Thomas Finger, Susan Folstein, Peter Fox, David Friedman, Claude Ghez, Alan Gibson, James Gordon, Peter Gouras, Suzanne Haber, Carol Hand, Wayne Hening, David Hubel, Thomas J. Imig, Michael Lehman, Marge Livingstone, Jane MacPherson, Ralph Norgren, Michael Potegal, Joseph L. Price, Carla Shatz, Ann-Judith Silverman, Celia Sladek, Larry Swanson, Roger Tootell, Terry Takahashi, Stanley Wiegand, and Torsten Wiesel.

I am greatly indebted to Sally Muir for reading, editing, and improving the clarity of much of the text. I would like to thank Jais Brennan for immeasurable help and encouragement, Lydia Kibiuk and Kathrin Hilten for help in preparing some of the art, and Erylin Riley for editorial assistance. I am grateful to Al Lamme and Bob Wooley for photographic assistance, and Pablo Garcia for preparation of the myelin-stained sections of the sacral spinal cord and visual cortex. I thank Christine Hastings and other members of the editorial staff and the design department at Elsevier for their assistance in the production of the book. I also thank Yale Altman for his encouragement and for maintaining a sense of humor throughout this endeavor. Lastly, a special note of gratitude and appreciation is extended to Susan Schmidler for all of her help and untiring patience in supervising the production of the art and for the book's extraordinary design and layout.

Introduction

Divided into three parts, this book first introduces the major concepts of central nervous system organization. Later chapters cover the functional neural systems, and appendices present an atlas of the surface anatomy of the brain and myelin-stained sections.

An overview of the general organization of the central nervous system and surface anatomy is presented in the first chapter. This material provides the background for the second chapter, where more complex aspects—in particular, the three-dimensional organization of brain structures—are presented from a developmental perspective. The functional organization of the central nervous system is surveyed in the third chapter. These three chapters are intended to provide a synthesis of the basic aspects of the functional architecture of the central nervous system and to establish a fundamental neuroanatomical vocabulary. The topic of the fourth chapter is the vasculature of the central nervous system. The study of vasculature is presented early in the book to enable integration of this information with later material on the functional organization of the central nervous system.

The remaining eleven chapters examine the major functional neural systems: sensory systems, motor systems, and the limbic system, a neural system that participates in learning, memory, and emotions. These chapters have a different organization from that of the introductory chapters. Each chapter on a particular neural system begins with a concise description of its functional organization. Here, neural circuits mediating specific sensory or motor functions are depicted in a standardized format. Representations of myelin-stained sections through selected levels of the spinal cord and brain stem are ordered in correct anatomical sequence with the neural circuit superimposed. Key features of the anatomy of the neural system are also considered in the first part of each chapter. The purpose of the first part of the chapter is to present an "overall view" of structure and function before getting down to the business of considering the detailed anatomical organization of the neural system, which is the focus of the latter part of each chapter. In keeping with the theme of the first part of the chapter, the relation between function and anatomy is emphasized in the latter part of the chapter. Here, myelin-stained sections are examined, usually in the sequence of the flow of information in the particular neural system. These sections are replicated in the atlas of myelin-stained sections. Since only the structures that are related to the particular neural system are identified in the chapters, the reader is encouraged to consult the atlas for more complete identification. To illustrate the close relation between anatomy and radiology, magnetic resonance imaging scans, positron emission tomography scans, and angiographs are included in many of the chapters.

This book has two appendices, which together are a reference of key anatomical structures. The first appendix is an atlas of the surface anatomy of the central nervous system. This is a collection of drawings that is based on specimens and brain models. Important features of the surface anatomy of the central nevous system are indicated. The second appendix is a complete photographic atlas of myelin-stained sections through the central nervous system in three anatomical planes. With few exceptions, I have chosen to use only the drawings and sections contained in the atlas for illustrating structure in the various chapters. In this way, the reader is better able to develop a thorough understanding of a limited (and complete) set of materials rather than to cope with anatomical variability.

NEUROANATOMY
Text and Atlas

Introduction to the Central Nervous System

1

Introduction to the Central Nervous System

The human nervous system carries out an enormous number of functions, and it does so by means of many subdivisions. Indeed, the complexity of the brain has traditionally made the study of neuroanatomy a notoriously demanding task. This task can be greatly simplified, however, by approaching the study of the nervous system from the dual perspectives of its functional and regional anatomy.

The functional approach considers sequentially those parts of the nervous system that work together to produce a behavior. It traces, for example, the route that sensory information travels from its origin in a sensory receptor, located at the periphery of the body, through the nervous system to the highest cognitive centers. There, a decision is made whether to ignore or to respond to the stimulus. A decision to respond will take the form of a motor command, which can then be traced down through the nervous system to its output on the appropriate skeletal muscles. An understanding of the anatomy falls into place more readily when it is tied to the functional interrelationships between various brain regions.

In contrast to functional neuroanatomy, the study of regional neuroanatomy focuses on the neighborhood relations of brain structures at any given level of the nervous system. Competence in understanding the regional anatomy of the brain facilitates clinical problem solving: determination of the site of a lesion on the basis of a constellation of behavioral signs. The traditional approach to the study of regional neuroanatomy has relied largely on the use of sections of the brain taken at different levels. A knowledge of the regional anatomy of the brain is essential to the clinician because damage to the brain is frequently not restricted to a single functional system. Structures that are functionally unrelated often lie next to one another, and damage of the sort caused by a stroke or tumor can affect a number of functional systems indiscriminately.

In this chapter, the organization and characteristic surface features of the nervous system are surveyed to establish a working knowledge of its structure and the vocabulary necessary to study its functional and regional organization. Later in the chapter we briefly consider techniques for examining the microscopic anatomy of the nervous system and functional anatomy of the human brain. In the next chapter, the development of the central nervous system will be considered, because a knowledge of its development can do much to clarify the complex anatomy of the mature brain. With this background, we will be in a good position to explore the functional organization of the central nervous system in the chapters that follow.

Neurons and Glia Are the Two Principal Cellular Constituents of the Nervous System

The nerve cell, or *neuron*, is the functional cellular unit of the nervous system. A major goal of neuroscience is to understand the myriad of complex functions of the nervous system in terms of the morphology, physiology, and biochemistry of neurons and their interconnections. Figure 1.1A illustrates a drawing of a neuron in the cerebral cortex, the brain region that mediates the most sophisticated aspects of human behavior, such as cognition, volition, and perception. This neuron was drawn by

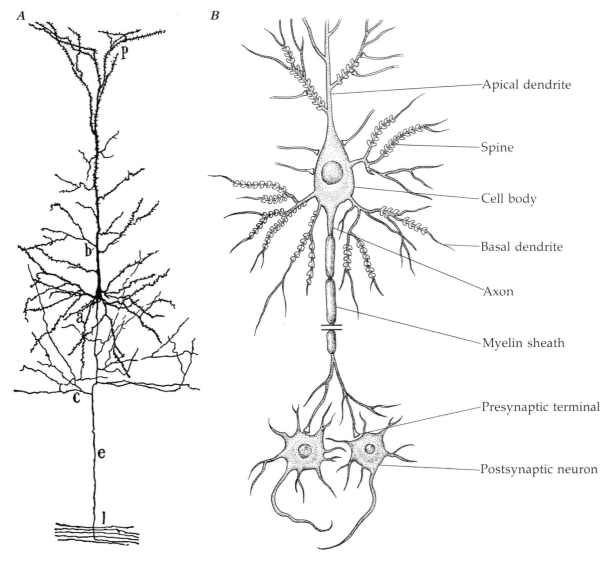

Figure 1.1 Pyramidal cells are the principal neurons of the cerebral cortex. **A.** Drawing of a pyramidal cell by the Spanish neuroanatomist Santiago Ramón y Cajal. **B.** Schematic nerve cell illustrating cell body, proximal portion of the apical and basal dendrites, and axon. Dendritic spines are located on the apical and basilar dendrites. These are sites of excitatory synapses. Inhibitory synapses are located on the shaft of the dendrites and the cell body. The axon can be seen to emerge from the cell. The presynaptic terminals of the neuron are shown synapsing on the cell bodies of the postsynaptic neurons. (*A,* Reproduced from Cajal, S. Ramon y. 1909, 1911. Histologie du système nerveux de l'homme et des vertèbres. 2 vols. Paris: Maloine; *B,* adapted from Kandel, E. R., and Schwartz, J. H. 1985. Principles of Neural Science. New York: Elsevier.)

the distinguished Spanish neuroanatomist, Santiago Ramón y Cajal in the beginning of the twentieth century. Neurons have four morphologically specialized regions, each of which subserves separate functions (Figure 1.1B). The *dendrites* (1) are the receiving portion of the neuron. The *cell body* (2) contains the nucleus and cellular organelles critical for the neuron's vitality. Similar to the dendrites, the cell body also receives and integrates incoming information. The *axon* (3) is specialized for the conduction of information—encoded in the form of action potentials—to the axon *terminal* (4). The terminal of the neuron in Figure 1.1A is not shown because it is located far from the cell body and could not be visualized by Cajal. Indeed, for this type of neuron the axon may be up to one meter from the cell body; the length of the axon may be up to 50,000 times the width of the cell body. The terminal lies in close apposition to the dendritic or somatic membrane of the neuron with which it contacts. The site where one neuron contacts another is termed the *synapse*. The synapse includes three key structures: 1) the terminal of the presynaptic neuron, termed the *presynaptic terminal*, 2) a small intercellular space, the *synaptic cleft*, and 3) the *postsynaptic neuronal membrane*. Into the synaptic cleft, the presynaptic neuron releases a chemical, termed a *neurotransmitter*, to communicate with the postsynaptic neuron. Whereas most forms of communication between neurons occur by means of chemical synaptic contacts, for some neurons, direct electrical communication also occurs. Neurons similar to the one shown in Figure 1.1A are specialized to transmit information to distant sites in the central nervous system because they have long axons. These neurons are termed *projection neurons*. Other neurons, termed *interneurons*, have short axons that serve communication within a local brain region. Instead of contacting postsynaptic neurons, the axon terminals of certain neurons contact muscle cells, such as striated limb muscle or smooth muscle of the blood vessel wall, or exocrine gland cells, such as those of the salivary gland.

The other major cellular constituent of the nervous system is the neuroglial cell, or *glia*, which does not participate directly in signaling of information. Rather, glia provide structural and metabolic support for neurons during development as well as in the mature brain. This must be a formidable task because glia outnumber neurons approximately 10 to one! There are two major classes of glia: (1) *microglia*, which subserve a phagocytic or scavenger role, responding to nervous system infection or damage, and (2) *macroglia*, which subserve a variety of support and nutritive functions. There are three types of macroglia: (1) oligodendrocytes, (2) astrocytes, and (3) ependymal cells, and each subserves different functions. *Oligodendrocytes* form a sheath around axons, termed the *myelin sheath* (Figure 1.1B); that is rich in a fatty substance called *myelin*.[1] The myelin sheath functions to increase the velocity of action potential conduction. *Astrocytes* subserve diverse structural and metabolic functions. An important function for astrocytes is in the developing nervous system, where they function as scaffolds for growing axons. *Ependymal cells* line fluid-filled cavities in the central nervous system (see later).

The Nervous System Has a Peripheral Component and a Central Component

The nervous system consists of two components, which are anatomically separate but closely related in function: the *central nervous system* and the *peripheral nervous system*. The central nervous system is composed of the *cerebral hemispheres*, the *brain stem*, and the *spinal cord*, and each

---

[1] Oligodendrocytes form the myelin sheath around axons in the central nervous system, whereas Schwann cells form the myelin sheath around peripheral axons.

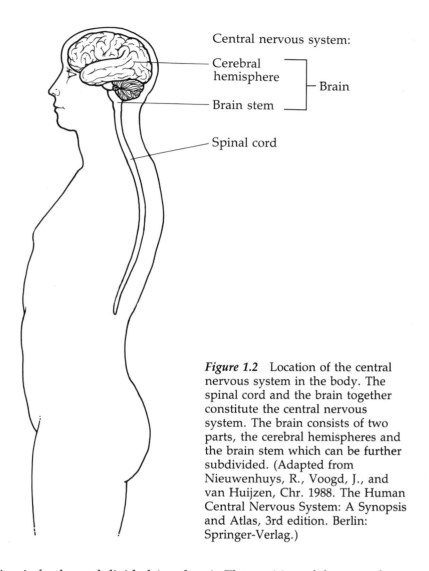

Central nervous system:

Cerebral hemisphere ⎤
⎥ Brain
Brain stem ⎦

Spinal cord

Figure 1.2 Location of the central nervous system in the body. The spinal cord and the brain together constitute the central nervous system. The brain consists of two parts, the cerebral hemispheres and the brain stem which can be further subdivided. (Adapted from Nieuwenhuys, R., Voogd, J., and van Huijzen, Chr. 1988. The Human Central Nervous System: A Synopsis and Atlas, 3rd edition. Berlin: Springer-Verlag.)

division is further subdivided (see later). The position of the central nervous system in the body is shown in Figure 1.2. The peripheral nervous system may be further subdivided into a *somatic* division and an *autonomic* division. As we will see in later chapters, these two divisions of the peripheral nervous system are under the control of separate, but overlapping, regions of the central nervous system. The somatic division includes axons that provide the motor innervation of skeletal musculature and the sensory innervation of the skin, the muscles, and the joints. This division of the peripheral nervous system mediates voluntary movement and much of perception. The autonomic nervous system provides innervation of the glands and the smooth muscle of the body's viscera and of blood vessels (see Chapter 14). The autonomic nervous system, with its separate *sympathetic, parasympathetic,* and *enteric* divisions, regulates body functions based on sensory information about the internal state of the organism. The autonomic nervous system was once thought not to be under conscious control. Now it is known that many autonomic functions can indeed be controlled, but with greater difficulty than control of skeletal musculature.

There Are Six Major Divisions of the Central Nervous System

The complexity of the central nervous system, with its hundreds of billions of neurons, can be reduced to six major divisions: (1) spinal cord, (2) medulla, (3) pons and cerebellum, (4) midbrain, (5) diencephalon, and (6) cerebral hemispheres. Whereas each division performs particular sets

Figure 1.3   A. Lateral surface of cerebral hemisphere and brain stem and a portion of the spinal cord. *B.* Medial surface. Boldface labeling indicates major brain divisions of the central nervous system or lobes of the cerebral cortex.

A

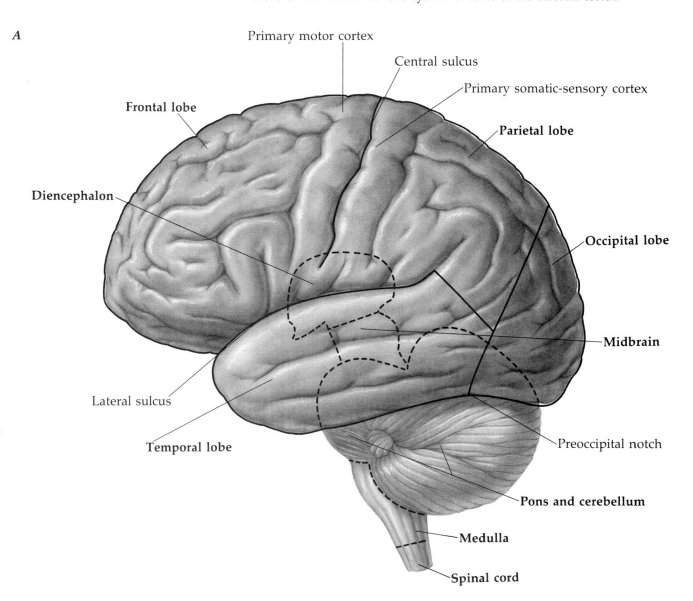

of functions, these functions are not unique and overlap with those of other brain regions. These divisions are shown in Figure 1.3, which presents a lateral view of the central nervous system (A) and a view of the midline (B). A portion of the spinal cord is illustrated in Figure 1.4 and the inset shows the entire spinal cord.

In each division of the central nervous system, there is a clear distinction between regions that contain predominantly neuronal cell bodies

B

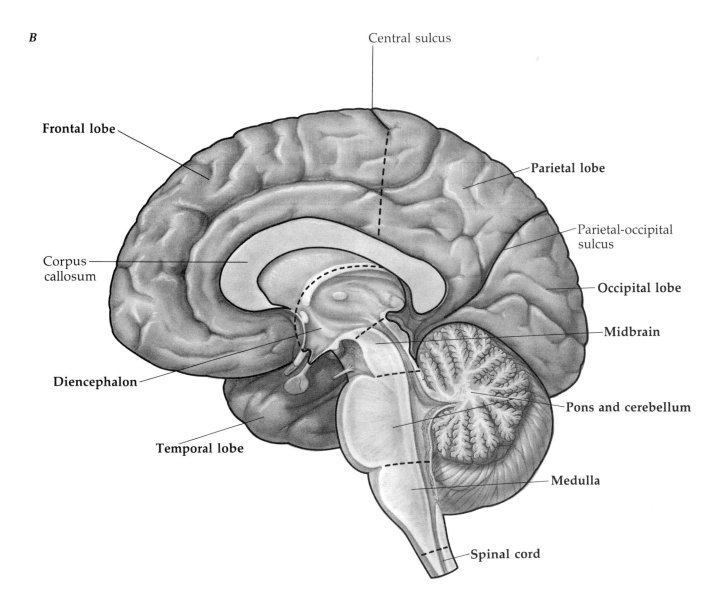

Figure 1.4 Surface topography and internal structure of the spinal cord. Inset shows the segmental arrangement of the spinal cord and vertebral column.

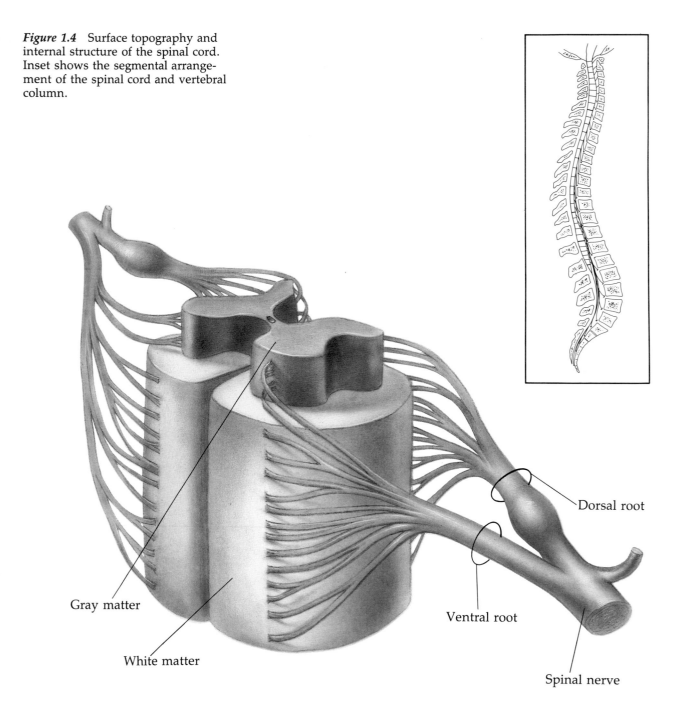

Gray matter

White matter

Dorsal root

Ventral root

Spinal nerve

and dendrites and regions that contain axons. Regions that contain the neuronal cell bodies and dendrites appear gray in fresh material, hence the familiar term *gray matter*. Neuronal cell bodies may be collected into sheets such as the cerebral cortex, or *nuclei*, which have a variety of shapes, such as a sphere or column. The gray matter of most of the spinal cord, brain stem, and diencephalon has a nuclear organization. Regions that contain axons appear white in fresh material, and as a consequence, these regions are termed *white matter*. This white appearance is due to the presence of the myelin sheath around axons (Figure 1.1B). Various terms are used to identify white matter structures. Commonly used terms are tract, column (or funiculus), lemniscus, capsule, and brachium.

The *spinal cord* (Figures 1.3 and 1.4) has the simplest organization of all six major divisions. It participates directly in the control of limb and trunk musculature, in visceral functions, and in the processing of sensory information from these structures. It also is a conduit for the flow of information to and from the brain. The spinal cord is the only portion of the central nervous system that has a clear external *segmental* organization (Figure 1.4 inset), reminiscent of its embryonic (Chapter 2) and phylogenetic origins. A dominant feature of the morphology of each spinal cord segment is the presence of a pair of roots (and associated branches or rootlets) called the dorsal and ventral roots. (The terms dorsal and ventral are commonly used to describe the spatial relations of structures. Dorsal and ventral, along with other anatomical terminology, are explained later.) The dorsal and ventral roots are a remarkable example of segregation of function in the nervous system. *The dorsal roots contain sensory axons whereas the ventral roots contain motor axons.* These sensory and motor axons, which are part of the peripheral nervous system, become intermingled in the *spinal nerves* (Figure 1.4) en route to their peripheral targets. The *spinal nerves*, which are also components of the peripheral nervous system, transmit sensory information to the spinal cord and motor commands to the muscles and viscera.

The next three divisions—medulla, pons and cerebellum, and midbrain—constitute the *brain stem* (Figures 1.3, 1.5, and 1.6). The brain stem has three general functions. First, the brain stem receives sensory information from cranial structures and controls muscles of the head. This function of the brain stem is similar to that of the spinal cord. The *cranial nerves* (nerve roots entering and exiting the brain stem in Figure 1.5) are the constituents of the peripheral nervous system that provide the sensory and motor innervation of the head and therefore are analogous to the spinal nerves. Second, the brain stem contains neural circuits that transmit information from the spinal cord to higher brain regions and back. Finally, the integrated actions of the medulla, pons, and midbrain regulate the levels of arousal. This function is mediated by the central portion, or core, of the brain stem, termed the *reticular formation*. In addition to these general functions, the various divisions of the brain stem subserve specific sensory and motor functions. The *medulla* and the *pons* participate in essential blood pressure and respiratory regulatory mechanisms. Indeed, damage to these parts of the brain is almost always life threatening. The *cerebellum* (Figure 1.6A) regulates body movements, and may do so by controlling the timing of skeletal muscle contractions. The cerebellum and pons are considered together because they develop from the same

A

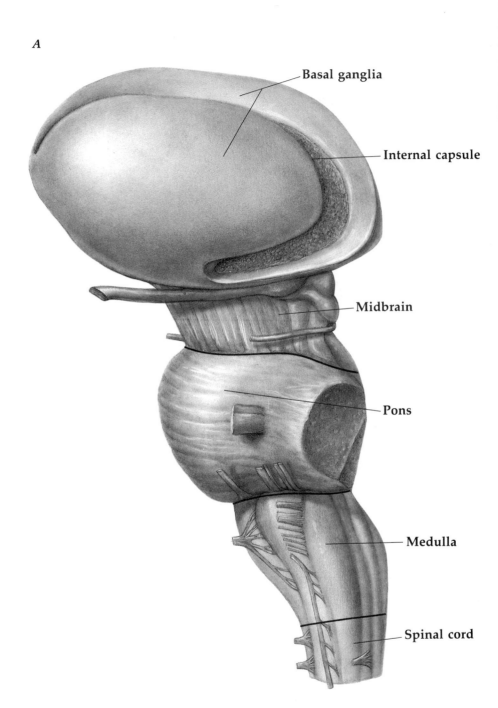

Basal ganglia

Internal capsule

Midbrain

Pons

Medulla

Spinal cord

Figure 1.5 ***A.*** Lateral surface of the brain stem. ***B.*** Ventral surface.

B

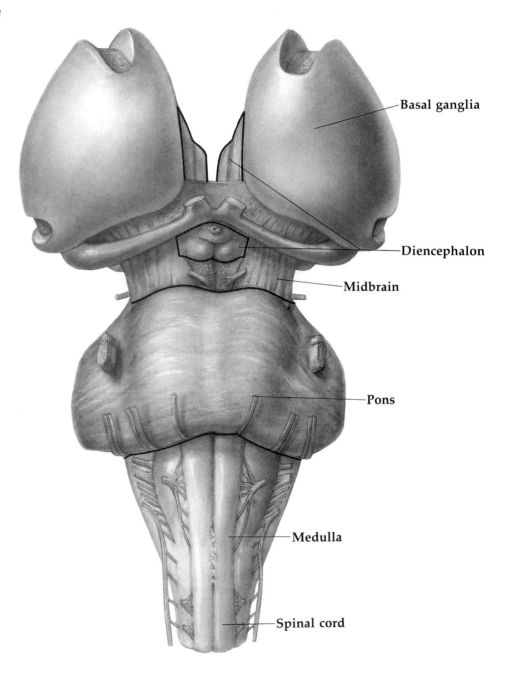

Basal ganglia

Diencephalon

Midbrain

Pons

Medulla

Spinal cord

A

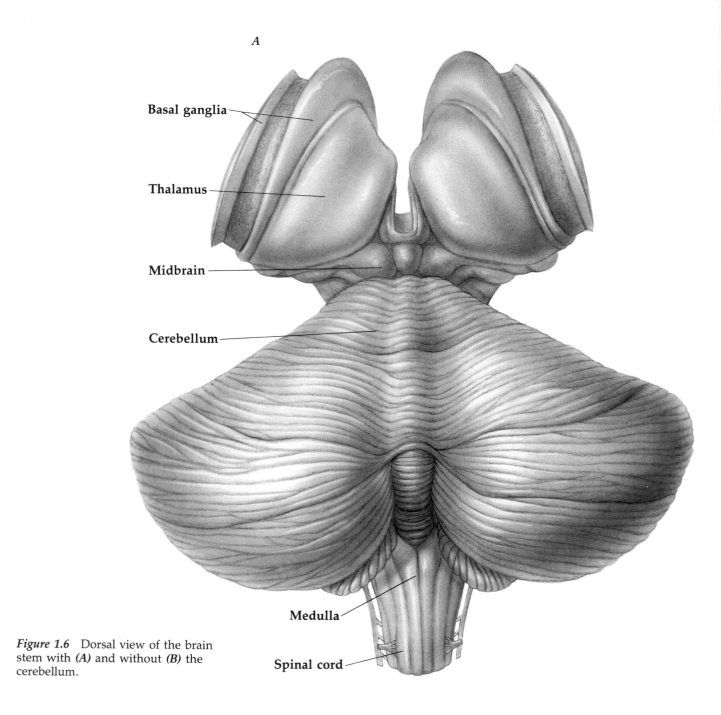

Basal ganglia

Thalamus

Midbrain

Cerebellum

Medulla

Spinal cord

Figure 1.6 Dorsal view of the brain stem with *(A)* and without *(B)* the cerebellum.

B

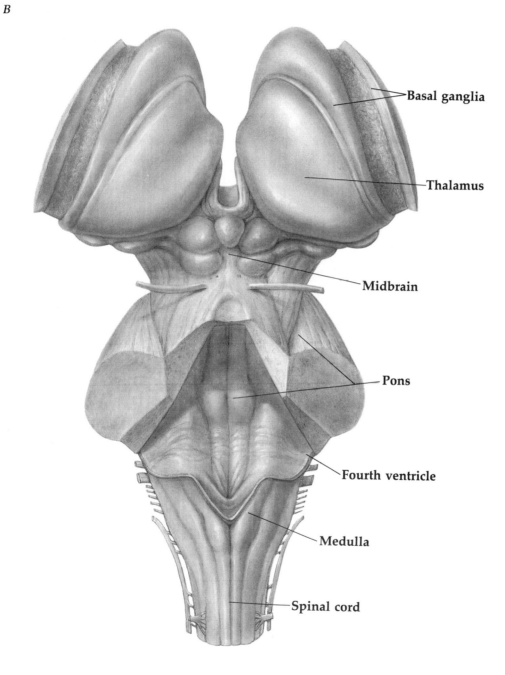

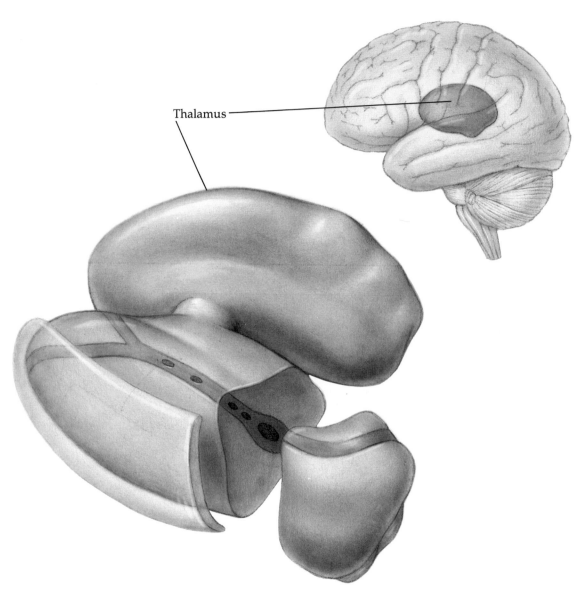

Thalamus

Figure 1.7 The thalamus, a bilaterally paired structure, has an egg-shaped configuration. The inset is a view of the lateral surface of the cerebral hemisphere and brain stem illustrating the location of the thalamus.

portion of the embryonic brain (see Chapter 2) and many of their motor control functions are closely related. The *midbrain* plays a key role in the control of eye movement.

The *diencephalon* and *cerebral hemispheres* are the most highly developed portions of the human central nervous system. The diencephalon consists of two major components. One, the *thalamus* (Figure 1.7), is a key structure for transmitting information to the cerebral hemispheres. The other component, the *hypothalamus* (Figure 1.8B), integrates the functions of the autonomic nervous system and endocrine hormone release from the pituitary gland. Technically, the diencephalon is part of the brain stem. It is discussed together with the cerebral hemispheres because of the important role diencephalic structures play in the functions of the cerebral hemispheres. The *cerebral hemispheres* are separated into two halves by the *sagittal* (or interhemispheric) *fissure* (Figure 1.8A). *Fissures* are deep grooves on the surface of the central nervous system that are consistently present from one brain to the next. The cerebral hemispheres have four major components: cerebral cortex, basal ganglia, hippocampal formation, and amygdala. The *cerebral cortex*, which is located on the surface (Figures 1.3 and 1.8), is highly convoluted. Convolutions are an evolutionary adaptation to fit a greater surface area within the confined space of the cranial cavity. These elevated convolutions are called *gyri* and are separated by folds called *sulci*. Sulci are not as deep as fissures, and their precise form and location are not reliably consistent as those of fissures. The cerebral cortex is divided into four *lobes* (Figures 1.3 and 1.8A), named after the cranial bones that overlie them: frontal, parietal, occipital, and temporal.

The frontal and parietal lobes are separated by the *central sulcus* (Figures 1.3 and 1.8A). This sulcus also separates two different functional regions of cortex: the primary motor cortex, which is located on the *precentral gyrus*, and the primary somatic sensory cortex, which is located on the *postcentral gyrus*. The occipital lobe subserves vision (see later). On the medial brain surface, the occipital lobe is separated from the parietal lobe by the *parietal–occipital sulcus* (Figure 1.3B), and laterally it is separated by an imaginary line connecting the tip of this sulcus with the *preoccipital notch* (Figure 1.3A). The temporal lobe, separated from frontal and parietal lobes by the *lateral sulcus* (or *Sylvian fissure*), subserves a variety of sensory functions. The auditory cortex is located on the lateral surface of the temporal lobe as well as within the lateral sulcus (Chapter 7). The *inferior* portion of the temporal lobe subserves visual function. Portions of the medial temporal lobe (Figure 1.3B) mediate olfaction (Chapter 8).

The second major component of the cerebral hemisphere is the *basal ganglia*, which are deeply located collections of neurons. A major portion of the basal ganglia called the *striatum* is illustrated in Figure 1.9 along with the lateral ventricle and third ventricle, which are fluid-filled cavities (see later). (The complex three-dimensional configuration of the striatum will be considered from a developmental perspective in Chapter 2.) The basal ganglia participate in many higher brain functions. For example, the role of the basal ganglia in the control of movement is clearly revealed when they become damaged, as in Parkinson's disease. Tremor and a slowing of movement are the most overt signs of this disease. The basal

A

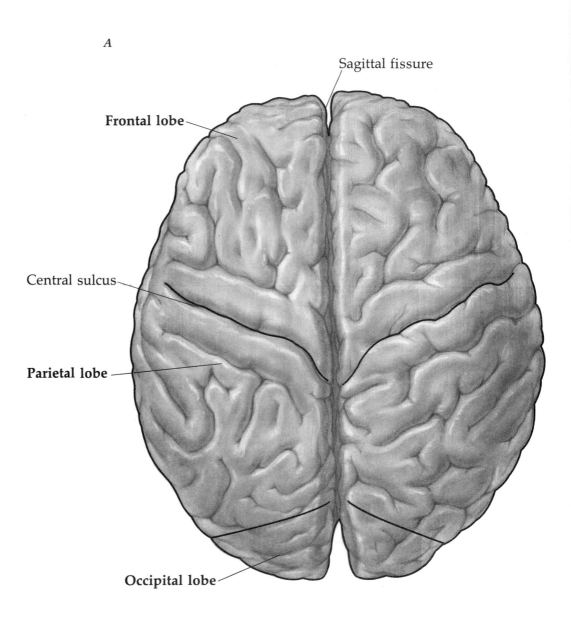

Sagittal fissure

Frontal lobe

Central sulcus

Parietal lobe

Occipital lobe

B

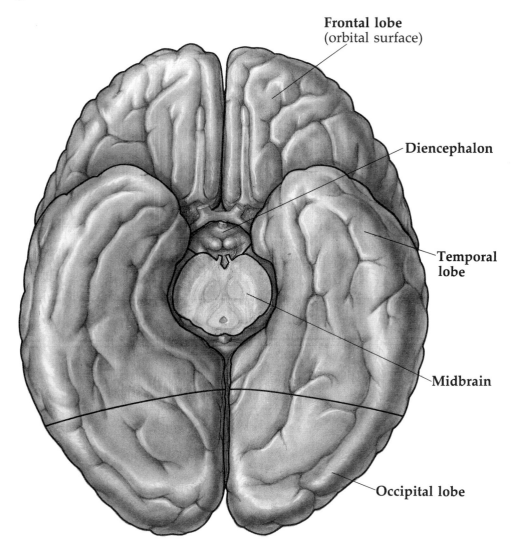

Frontal lobe
(orbital surface)

Diencephalon

Temporal
lobe

Midbrain

Occipital lobe

A

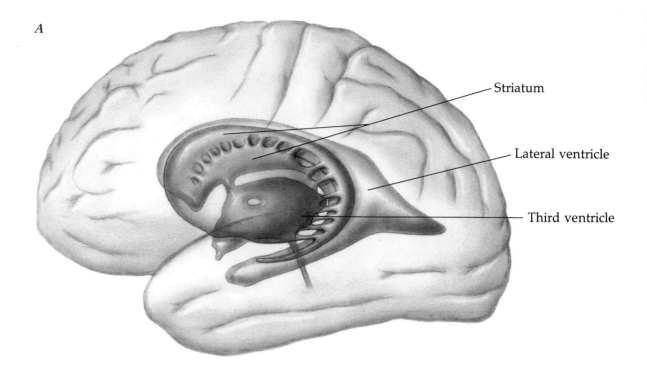

Striatum

Lateral ventricle

Third ventricle

B

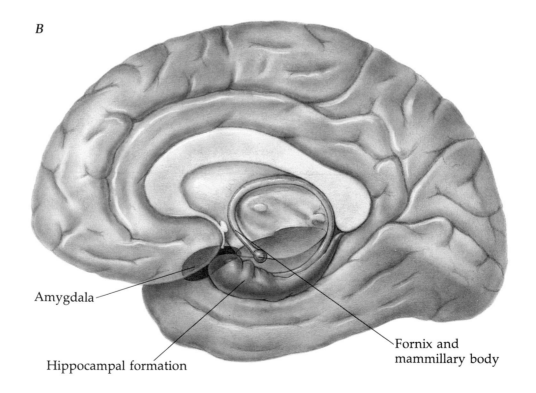

Amygdala

Hippocampal formation

Fornix and
mammillary body

◁ *Figure 1.9* Three-dimensional views of deep structures of the cerebral hemisphere. *A.* Striatum, a component of the basal ganglia. The lateral ventricle and third ventricle are also illustrated. Note the similarity in overall shape of the striatum and the lateral ventricle. *B.* The hippocampal formation and amygdala. The fornix and mammillary body are structures that are anatomically and functionally related to the hippocampal formation.

ganglia participate in other aspects of behavior, including emotion and cognition.

The third and fourth major components of the cerebral hemisphere are also located beneath the cortical surface: the *hippocampus* and the *amygdala* (Figure 1.9B). The hippocampus is believed to participate in memory, whereas the amygdala may coordinate the actions of the autonomic nervous system and hormone release as well as participate in emotions. These two structures are part of the *limbic system*, which includes additional components of the cerebral hemisphere as well as parts of the diencephalon and midbrain (Chapter 15). Together the various components of the limbic system play a key role in thought and mood. Not surprisingly, psychiatric disorders are typically associated with limbic system dysfunction.

The Central Nervous System Is Covered by Three Meningeal Layers

The brain and spinal cord are covered by three separate membranes collectively termed the *meninges*, which have important protective and circulatory functions. The meninges consist of the dura mater, the arachnoid mater, and the pia mater (Figure 1.10). *Dura mater* is the thickest and outermost of these membranes. The dura overlying the cerebral hemispheres and brain stem actually contains two layers: an outer *periosteal layer* and an inner *meningeal layer*. The periosteal layer is attached to the inner surface of the skull. Within the dura are large, low-pressure blood vessels, which are part of the return path for cerebral venous blood, termed the *dural sinuses* (Chapter 4). Two important partitions arise from the meningeal layer and separate different components of the cerebral hemispheres and brain stem (Figure 1.10B). The *falx cerebri* (1) separates the two cerebral hemispheres. The *tentorium cerebelli* (2) separates the cerebellum from the cerebral hemispheres. The dura mater that covers the spinal cord is continuous with both the meningeal layer of the cranial dura and the epineurium of peripheral nerves.

The *arachnoid mater* adjoins but is not tightly bound to the dura mater, thus allowing a potential space to exist between them. This potential space, called the *subdural space*, is important clinically. Because the dura mater contains blood vessels, breakage of one of its vessels can lead to subdural bleeding and to the formation of a blood clot (a *subdural hematoma*). In this condition the blood clot pushes the arachnoid away from the dura mater, fills the subdural space, and compresses the underlying

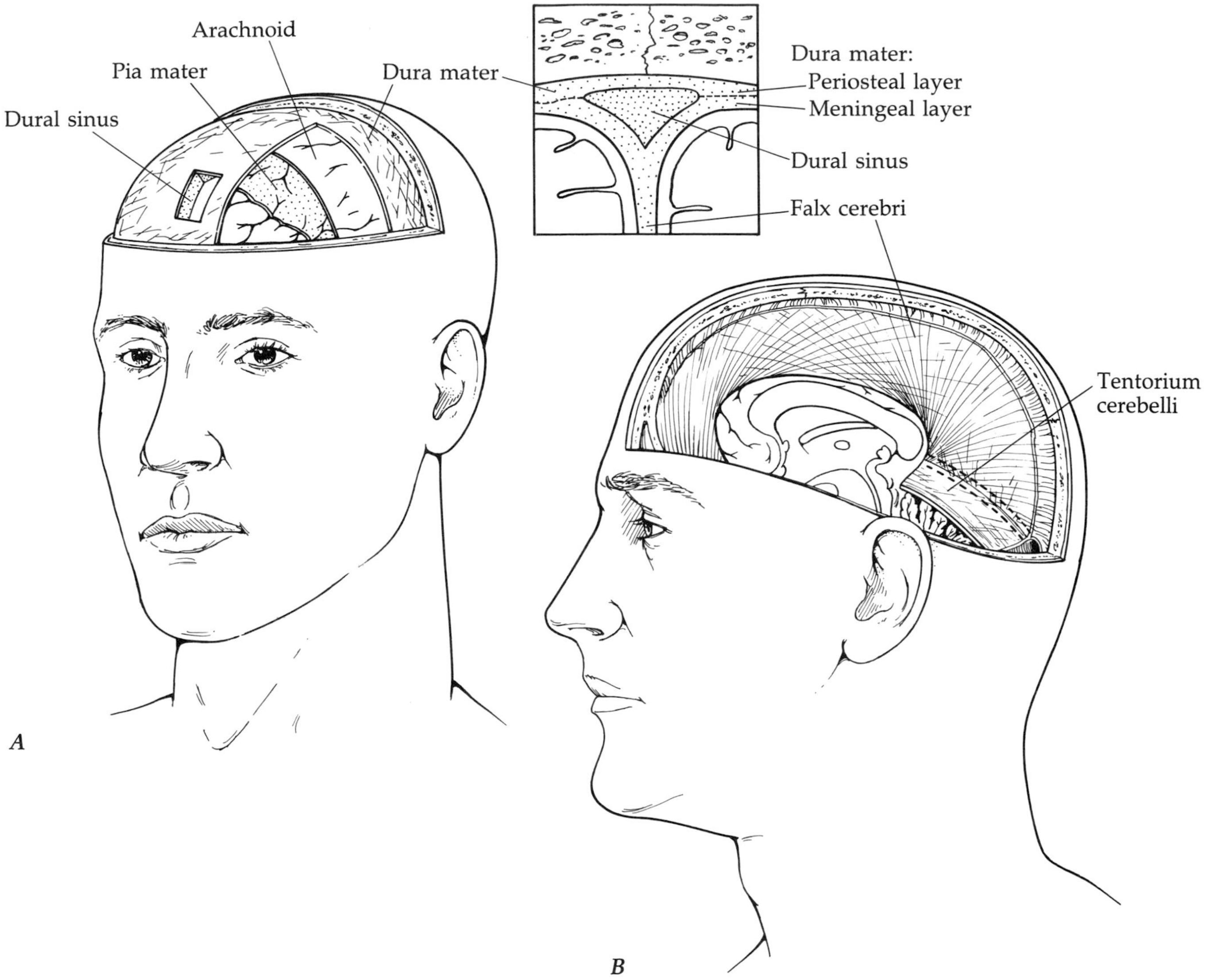

Figure 1.10 **A.** The meninges, which consist of the dura mater, arachnoid mater, and the pia mater. **B.** The two major dural flaps are the falx cerebri, which incompletely separates the two cerebral hemispheres, and the tentorium cerebelli, which separates the cerebellum from the cerebral hemisphere. The inset shows the dural layers. The dashed line at the junction of the falx cerebri and tentorium cerebelli indicates the location of a dural sinus. (*A*, Adapted from Snell, R. S. 1987. Clinical Neuroanatomy for Medical Students. Boston: Little-Brown.)

neural tissue. An actual space, called the *subarachnoid space*, separates the arachnoid mater from the innermost meningeal layer, the *pia mater*. Filaments of arachnoid mater pass through the subarachnoid space and connect to the pia mater, giving this space the appearance of a spider's web. (Hence the name *arachnoid*, which is from the Greek word *arachne*, meaning "spider.") The subarachnoid space is filled with cerebrospinal fluid (see later); it also contains the veins and arteries that overlie the surface of the central nervous system. The pia mater is very delicate and adheres to the surface of the brain and spinal cord.

A

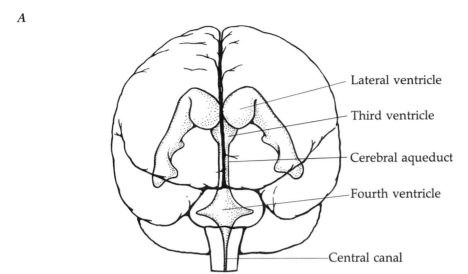

Lateral ventricle

Third ventricle

Cerebral aqueduct

Fourth ventricle

Central canal

B

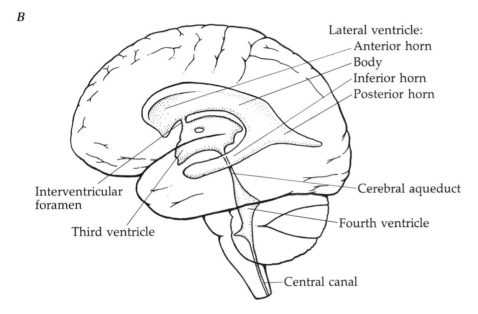

Lateral ventricle:
Anterior horn
Body
Inferior horn
Posterior horn

Interventricular
foramen

Third ventricle

Cerebral aqueduct

Fourth ventricle

Central canal

Figure 1.11   Ventricular system.
A. The lateral ventricles, third ventricle, cerebral aqueduct, and fourth
ventricle are seen from the rostral
(and ventral) brain surface. *B.* The
ventricular system is shown from the
lateral brain surface. The lateral
ventricle is divided into four main
components: anterior (or frontal)
horn, body, inferior (or temporal)
horn, and the posterior (or occipital)
horn. The interventricular foramen
(of Monro) connects the lateral
ventricle and the third ventricle.
(Adapted from Noback, C., and
Demarest, R. J. 1981. The Human
Nervous System: Basic Principles of
Neurobiology, 3rd ed. New York:
McGraw-Hill.)

Cavities within the Central Nervous System Contain Cerebrospinal Fluid

The central nervous system is basically tubular in its organization
(Chapters 2 and 3). Within it are cavities that are collectively termed the
ventricular system (Figure 1.11). The ventricular system contains *cerebrospinal fluid* which is produced mainly by the *choroid plexus*, an intraven-
tricular structure. The mechanism by which the choroid plexus secretes
cerebrospinal fluid is not well understood. It was once thought to be an
ultrafiltrate of the blood, but because the ionic constituents of cerebrospinal fluid differ from those of blood it is now believed to involve active
secretory and ion reuptake mechanisms.

Cerebrospinal fluid not only bathes the interior of the brain via the
ventricular system, but flows over the surface of the entire central nervous

system through the subarachnoid space. It cushions the central nervous system from physical shocks and is a medium for chemical communication. The brain has no known lymphatic system. By way of the cerebrospinal fluid and the ventricular system, water is returned to the venous system.

The brain ventricles are illustrated in Figure 1.11. The two *lateral ventricles* are located within the two halves of the cerebral hemisphere, and each lateral ventricle is further subdivided (Chapter 2). The third ventricle is unpaired; it lies along the midline between the two halves of the diencephalon (Figure 1.9A). The fourth ventricle is located in the brain stem. The central canal is the portion of the ventricular system that extends into the spinal cord. The ventricles are interconnected: the *interventricular foramina* (of Monro) connect the lateral ventricles with the third ventricle and the *cerebral aqueduct* (of Sylvius) connects the third and fourth ventricles. The central canal of the spinal cord is continuous with the fourth ventricle. Cerebrospinal fluid exits the ventricular system through three small apertures in the roof of the fourth ventricle: the two laterally placed *foramina of Luschka* and the *foramen of Magendie*, which is located at the midline. After leaving the fourth ventricle, cerebrospinal fluid circulates around the brain and spinal cord, within the *subarachnoid space*. In Chapter 4 we will see the path through which cerebrospinal fluid is returned to the venous circulation.

An Introduction to Neuroanatomical Terms

The complex three-dimensional organization of the brain requires a precise method for describing both the absolute position of particular structures and their relative position with reference to other structures and major spatial axes. The terminology of neuroanatomy is specialized to meet this need. Although the use of more intuitive descriptions of the positions of structures may at first make neuroanatomy easier to understand, their lack of precision quickly results in confusion. The major axes of the nervous system and those terms describing spatial relations are briefly described next. These terms may seem arbitrary at first, but in Chapter 2 we will see that they follow logically from the developmental plan of the central nervous system.

Two Major Axes Describe the Organization of the Central Nervous System

The *rostral–caudal* axis and the *dorsal–ventral* axis (Figure 1.12) are the principal axes along which the central nervous system is organized. These axes are most easily understood in mammals with a central nervous system that is more simple than that of humans, for example, the rat. Here, the rostral–caudal axis runs approximately in a straight line from the nose to the tail. This axis is also the *longitudinal axis* of the nervous system, and is often termed the *neuraxis* because the central nervous system has a predominant longitudinal organization. In Chapter 3, major neural systems that have a longitudinal organization are examined. The dorsal–ventral axis, which is perpendicular to the rostral–caudal axis, runs from the back to the abdomen. The terms *posterior* and *anterior* are synonymous with dorsal and ventral, respectively.

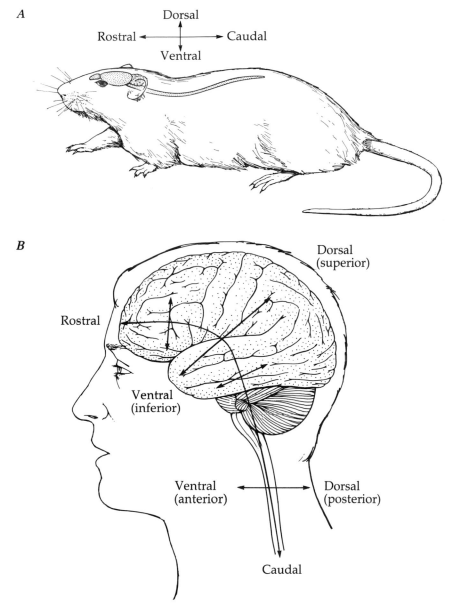

A

Dorsal

Rostral ← → Caudal

Ventral

B

Dorsal
(superior)

Rostral

Ventral
(inferior)

Ventral
(anterior) ← → Dorsal
(posterior)

Caudal

Figure 1.12 The axes of central nervous system are illustrated for the rat *(A)*, an animal whose central nervous system is organized in a linear fashion, and the human *(B)*, whose central nervous system has a prominent flexure at the mid-brain. (Adapted from Kandel, E. R., and Schwartz, J. H. 1985. Principles of Neural Science. New York: Elsevier.)

The longitudinal axis of the human nervous system is not straight as it is in the rat. During development, the brain—and therefore the longitudinal axis—undergoes a prominent bend, or *flexure*. This flexure occurs at the midbrain. Superior and inferior are also descriptive terms analogous to the usage of the terms dorsal and ventral, rostral to the flexure. Posterior and anterior are descriptive terms more commonly used for structures located caudal to the flexure.

A   Horizontal plane

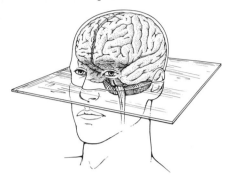

B   Coronal plane

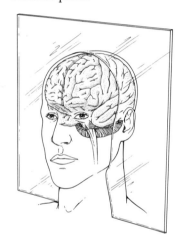

C   Sagittal plane

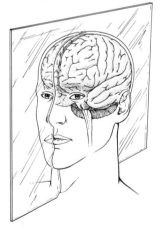

Figure 1.13 The three main anatomical planes: *(A)* horizontal, *(B)* coronal, and *(C)* sagittal.

There Are Three Major Planes of Section through the Central Nervous System

A specific terminology also exists for the planes in which anatomical sections, or slices, are made through the brain and spinal cord (Figure 1.13). Sections are cut in one of three principal planes that are topographically related to the longitudinal axis of the nervous system. *Horizontal* sections (1) are parallel to the longitudinal axis, and cut from one side to the other. *Transverse* sections (2) are perpendicular to the longitudinal axis and cut between the dorsal and ventral surfaces. Transverse sections through the cerebral hemisphere are roughly parallel to the coronal suture and, as a consequence, are also termed *coronal* sections. *Sagittal* sections (3) are cut in the vertical plane, parallel both to the longitudinal axis of the central nervous system and to the midline. A *midsagittal* section divides the central nervous system into two symmetrical halves, whereas a *parasagittal* section is cut off the midline.

Techniques for Studying the Regional Anatomy and Interconnections of the Central Nervous System

Historically, the earliest methods for studying normal regional anatomy involved selective staining of different portions of the neuron: either the cell body and dendrites, or the axon. Cell stains principally reveal the locations of neuronal cell bodies. There are numerous methods for staining neuronal cell bodies. The Nissl method utilizes a dye that binds to acid groups, in particular to ribonucleic acids of the ribosomes, which are located within the cell body. Staining methods that reveal the location of axons use dyes that bind to the myelin sheath, for example the Weigert method. Tissues prepared with either a *cell stain* or a *myelin stain* have a different appearance (Figure 1.14). This is because axons that conduct neural signals from one region of the nervous system to another region often collect in areas (for example, a tract) that are separate from those containing neuronal cell bodies (for example, a nucleus). Stains that use silver, for example the Golgi method (see Figure 10.11), may show not only the neuron's cell body but its dendrites and axon as well. Silver is thought to bind to filamentous proteins within the cytoplasm. Unlike the Nissl and Weigert methods, which stain the appropriate parts of all neurons exposed to the dye, silver stains an entire neuron (or glial cell) but, curiously, only a small number of cells in an area. Clearly, the different staining methods are used for different purposes. A myelin stain is used to distinguish white matter from gray matter, and a cell stain to identify the cellular organization of gray matter. Silver stains are used to study the detailed morphology of neurons.

Recently developed staining methods reveal the presence of specific neuronal chemicals, such as neurotransmitters, receptor molecules, or enzymes. By exploiting their capacity to fluoresce, the presence of monoamine neurotransmitters (for example, dopamine) is determined. Immunohistochemical methods have been developed in which a variety of neurotransmitters, enzymes, and other proteins can be localized (see Figure 11.16). Most recently, the capacity of a neuron to manufacture a specific gene product, for example a hormone, has been probed with in situ hybridization. This is a method in which neurons are exposed to specially

A Cell stain

B Myelin stain

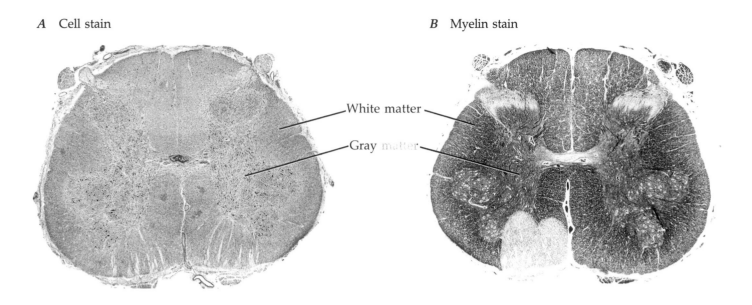

White matter

Gray matter

designed DNA—and labeled with ³H—which binds to the messenger RNA that specifies the composition of the chemical.

The connections between regions of the nervous system have been examined anatomically in two fundamentally different ways. The first approach exploits neuronal structural changes following *axon transection*. The portion of the axon distal to the cut, now isolated from the neuronal cell body, degenerates because it is deprived of nourishment. This process is termed *Wallerian* (or *anterograde*) *degeneration*. The degenerating axons and terminals can be selectively stained, thereby directly revealing their location. Alternatively, the tissue can be stained for the presence of normal myelin, in which case the axons that have previously degenerated will not be visualized. Myelin staining has been commonly used to examine human tissue (for example, Figure 5.7A). (The cell body also undergoes characteristic changes that can be recognized microscopically.) The second approach relies on the process of *axonal transport*. Certain materials, when injected into regions of the central nervous system, are taken up by axon terminals in the vicinity of the injected material and *retrogradely transported* to the cell body. Horseradish peroxidase, the plant lectin wheat germ agglutinin, and certain fluorescent dyes are chemicals commonly used for retrograde transport. Alternatively, the *anterograde transport* of materials, for example ³H-labeled amino acids, from the cell body to the terminals can be used to trace connections (for example, Figure 6.8). The agents that are taken up at the neuron terminals or cell body and transported are visualized by special histochemical reactions, fluorescence microscopy, or autoradiography depending on the specific materials used. Certain compounds used for axon tracing are transneuronally transported and thereby offer the opportunity to probe the anatomical organization of neural pathways. Moreover, the transneuronal transport of some of these compounds is believed to be dependent on the activity of neurons in the pathway. While still in its infancy, this activity-dependent transport has been used to reveal the anatomy of particular sets of functional connections.

Figure 1.14 *A.* Cell-stained section through the spinal cord showing the locations of neuronal cell bodies in the gray matter. *B.* Myelin-stained section showing the location of myelinated axons in the white matter. (Photograph by Al Lamme, Department of Pathology, Columbia University.)

Structure and Function Can Be Imaged in the Living Brain

Modern radiological techniques now permit precise examination of the regional anatomy of the living human brain as well as its functional anatomy. This is done with two recently-developed techniques. The first, *magnetic resonance imaging* (MRI), probes the regional anatomy of the brain principally by distinguishing differences in the water content of tissues. The second technique, *positron emission tomography* (PET), provides an image of brain function by showing the distribution of radiolabeled compounds involved in neuronal metabolism or cerebral blood flow. Here, selected examples of these two techniques are used to explore, in a very general way, a component of the central nervous system that participates in *visual perception*.

The components of the nervous system that are important for visual perception are schematically illustrated in Figure 1.15A. (The visual system is discussed in detail in Chapter 6.) Briefly, the visual pathway begins in the *retina*, the portion of the eye where sensory receptors that convert visual energy to neuronal events are located. Receptors synapse on interneurons, which, in turn, synapse on projection neurons. The axons of projection neurons terminate in a specific location in the *thalamus*. The thalamus functions as a gateway for the flow of information to the cerebral cortex. This function is subserved not only for visual information but for information from other sensory modalities as well as neural signals that are important for the control of movement, cognition, and emotions. However, the thalamus does not simply route information passively to the cerebral cortex. Rather, incoming information is transformed. From the thalamus, the next processing stage in the visual path is the *primary visual cortex*. Each sensory modality has a *primary* cortical area, so termed because it receives sensory information directly from the thalamus. A cascade of intracortical projections that are important for perception is initiated from the primary sensory cortex. These projections terminate in the *secondary sensory cortex* where another set of connections lead to the *tertiary sensory cortex*. Each sensory modality, in addition to having a primary area, has numerous higher-order areas. In the human brain, the primary visual cortex is located in the occipital lobe, in the banks and depth of the *calcarine fissure* (Figure 1.15A).

Regional anatomy can be viewed with extraordinary precision by examining a MRI scan of the midsagittal plane of the central nervous system (Figure 1.15B). The key structures of the path for visual perception, including the thalamus and the cortex adjacent to the calcarine fissure, are clearly revealed in the MRI scan. The PET scan in Figure 1.15C presents an image of the function of the primary visual cortex in the human brain. This PET scan reflects the increase in cerebral blood flow (probed by measuring the distribution of ^{15}O-labeled water) that accompanies neuronal activation. The bright region corresponds to the part of the primary visual cortex that is active when a visual stimulus is presented to a particular portion of the retina.

The degree to which the structure of the living brain can be visualized with MRI underscores the importance of studying regional neuroanatomy. PET permits direct examination of brain function. PET is also used to map the distribution of a variety of biologically active compounds.

A

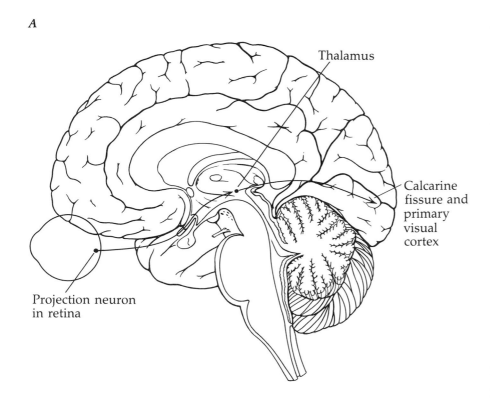

Thalamus

Calcarine fissure and primary visual cortex

Projection neuron in retina

Figure 1.15 Structures that are important for visual perception are illustrated in this figure. *A.* Line drawing of the medial surface of the cerebral hemisphere schematically illustrating the visual path from the retina to the cerebral cortex.
B. Magnetic resonance image (MRI) of the midsagittal human central nervous system is illustrated.
C. Positron emission tomograph (PET scan) of the human brain. This is a ^{15}O-labeled water PET scan of a midsagittal slice. The scan was obtained while the subject viewed a visual stimulus (presented to the macular region of the retina). The distribution of ^{15}O-labeled water approximates that of cerebral blood flow, which correlates with neuronal activity. This image reflects the calculated difference between cerebral blood flow at rest and cerebral blood flow during visual stimulation. (*B,* Courtesy of Dr. Neal Rutledge, University of Texas at Austin; *C,* Courtesy of Dr. Peter Fox, Washington University; adapted from Fox et al. 1987. J. Neurosci. 7:913–922.)

Thalamus   Calcarine fissure

B   *C*

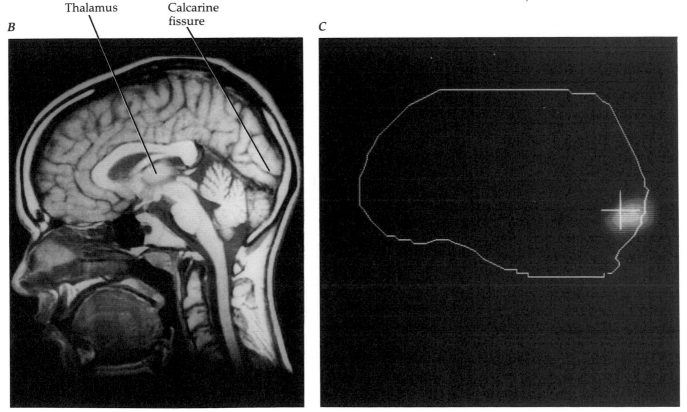

For example, radiolabeled neurotransmitters or drugs can be administered intravenously and permitted to bind to receptors on the neuronal membrane. By use of the same methodology employed in determining the distribution of radiolabeled oxygen, the localization of the labeled neurotransmitter is determined.

Summary

The cellular constituents of the nervous system are the *neurons* (Figure 1.1) and the *glia*. The nervous system contains two separate divisions, the *peripheral nervous system* and the *central nervous system* (Figure 1.2). Each may be further subdivided. The *autonomic* component of the peripheral nervous system controls the glands and smooth muscle of the viscera and blood vessels, whereas the *somatic* component provides the sensory innervation of body tissues and the motor innervation of skeletal muscle. There are six separate components of the central nervous system (Figures 1.3–1.9): (1) *spinal cord*, (2) *medulla*, (3) *pons and cerebellum*, (4) *midbrain*, (5) *diencephalon*, which contains the *hypothalamus* and *thalamus*, and (6) *cerebral hemispheres*, which contain the *basal ganglia*, *amygdala, hippocampus formation*, and *cerebral cortex*. The external surface of the cerebral cortex is characterized by *sulci* (grooves) and *gyri* (convolutions). The central nervous system is covered by three meningeal layers (Figure 1.10), from outermost to innermost: *dura mater, arachnoid mater*, and *pia mater*. Arachnoid mater and pia mater are separated by the *subarachnoid space*, which is filled with *cerebrospinal fluid*, a watery fluid that derives from the blood but has different ionic constituents. Cerebrospinal fluid also flows within cavities in the central nervous system termed the *ventricular system* (Figure 1.11). Two *lateral ventricles* are located in each of the cerebral hemispheres, the *third ventricle* is located in the diencephalon, and the *fourth ventricle* is in the pons and medulla. The *central canal* is the component of the ventricular system in the spinal cord. The *interventricular foramina* (of Monro) connect the two lateral ventricles with the third ventricle. The *cerebral aqueduct* connects the third and fourth ventricles. Cerebrospinal fluid exits from the ventricular system, to the subarachnoid space, via three apertures in the roof of the fourth ventricle, the two lateral foramina of *Luschka* and the foramen of *Magendie*, located at the midline.

The central nervous system is oriented along two major axes (Figure 1.12): the *rostral–caudal axis*, which is also termed the *longitudinal axis*, and the *dorsal–ventral axis*, which is perpendicular to the longitudinal axis. Sections through the central nervous system are cut in relation to the rostral–caudal axis (Figure 1.13). *Horizontal* sections (1) are cut parallel to the rostral–caudal axis, from one side to the other. *Transverse* or *coronal* sections (2) are cut perpendicular to the rostral–caudal axis, between the dorsal and ventral surfaces. *Sagittal* sections (3) are cut vertically and parallel to the longitudinal axis and the midline.

Cell staining methods (e.g., Nissl stain) demonstrate the cellular organization of gray matter (Figure 1.14A), *myelin staining* methods (e.g., Weigert) distinguish white matter from gray matter (Figure 1.14B), and silver staining methods (e.g., Golgi) reveal the detailed morphology of neurons. Recently developed staining methods reveal the locations of *specific neuronal chemicals.* Anatomical connections are demonstrated by *degeneration* techniques as well as *axonal transport* (anterograde and retrograde). The structure of the living brain can be probed with *magnetic resonance imaging* (Figure 1.15B), whereas brain function is probed with *positron emission tomography* (Figure 1.15C). ■

References

Berne, R. M., and Levy, M. N. 1983. Physiology. St. Louis: Mosby.

Cajal, S. Ramon y. 1909, 1911. Histologie du système nerveux de l'homme et des vertèbres. 2 vols. Paris: Maloine.

Fox, P. T., Miezin, F. M., Allman, J. M., et al. 1987. Retinotopic organization of human visual cortex mapped with positron emission tomography. J. Neurosci. 7:913–922.

Nieuwenhuys, R., Voogd, J., and Van Huijzen, Chr. 1988. The Human Central Nervous System: A Synopsis and Atlas, 3rd edition. Berlin: Springer-Verlag.

Noback, C., and Demarest, R. J. 1981. The Human Nervous System: Basic Principles of Neurobiology, 3rd ed. New York: McGraw-Hill.

Selected Readings

Carpenter, M. B., and Sutin, J. 1983. Human Neuroanatomy. Baltimore: Williams & Wilkins.

Heimer, L. 1983. The Human Brain and Spinal Cord. New York: Springer-Verlag.

Jones, E. G., and Cowan, W. M. 1983. Nervous tissue. In Weiss, L. (ed.), Histology: Cell and Tissue Biology, 5th ed. New York: Elsevier Biomedical, pp. 283–370.

Kandel, E. R., and Schwartz, J. H. 1985. Principles of Neural Science. New York: Elsevier.

Nauta, W. J., and Feirtag, M. 1986. Fundamental Neuroanatomy. New York: W. H. Freeman & Co.

Oldendorf, W. H. 1980. The Quest for an Image of Brain. New York: Raven Press.

Sawchenko, P. E., and Gerfen, C. R. 1985. Plant lectins and bacterial toxins as tools for tracing neuronal connections. Trends in Neurosci. 8:378–384.

Development of the Central Nervous System

2

Development of the Central Nervous System

The key to understanding the complex anatomy of the mature brain is to understand how it develops. Principles that govern the regional anatomy of the brain are more easily appreciated in its simpler, embryonic form. In this chapter we examine those aspects of central nervous system development that provide insight into the complex three-dimensional structure of the mature brain. First we consider how the nervous system forms from the ectoderm of the embryo. Then the development of key components of each major division of the central nervous system and the ventricular system is surveyed from their earliest stages through maturity.

The Neural Tube Forms Five Brain Vesicles and the Spinal Cord

The human embryo has three principal cell layers: *ectoderm*, the outermost layer, *mesoderm*, the middle layer, and *entoderm*, the innermost layer. The cellular constituents of the central nervous system, neurons and glial cells, are formed from a specialized region of the ectoderm called the *neural plate*. The process by which the neural plate becomes committed to the formation of the nervous system is termed *neural induction*. The neural plate lies along the *dorsal* midline of the embryo (Figure 2.1). The proliferation of cells is greater along the margin of the neural plate than along the midline. This results in the formation of a midline indentation that deepens gradually, termed the *neural groove*, and closes to form a hollow structure, termed the *neural tube* (Figure 2.1). Closure of the neural plate to form the neural tube occurs first at the location where the neck will form, then proceeds both caudally and rostrally. All of the major components of the central nervous system are represented at this early developmental stage: the caudal portion becomes the *spinal cord*, and the intermediate and rostral portions differentiate into the *brain stem* and *cerebral hemispheres*, respectively. The ventricular system of the central nervous system is derived from the cavity inside the neural tube.

There are important clinical correlates of neural tube formation. Occasionally, during early development, the neural plate fails to close completely. When this occurs in the caudal portion of the neural plate, the functions subserved by the lumbar and sacral spinal cord are severely disrupted, resulting in varying degrees of lower limb paralysis and defective bladder control. This developmental abnormality is one of a wide range of neural tube deficits, collectively termed *spina bifida*, that are often associated with herniation of the meninges and neural tissue to the body surface. When the neural plate fails to close at rostral levels *anencephaly* may occur, and the overall structure of the brain is grossly disturbed.

Figure 2.1 The neural tube forms from the dorsal surface of the embryo. The left side of the figure presents dorsal views of the developing embryo during the third and fourth weeks after conception. The right side illustrates transverse sections through the developing nervous system. The levels at which the sections are taken are indicated by the bold lines on the left. (Adapted from Cowan, W. M. 1979. The development of the brain. Sci. Am. 241:112–133.) ▷

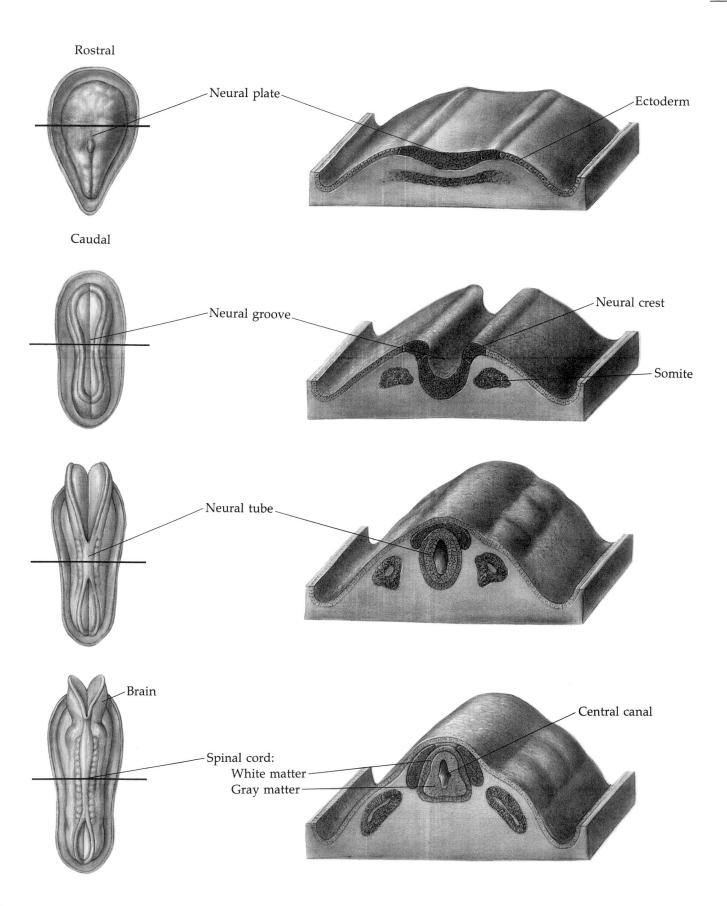

Rostral

Neural plate

Ectoderm

Caudal

Neural groove

Neural crest

Somite

Neural tube

Brain

Central canal

Spinal cord:
White matter
Gray matter

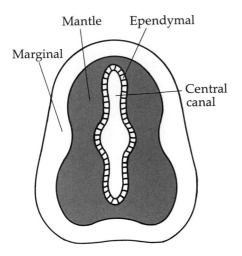

Figure 2.2 Schematic diagram of a transverse section through the developing spinal cord illustrating the three cell layers of neural tube.

Neurons of the Central Nervous System Derive from the Neuroepithelium

Virtually all the neurons and glial cells (macroglia) of the *central nervous system* are generated by the *neuroepithelium*, the epithelial cells lining the neural tube. By contrast, neurons whose cell bodies lie outside the central nervous system, such as *dorsal root ganglion cells* (the cells that provide the sensory innervation of the limbs and trunk) are derived from the *neural crest*, a population of cells originally located at the lateral margins of the neural plate (Figure 2.1). Other constituents of the nervous system that derive from the neural crest include (1) the arachnoid and pia mater (the outermost meningeal layer, the dura mater, is derived from the mesoderm), (2) the chromaffin cells of the adrenal medulla, (3) the postganglionic autonomic neurons (Chapter 14) and (4) Schwann cells, which form the myelin sheath of peripheral nerves (oligodendrocytes, which are the glial cells that form the myelin sheath over axons in the central nervous system, are derived from the neuroepithelium).

The developing central nervous system is laminated, as are many regions of the mature central nervous system. Progressing outward from the cavity within the neural tube, there are three principal layers (Figure 2.2). The neuroepithelium is located in the *ependymal layer* (1). The cells of the neuroepithelium divide repeatedly and differentiate into the neurons and glial cells of the central nervous system. Immature nerve cells arise from the division of neuroependymal cells and migrate to the *mantle layer* (2). Within the mantle layer specialized glial cells form a scaffolding along which much of this migration takes place. The *marginal layer* (3) contains the axonal processes of developing neurons. In the mature brain, the ependymal layer remains one cell thick, is ciliated, and lines the ventricular system. The mantle layer becomes the gray matter and the marginal layer, the white matter.

The Brain Vesicles Form the Brain Stem and Cerebral Hemispheres

In early stages of development, the rostral portion of the neural tube forms three vesicles, called the *prosencephalon* or *forebrain*, the *mesencephalon* or *midbrain*, and the *rhombencephalon* or *hindbrain* (Figure 2.3A). Later in development two structures emerge from the primitive forebrain: the *telencephalon* (or end brain), which gives rise to the *cerebral hemispheres*, and the *diencephalon* (or between brain), composed primarily of the *thalamus* and the *hypothalamus*. In this later stage of development, the *mesencephalon* remains undivided. The rhombencephalon gives rise to two structures: the *metencephalon* (or afterbrain), consisting of the *pons* and the *cerebellum*, and the *myelencephalon* or medulla. The caudal portion of the neural tube remains undivided and becomes the *spinal cord*. Thus, the five brain vesicles and the spinal cord define the six major divisions of the mature central nervous system and are identifiable by the sixth week of fetal life.[1]

---

[1] The retina, the peripheral visual apparatus, also develops from the diencephalon (Figure 2.3, right). Despite its peripheral location, the retina is a portion of the central nervous system.

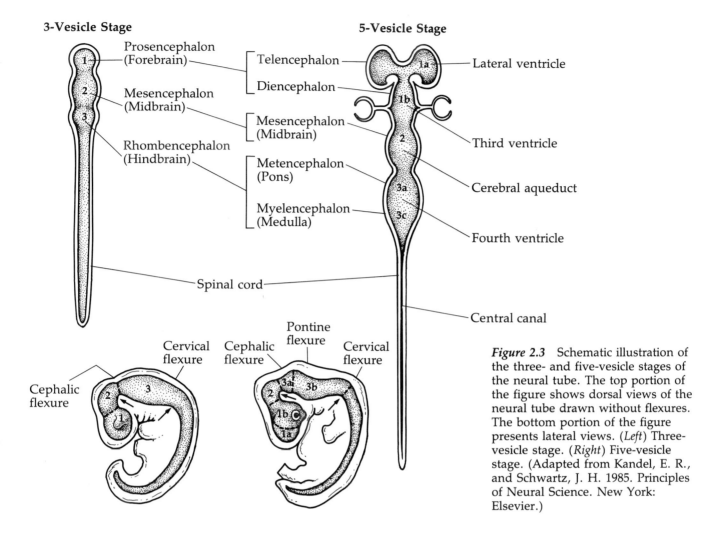

3-Vesicle Stage

5-Vesicle Stage

Prosencephalon (Forebrain)

Telencephalon — Lateral ventricle

Diencephalon

Mesencephalon (Midbrain)

Mesencephalon (Midbrain) — Third ventricle

Rhombencephalon (Hindbrain)

Metencephalon (Pons)

Myelencephalon (Medulla) — Cerebral aqueduct

— Fourth ventricle

Spinal cord

— Central canal

Cephalic flexure

Cervical flexure Cephalic flexure Pontine flexure Cervical flexure

Figure 2.3 Schematic illustration of the three- and five-vesicle stages of the neural tube. The top portion of the figure shows dorsal views of the neural tube drawn without flexures. The bottom portion of the figure presents lateral views. (*Left*) Three-vesicle stage. (*Right*) Five-vesicle stage. (Adapted from Kandel, E. R., and Schwartz, J. H. 1985. Principles of Neural Science. New York: Elsevier.)

The Longitudinal Axis of the Developing Brain Bends at the Midbrain–Diencephalic Juncture

The manner in which the developing brain bends, or *flexes*, provides the basis for a better understanding of the organization of the mature brain. The flexures occur as a consequence of the enormous proliferation of cells in the brain stem and cerebral hemispheres. At the three-vesicle stage there are two prominent flexures: the *cervical flexure*, at the junction of the spinal cord and the hindbrain, and the *cephalic flexure*, at the level of the midbrain (Figure 2.3). At the five-vesicle stage a third flexure becomes prominent, the *pontine flexure*. As the pontine flexure increases, a deep fissure is formed. The region immediately caudal to this fissure becomes approximated with the region located immediately rostral, thereby canceling out any net effect that the pontine flexure might have on the longitudinal axis. At birth, the cervical flexure is no longer apparent. In contrast to the cervical and pontine flexures, the cephalic flexure remains prominent, and actually causes the longitudinal axis of the forebrain to deviate from the longitudinal axis of the midbrain, hindbrain, and spinal cord.

The Ventricular System Develops from the Cavities in the Neural Tube

The large cavities within the cerebral vesicles develop into the ventricular system of the brain, and the caudal cavity becomes the central canal of the spinal cord (Figures 2.2 and 2.3). The ventricular system contains *cerebrospinal fluid* which is produced mainly by the *choroid plexus*. The choroid plexus forms in the ventricles (but not the cerebral aqueduct and the central canal) of the developing brain from the apposition of highly vascular mesodermal tissue with the ependymal lining of the neural tube. Here we examine the development of the general organization of the ventricular system. In a later section we will consider in detail the component of the ventricular system with the most complex three-dimensional configuration, the lateral ventricle.

As the five brain vesicles develop, the cavity in the forebrain differentiates into the two *lateral ventricles* (named the first and second ventricles by early anatomists) and the *third ventricle* (Figure 2.3). The lateral ventricles develop as outpouchings from the third ventricle. This evagination occurs in the region immediately caudal to the rostral wall of the third ventricle, which is also the location of the anterior neural tube closure, termed the *lamina terminalis*. The *interventricular foramina* (of *Monro*) interconnect each lateral ventricle with the third ventricle.

Figure 2.4 A. Schematic drawing of transverse sections of the spinal cord at three stages of development. *B.* Myelin-stained section through spinal cord of mature nervous system.

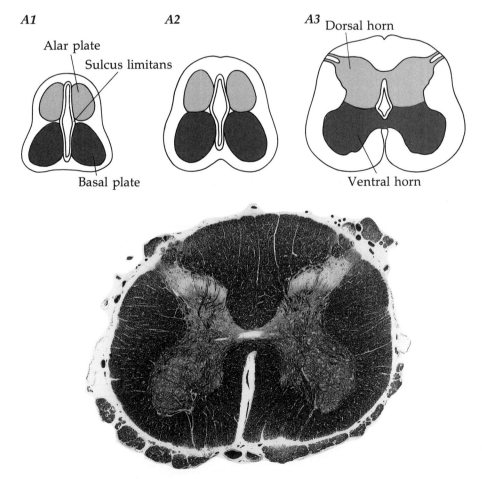

A1 Alar plate, Sulcus limitans, Basal plate

A2

A3 Dorsal horn, Ventral horn

The *fourth ventricle*, the most caudal ventricle, develops from the cavity within the rhombencephalon. It is connected to the third ventricle by the *cerebral aqueduct* (of *Sylvius*). The cerebral aqueduct is more dilated in the embryonic brain than in the mature brain. Throughout development, proliferation of cells in the dorsal region of the midbrain, which is termed the *tectum*, compresses the cerebral aqueduct and constricts its diameter (for example, compare Figures 2.8A1, A3, and B). The midbrain tectum of the mature brain, as we will see in the next chapter, contains separate collections of neurons that are important in processing auditory information and controlling rapid eye movements. Similar to the cerebral aqueduct, the central canal becomes much smaller during development (see Figure 2.4).

The interventricular foramina and the cerebral aqueduct are more vulnerable than other components of the ventricular system to the constricting effects of tumors, inflammation, or swelling from trauma. Two factors contribute to this vulnerabilty: the interventricular foramina and cerebral aqueduct (1) have small diameters and (2) are conduits for the flow of cerebrospinal fluid. (Cerebrospinal fluid does not flow through the central canal because it has no aperture for its exit to the subarachnoid space.) Pathological processes can close the interventricular foramina or the cerebral aqueduct, effectively damming the flow of cerebrospinal fluid, which continues to be produced by the choroid plexus. If occlusion occurs before the bones of the skull are fused—in embryonic life or in infancy—the increasing ventricular size will cause head size to increase, a condition called *hydrocephalus*. In contrast, if occlusion of the interventricular foramina or the cerebral aqueduct occurs after the bones of the skull are fused, ventricular size cannot increase without increasing intracranial pressure, a life-threatening condition.

The Spinal Cord and Brain Stem Develop from the Caudal and Intermediate Portions of the Neural Tube

The spinal cord receives sensory information from the limbs and trunk and provides the motor innervation of the muscles of these structures via the *spinal nerves*. The sensory and motor innervation of the head is provided by the *cranial nerves*, which enter and exit from the brain stem. An important principle governs the organization of the gray matter—the cellular regions—of the spinal cord and the brain stem. Nuclei in these regions that directly mediate sensory and motor functions form longitudinally oriented columns of cells. In this section, the development of the spinal cord is considered first, followed by the development of key components of the brain stem.

Dorsal and Ventral Regions of the Spinal Cord Mediate Somatic Sensation and Motor Control of the Limbs and Trunk

During development, two zones of proliferating neuroblasts in the mantle cell layer of the embryonic spinal cord form columns that extend its full length. One zone, termed the *alar plate*, is located in the dorsal portion of the wall of the neural tube, and the second zone, the *basal plate*, is located in the ventral portion (Figure 2.4A). These plates are separated by a shallow groove, the *sulcus limitans*. The major principle of

Table 2.1 Functional Classes of Spinal Nerves

Classification	Function	Structure Innervated
Afferent fibers		
General somatic	Tactile, pain/ temperature proprioception	Skin, mucous membranes, skeletal muscles
General visceral	Mechanical, pain/ temperature	Viscera, cardiovascular, respiratory, genitourinary tract
Motor fibers		
General somatic	Skeletal muscle control (somites)	Limb and axial musculature
General visceral	Autonomic control	Sweat glands, gut

spinal cord development is that the dorsally located cell column (the alar plate) and the ventrally located column (the basal plate) mediate sensory and motor function, respectively. Developing neurons from the alar plate form the *dorsal horn* of the mature spinal cord (Figure 2.4B). The dorsal horn mediates somatic and visceral sensations, such as pressure and pain. Dorsal horn neurons receive their input from sensory neurons that are part of the peripheral nervous system, termed *primary sensory neurons*. The axons of these sensory neurons enter the spinal cord through the dorsal roots (see Figure 1.4). As we will see in Chapter 5, the primary sensory neurons are specialized to receive sensory information from the body surface and peripheral organs and to transmit this information to the spinal cord.

Developing neurons of the basal plate mediate *motor* function in the mature central nervous system. These neurons are located in the *ventral horn* of the spinal cord gray matter (Figure 2.4), and they send their axons to the periphery via the *ventral root* (Figure 1.4). Somatic motor neurons innervate striated muscle. Visceral motor neurons[2] innervate neurons of the autonomic nervous system that are located in the periphery. These peripheral autonomic neurons, in turn, innervate visceral structures (Chapter 14). Other developing neurons of the basal plate become interneurons. Unlike motor neurons, whose axons leave the spinal cord, the axon of the interneurons remains in the spinal cord.

The sensory and motor innervation of somatic and visceral structures is mediated by separate primary sensory neurons and motor neurons. The axons of these neurons travel in peripheral nerves, which collect in the spinal nerves before approaching the spinal cord. The axons of the primary sensory neurons and motor neurons that innervate somatic and visceral structures, such as the skin and blood vessels respectively, have different anatomical characteristics and functional properties. There is a special nomenclature for the different functional categories of axons in peripheral nerves based on whether the axon is sensory or motor and whether it innervates somatic or visceral structures. For this nomenclature, the term *afferent* is used instead of sensory. The distinction between

---

[2] Visceral motor neurons are actually located at the junction of the dorsal and ventral horns, in a nucleus called the intermediolateral cell column (or nucleus). This region is sometimes called the lateral horn because it protrudes into the white matter of the spinal cord at certain levels.

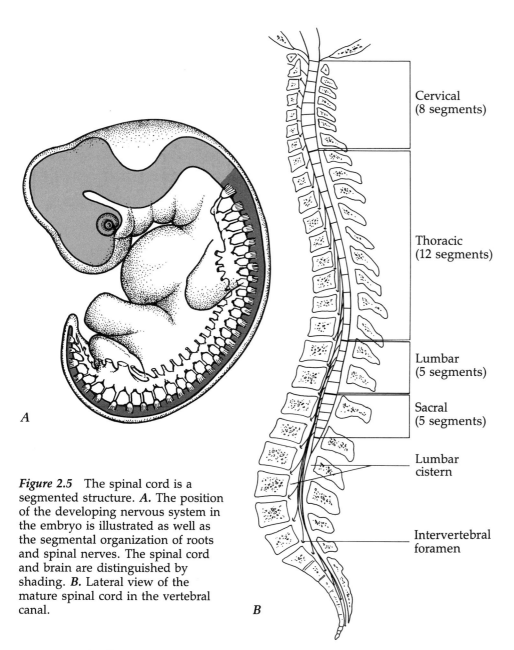

Figure 2.5 The spinal cord is a segmented structure. *A.* The position of the developing nervous system in the embryo is illustrated as well as the segmental organization of roots and spinal nerves. The spinal cord and brain are distinguished by shading. *B.* Lateral view of the mature spinal cord in the vertebral canal.

Cervical
(8 segments)

Thoracic
(12 segments)

Lumbar
(5 segments)

Sacral
(5 segments)

Lumbar
cistern

Intervertebral
foramen

A

B

sensory and afferent is subtle and when applied to functional categories of axons in peripheral nerves these two terms are essentially synonymous. (In Chapter 3, a more general definition of afferent is presented.) These four categories are: (1) *somatic afferent*, (2) *visceral afferent*, (3) *somatic motor*, and (4) *visceral motor*. Table 2.1 summarizes these functional categories. As we will see later (Table 2.2), there are a greater number of cranial nerve categories.

The Spinal Cord Has a Segmented Structure

The spinal cord has a *segmental* organization. In the embryo (Figure 2.5A), there are 38–40 pairs of *somites* from which the muscles, bones, and other structures of the neck, limbs, and trunk develop: 8 cervical, 12 thoracic, 5 lumbar, 5 sacral, and 8–10 coccygeal—most of which disappear later in development. (There are 4 occipital somites that form structures of the head, not shown.) As the somites form different portions of the body, separate spinal cord segments subserve sensation and movement of different portions of the body. The cervical spinal cord innervates the skin and muscles of the back of the head, neck, and arms. The thoracic spinal cord innervates the trunk, and the lumbar and sacral segments innervate the legs and perineal region. (The cranial nerves provide the sensory and motor innervation of the head—see later.)

Each somite has direct neural connections with a separate spinal cord segment. These connections provide the sensory and motor innervation of the skin and muscle. The neural connections between the developing somite and spinal cord are made by the axons of primary sensory neurons and motor neurons. Traveling together in spinal nerves, the sensory and motor axons enter and leave the spinal cord via the dorsal and ventral roots respectively. The mature spinal cord is shown in Figure 2.5B. Segmentation of the spinal cord in the mature central nervous system is apparent as the series of dorsal and ventral roots emerging from its lateral surface.

Throughout the first three months of development the length of the spinal cord increases in parallel with the enlargement of the vertebral column. During this period the spinal cord occupies the entire *vertebral canal*, the space within the vertebral column. The dorsal and ventral roots associated with each segment pass directly through the intervertebral foramina (Figure 2.5B) to reach their target structures. Later, the growth of the vertebral column exceeds that of the spinal cord, with two important anatomical consequences. First, a space forms within the caudal portion of the spinal canal that is part of the subarachnoid space and is termed the *lumbar cistern* (Figure 2.5B; see Figure 4.11). Cerebrospinal fluid can be withdrawn from the lumbar cistern by inserting a needle through the space between the third and fourth (or the fourth and fifth) vertebrae. This procedure is known as a *spinal* or *lumbar tap*. Second, the dorsal and ventral roots subserving sensation and movement of the legs must travel a long distance before exiting the vertebral canal (Figure 2.5B). These roots resemble a horse's tail, hence the name *cauda equina*.

The Somatic and Visceral Cell Columns in the Brain Stem Are Separate and Subdivided

The brain stem follows a developmental plan that is much like that of the spinal cord. Specific features of the development of the medulla, pons, and midbrain are illustrated in Figures 2.6–2.8, along with myelin-stained sections through the mature brain stem. Here, we will briefly consider the organization of the cranial nerve nuclei from a developmental perspective. The various cranial nerves are introduced in Chapter 3 and the cranial nerve nuclei will be considered in greater detail in Chapters 12 and 13. The gray matter of the brain stem consists of separate alar and basal plates extending from the medulla to the midbrain that form columns of neurons. Similar to the spinal cord, many immature neurons of the alar plate of the brain stem will function as neurons that process and relay sensory information in the mature central nervous system. Similarly, many neurons of the basal plate will develop into somatic and visceral motor neurons. In the brain stem, the alar and basal plates are also sep-

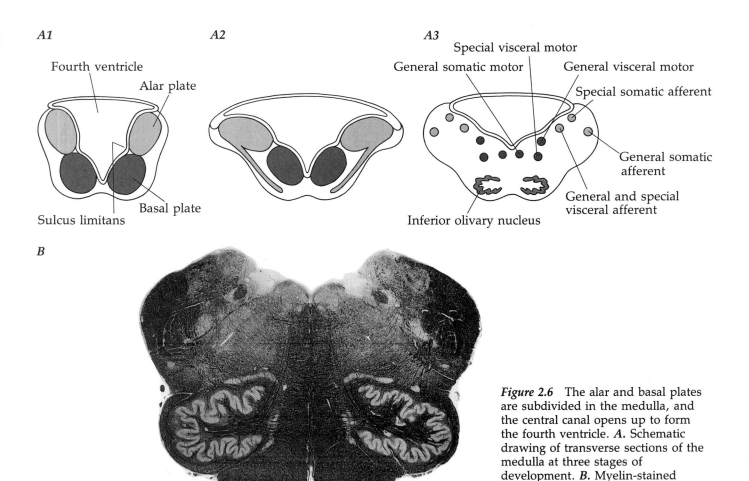

Figure 2.6 The alar and basal plates are subdivided in the medulla, and the central canal opens up to form the fourth ventricle. *A.* Schematic drawing of transverse sections of the medulla at three stages of development. *B.* Myelin-stained section through medulla of mature nervous system.

arated by the sulcus limitans. *Cranial nerve motor nuclei* contain motor neurons that innervate cranial muscle; *cranial nerve sensory nuclei* contain neurons that receive sensory information from cranial structures. The cranial nerve nuclei are connected with peripheral structures, such as muscles or sensory receptors, by the *cranial nerves*. The cranial nerve nuclei are analogous to the dorsal and ventral horns of the spinal cord and the cranial nerves are analogous to the spinal nerves. The key difference between the developmental plan of the spinal cord and that of the brain stem is that the visceral and somatic cell columns of the alar and basal plates of the brain stem are separate and each column is subdivided. In addition, compared with spinal nerves there are more functional categories of cranial nerves. There are seven functional categories of axons in cranial nerves (Table 2.2) and there are separate cranial nerve nuclei with which these nerves are associated (Figure 2.6). The reason for the additional three categories is that there are sensory and motor structures unique to the head. These structures are innervated by axons of the *special afferent* and *special motor* categories. The special sensory (afferent) structures are[3] the olfactory epithelium, the retina, the cochlea, the labyrinth,

---

[3] The olfactory epithelium and the retina are further distinguished because they connect to the telencephalon and diencephalon directly.

Table 2.2 Functional Classes of Cranial Nerves[a]

Classification	Function	Structure Innervated	Cranial Nerve
Afferent fibers			
General somatic	Tactile, pain/temperature proprioception	Skin, mucous membranes, skeletal muscles of head and neck	V, VII, IX, X
General visceral	Mechanical, pain/temperature proprioception	Oral cavity, pharynx, larynx	V, VII, IX, X
Special somatic	Audition, balance	Cochlea, labyrinth	VIII
Special visceral	Taste, olfaction	Taste buds, olfactory epithelium	I, VII, IX, X
Motor fibers			
General somatic	Skeletal muscle control (somites)	Extraocular and tongue muscles	III, IV, VI, XII
General visceral	Autonomic control	Tear glands, sweat glands, gut	III, VII, IX, X
Special visceral	Skeletal muscle (branchiomeric)	Facial expression, jaw	V, VII

[a] The optic nerve (II) is not considered in this table because it does not contain the axons of primary sensory neurons but rather those of third-order neurons in the visual pathway. The visual system is, however, considered to be part of the special somatic afferent class.

Figure 2.7 Immature neurons migrate from the alar plate and form the pontine nuclei. *A.* Schematic drawing of transverse sections of the pons at three stages of development. *B.* Myelin-stained section through pons of mature nervous system.

and the taste buds. The special motor structures are the muscles of banchiomeric origin (Table 2.2).

Rather than being oriented in the dorsal–ventral axis, as in the spinal cord, the visceral and somatic cell columns of the brain stem cranial nerve nuclei are aligned roughly from the midline to the lateral brain stem margin. This is because the roof of the fourth ventricle expands more laterally than the ventricular floor (Figure 2.6). The cell column that contains the cranial nerve nuclei that innervate skeletal muscles that are derived from

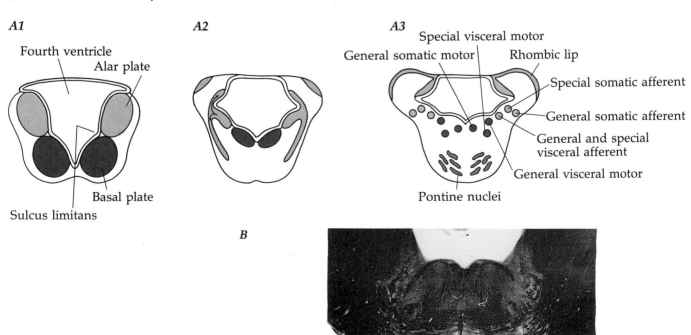

A1
- Fourth ventricle
- Alar plate
- Basal plate
- Sulcus limitans

A2

A3
- General somatic motor
- Special visceral motor
- Rhombic lip
- Special somatic afferent
- General somatic afferent
- General and special visceral afferent
- General visceral motor
- Pontine nuclei

B

body somites is located most medially. This column is called the *general somatic motor* column. The next two cell columns contain neurons that mediate the *special* and *general visceral motor* projections. Because of their visceral origin, motor neurons that innervate the branchiomeric skeletal muscle are located in the special visceral motor column. The general visceral motor column contains autonomic preganglionic neurons. The sulcus limitans separates the motor columns from the afferent columns, which are located more laterally. The afferent column closest to the sulcus limitans contains neurons that process *general* and *special visceral afferent information*, visceral chemoreception and taste, respectively. The most lateral afferent cell columns mediate sensation from structures of somatic origin, for example tactile stimulation of the face (*general somatic afferent*), audition, and balance (*special somatic afferent*). In the adult, the sulcus limitans remains as a landmark on the floor of the fourth ventricle.

There is a second major difference between the developmental plans of the spinal cord and the brain stem. Other nuclei that are not cranial nerve nuclei, and therefore not analogous to the dorsal and ventral horns of the spinal cord, are derived from the alar and basal plates of the brain stem. These nuclei develop from immature neurons that *migrate* farther from the mantle layer than those forming the cranial nerve nuclei. The immature neurons reach their final destinations in the ventral portion of the brain stem or in regions dorsal to the ventricular system (Figures 2.6–2.8). Some of the nuclei that develop from migrating immature neurons include the inferior olivary nucleus (Figure 2.6A3) and the pontine nuclei (Figure 2.7A3), which relay information from the medulla and pons to the cerebellum. The red nucleus and substantia nigra (Figure 2.8A3) also develop from immature neurons that migrate from more dorsal portions

Figure 2.8 The tectum of the midbrain develops from the alar plate *A*. Schematic drawing of transverse sections of the midbrain at three stages of development. *B*. Myelin-stained section through midbrain of mature nervous system.

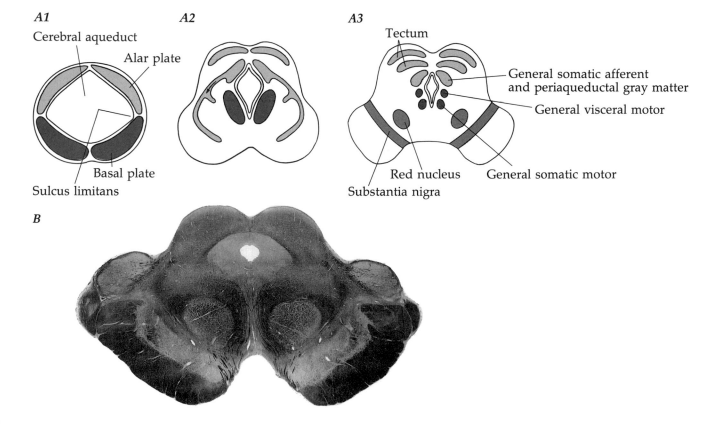

A1
Cerebral aqueduct
Alar plate
Basal plate
Sulcus limitans

A2

A3
Tectum
General somatic afferent and periaqueductal gray matter
General visceral motor
Red nucleus
General somatic motor
Substantia nigra

B

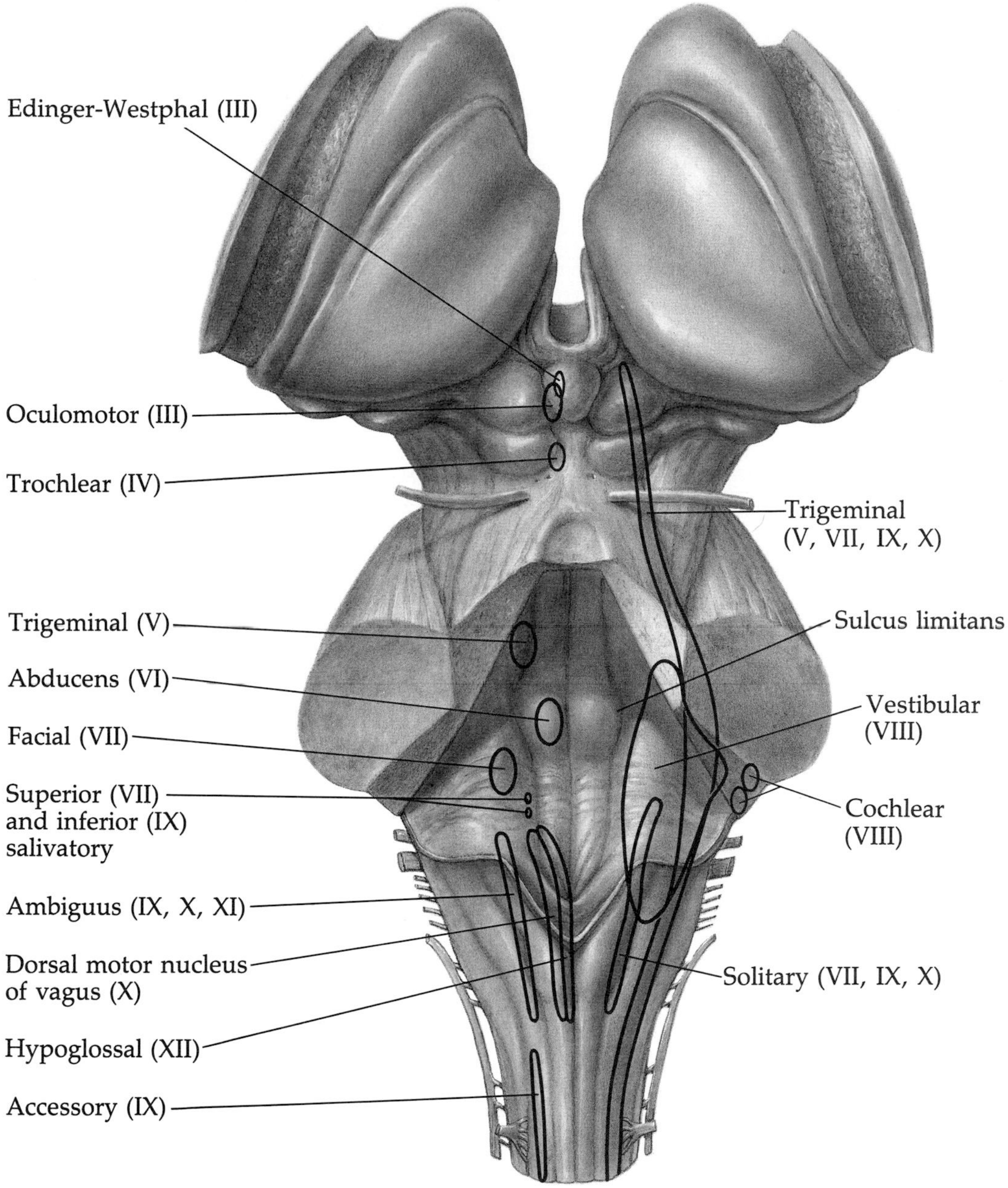

Edinger-Westphal (III)

Oculomotor (III)

Trochlear (IV)

Trigeminal (V, VII, IX, X)

Trigeminal (V)

Abducens (VI)

Facial (VII)

Superior (VII) and inferior (IX) salivatory

Sulcus limitans

Vestibular (VIII)

Cochlear (VIII)

Ambiguus (IX, X, XI)

Dorsal motor nucleus of vagus (X)

Solitary (VII, IX, X)

Hypoglossal (XII)

Accessory (IX)

Figure 2.9 The cranial nerve nuclei have a longitudinal organization. A dorsal view of the brain stem of the mature central nervous system is illustrated with the locations of the various cranial nerve nuclei indicated.

of the midbrain. These two structures are part of the motor system in the mature brain. The cerebellum also develops from migrating immature neurons of the alar plate neuroblasts (see later).

Knowledge of the organization of the brain stem alar and basal plates provides a framework for understanding the mature brain stem. Compare the general configuration of the schematic sections through the developing brain stem with myelin-stained sections through the mature brain stem (Parts B in Figures 2.6–2.8). In later chapters, we will have the opportunity to examine the detailed structure of the brain stem. During development, the visceral and somatic cell columns maintain constant relative positions with respect to the midline and the floor of the fourth ventricle. Because cranial nerve nuclei that serve similar functions are aligned in rostral–caudal columns, knowledge of the locations of these nuclei will aid in understanding their function. The longitudinal organization of the various cell columns forming the cranial nerve nuclei in the mature brain stem is shown in Figure 2.9.

The Cerebellum Develops from the Rhombic Lips

The cerebellum plays a key role in the control of movement. Without the cerebellum, even simple movements are uncoordinated. In the mature central nervous system, the cerebellum has numerous anatomical and functional subdivisions. Understanding how the cerebellum develops makes its adult structure less mysterious. The cerebellum develops from immature neurons of the *rhombic lips*, a specialized region of the alar plate of the metencephalon (Figure 2.7). The rhombic lips are located in the dorsolateral metencephalon, initially widely separated from each other. These two dorsolateral sites of proliferating cells eventually fuse at the midline, forming the *vermis* of the cerebellum (Figure 2.10). This region of the cerebellum is most concerned with balance and posture. The paired

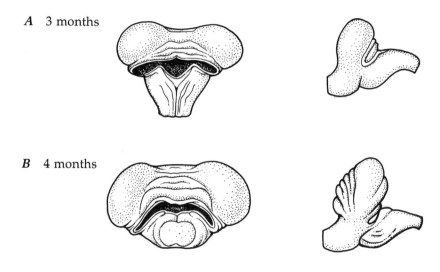

A 3 months

B 4 months

Figure 2.10 The cerebellum develops from the dorsal portion of the metencephalon, a region termed the rhombic lip. Caudal views (*left*) and lateral views (*right*) are shown at three stages of development. (Adapted from Keibel, F., and Mall, F. P. (eds.). 1910–1912. Manual of Human Embryology. 2 vols. Philadelphia: Lippincott.)

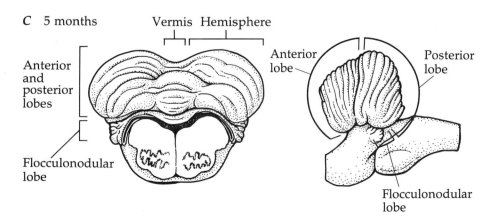

C 5 months

Vermis Hemisphere

Anterior and posterior lobes

Flocculonodular lobe

Anterior lobe

Posterior lobe

Flocculonodular lobe

lateral regions form the *cerebellar hemispheres*, which participate in the control of limb movements, such as reaching. Later in development, fissures develop. The most prominent of these fissures are oriented from medial to lateral, and divide the cerebellum into three lobes: anterior, posterior, and flocculonodular. The functional organization of the cerebellum will be considered in Chapter 11.

As the cerebellum develops from immature neurons that migrate from the alar plate, two prominent brain stem nuclei have neurons that send their axons to the cerebellum also develop from the alar plate. However, these immature neurons migrate to the ventral brain stem. The *inferior olivary nucleus* (1) are located in the medulla (Figure 2.6), and the *pontine nuclei* (2), in the pons (Figure 2.7). These nuclei, which form important circuits for the learning of motor skills, will be considered in greater detail in Chapter 10.

The Rostral Portion of the Neural Tube Gives Rise to the Diencephalon and Cerebral Hemispheres

More than any other brain region, the structure of the cerebral hemispheres is markedly transformed during development (Figure 2.11). Whereas the brain stem and spinal cord retain their longitudinal organization in the mature brain, the cerebral hemispheres have a more complex three-dimensional shape. This is largely the result of the enormous proliferation of cells of the cerebral cortex. As we saw in Chapter 1, the cerebral hemisphere contains four major components: (1) cerebral cortex, (2) basal ganglia, (3) hippocampal formation, and (4) amygdala. The development of the diencephalon, a separate division of the central nervous system, is considered along with the cerebral hemispheres for two reasons. First, one component of the diencephalon, the thalamus, relays information to the cerebral cortex and its development parallels that of the cerebral cortex. Second, because sections of the mature cerebral hemispheres transect the cerebral cortex, basal ganglia, and diencephalon, it is important to understand the ontogenic basis of their relative spatial relationships. The development of the cerebral hemispheres and diencephalon is examined by referring to their gross anatomy and to transverse sections through both the developing and mature brain. Familiarity with sections through the developing brain makes it easier to understand sections through the mature cerebral hemispheres.

The Lateral Margin of the Diencephalon Fuses with the Telencephalon

The diencephalon and third ventricle lie medial to the cerebral hemispheres and lateral ventricles when the five-vesicle stage is first achieved early in development. At this stage, three components of the diencephalon are apparent: the *epithalamus*, from which the pineal gland forms, the *thalamus*, a collection of nuclei that communicate with the cerebral cortex, and the *hypothalamus*, the structure important in regulating visceral functions and their emotional counterparts. These components are shown in Figure 2.12, at an earlier stage and a later stage of devel-

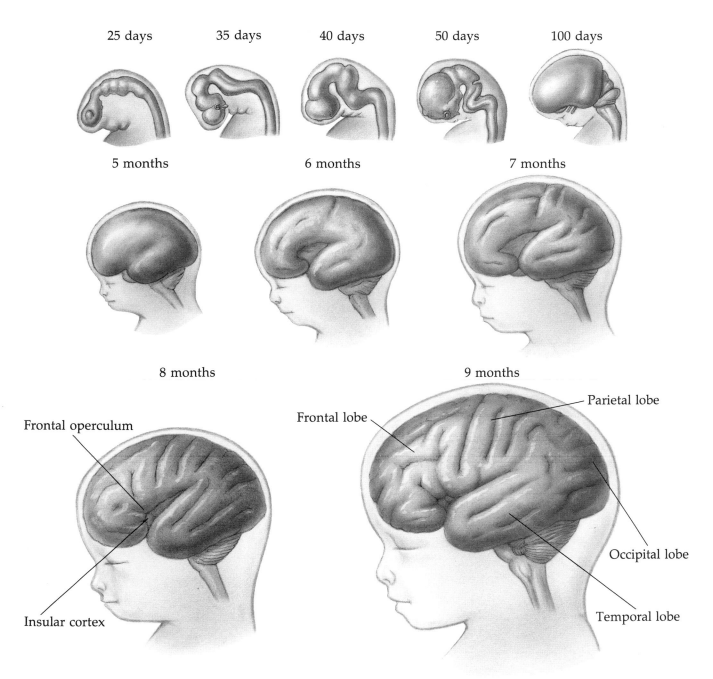

Figure 2.11 The development of human brain is shown from the lateral surface in relation to the face and the general shape of the cranium. (Adapted from Cowan, W. M. 1979. The development of the brain. Sci. Am. 241:112–133.)

opment. The transverse sections (Figure 2.12A2) reveal the thalamus and hypothalamus.

In Figure 2.12 we can also see components of the developing telencephalon and their spatial relations with those of the diencephalon. The cerebral cortex and the basal ganglia are two principal neural structures

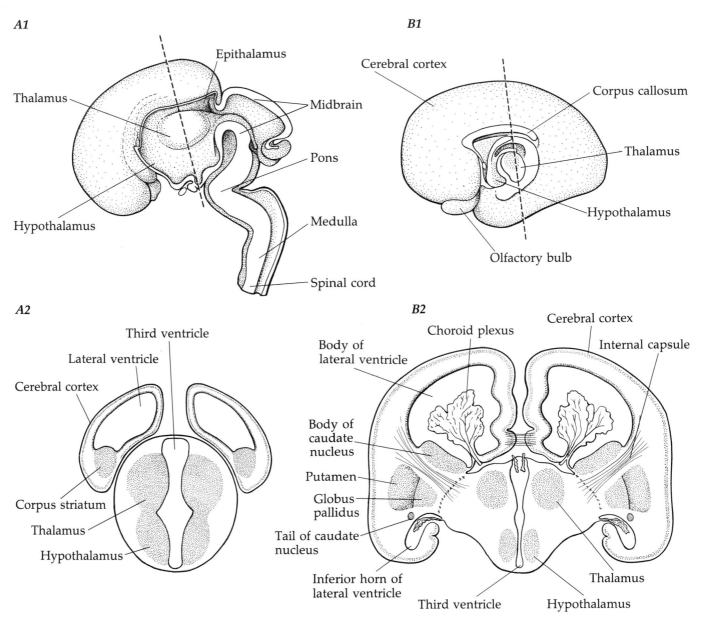

Figure 2.12 Portions of the cerebral hemispheres fuse with the diencephalon. The top portions of this figure illustrate medial views of brain during an early *(A)* and a later *(B)* stage of development. The bottom portion of the figure shows schematic transverse sections through the brain in the planes indicated on top (*dashed lines*). (Adapted from Patten, B. M. 1968. Human Embryology. New York: McGraw-Hill (Blackston Division).)

of the cerebral hemispheres. The developing cerebral cortex consists of a thin sheet of immature neurons and their axonal processes overlying the lateral ventricle. Two of the components of the basal ganglia develop from immature neurons of the *corpus striatum*, in the floor of the lateral ventricle: the *caudate nucleus* and the *putamen*. The third component of the basal ganglia, the *globus pallidus*, is of diencephalic origin. Immature neurons of the developing globus pallidus migrate from the ventricular surface, near the interventricular foramen, to a more lateral location.

The expansion of the cerebral cortex (see later) results in the apposition and fusion of a portion of the medial surface of the telencephalon and the lateral surface of the diencephalon (Figure 2.12B2). There are two important consequences of this fusion. First, the caudate nucleus and the thalamus appose, a spatial arrangement that continues into brain maturity. Second, the caudate nucleus and the putamen are incompletely separated by fiber tracts formed by axons of thalamic neurons that project to the cerebral cortex and axons that descend from the cortex. These ascending and descending fibers form the *internal capsule* (see Figure 3.10). The fibers course to and from the cortex through this region of apposition (Figure 2.12B2). In the mature brain, the caudate nucleus and putamen are collectively called the *striatum* because the passing axons give these structures a striated appearance.

Two additional structures once considered components of the basal ganglia are the amygdala and claustrum. Although both the *amygdala* and the striatum share a developmental history (the amygdala develops from the corpus striatum) and a close spatial relationship, their functions are quite dissimilar. Whereas the striatum participates in cognition and motor function, the amygdala is important in visceral function and emotions. The *claustrum* does not develop from the corpus striatum, but is thought instead to derive from the cerebral cortex that overlies it. Although we understand many of the anatomical connections of the claustrum, we understand little of its function.

The Cerebral Cortex Encircles the Diencephalon

The expansion of the cerebral cortex (Figure 2.11) forces many of the underlying structures to assume a more complex three-dimensional configuration. The portion of the cerebral cortex to develop earliest will become the parietal lobe. As the cortex develops, it expands first rostrally to form the frontal lobes, then posteriorly to form the occipital lobe and inferiorly to form the temporal lobe (Figure 2.11). As a result of this inferior and posterior expansion, the cortex takes on a *C-shaped configuration*. Many structures on the medial surface of the cerebral hemisphere have a C-shaped configuration and these structures constitute a major portion of the limbic system (Chapter 15).

Even before the cerebral cortex develops its characteristic surface convolutions, the gyri and sulci, a region of the lateral surface of the frontal, parietal, and temporal lobes becomes buried during development (Figures 2.11 and 2.13). This region, termed the *insular cortex*, is located deep within the lateral (Sylvian) fissure in the mature brain and therefore is revealed only in sections through the cerebral hemisphere. The portions of the frontal, parietal, and temporal cortices that cover the insular cortex are termed the *operculum*. The *frontal operculum* (Figure 2.11) of the dominant hemisphere (typically the left hemisphere in right-handed individuals) is important in motor mechanisms for speech. The parietal and temporal opercular regions and the insular cortex are important in sensory function.

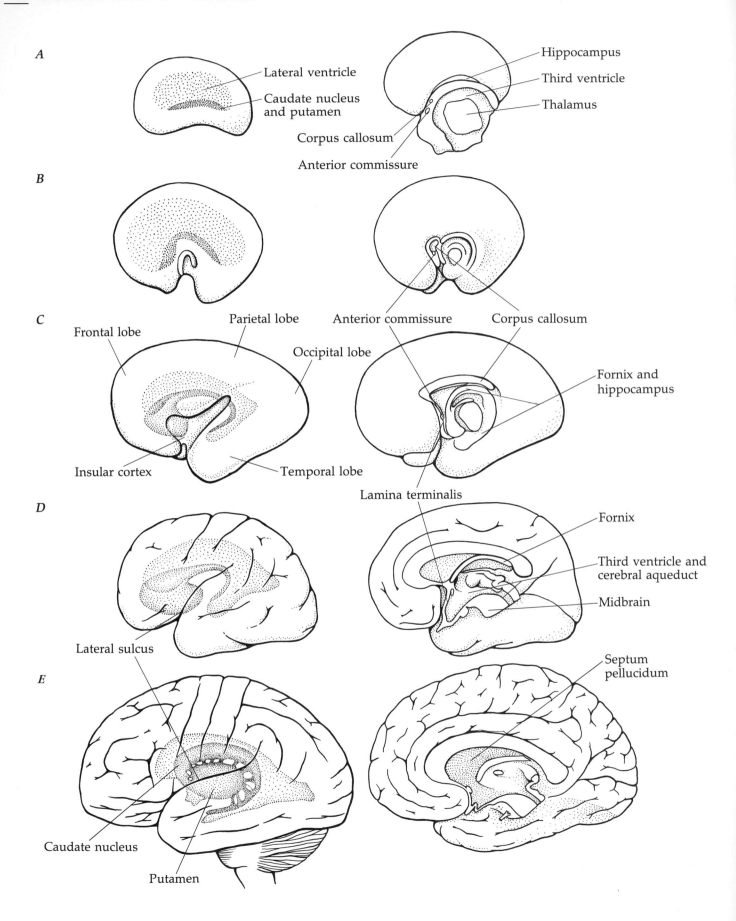

A

Lateral ventricle

Caudate nucleus and putamen

Hippocampus

Third ventricle

Thalamus

Corpus callosum

Anterior commissure

B

C

Parietal lobe

Frontal lobe

Occipital lobe

Anterior commissure

Corpus callosum

Fornix and hippocampus

Insular cortex

Temporal lobe

Lamina terminalis

D

Fornix

Third ventricle and cerebral aqueduct

Midbrain

Lateral sulcus

E

Septum pellucidum

Caudate nucleus

Putamen

◁ *Figure 2.13* Various components of the telencephalon acquire a C-shape during development. Lateral views of the cerebral hemisphere, with lateral ventricle lightly stippled and the caudate nucleus densely stippled, are shown on the left; medial views are shown on the right. Five stages of development are illustrated: 2, 3, 5, 7, and 9 months. (Adapted from Keibel, F., and Mall, F. P. (eds.). 1910–1912. Manual of Human Embryology. 2 vols. Philadelphia: Lippincott.)

As development of the cerebral cortex proceeds, so too does the large fiber path that interconnects the cerebral cortex of the two hemispheres, the *corpus callosum* (Figure 2.13, right). Collections of axons that interconnect the two halves of the central nervous system are termed *commissures* and the corpus callosum is the largest brain commissure. Remarkably, when this structure is surgically transected, for amelioration of the most severe symptoms of epilepsy, the two halves of the cerebral hemisphere function independently. The right hand may reach for an item only to be intercepted by the left hand!

The Lateral Ventricle and the Caudate Nucleus Are Subcortical C-Shaped Structures

As the cerebral cortex develops a C-shaped configuration, so too do two major subcortical structures: the lateral ventricle and a component of the basal ganglia, the caudate nucleus (Figure 2.13, left). The hippocampal formation and its efferent pathway, the fornix, also have a C-shape (Figure 1.9B). These structures are considered in Chapter 15. At 2 months of intrauterine life the lateral ventricle is roughly spherical in shape and the caudate nucleus lies in its floor. The transformation of the lateral ventricle and caudate nucleus into the characteristic C-shape of the mature brain begins at about 3 months. The three-dimensional configuration of the lateral ventricle in the mature brain is shown in the bottom row of Figure 2.13. It should be recalled that the lateral ventricle has four component parts: the *anterior* (or frontal) *horn*, the *body*, the *posterior* (or occipital) *horn*, and the *inferior* (or temporal) *horn* (see Figure 1.11B). The anterior horn and body of the two lateral ventricles remain close to the midline and are separated by the *septum pellucidum*, which can be seen on the medial brain surface (Figure 2.13, right). The anterior horn, body, and inferior horn collectively describe a C-shaped arc. The choroid plexus also has a C-shape configuration (see Figure 4.11). It forms a continuous band of tissue running from the inferior horn to the body of the lateral ventricle, through the interventricular foramen, and into the roof of the third ventricle. The three-dimensional configuration of the caudate nucleus in the mature brain is also shown in Figure 2.13. The rostral portion of the caudate nucleus is not separated from the putamen (Figure 2.13) because the internal capsule is located more caudal.

The lateral ventricle and caudate nucleus are important landmarks in sections through the mature brain and the key to understanding their locations in the two-dimensional slices is that they are located *dorsally* and *ventrally*. A myelin-stained transverse section through the mature brain is shown in Figure 2.14. The body of the lateral ventricle is seen in the dorsal portion of the section, in the frontal lobe; ventrally, the tem-

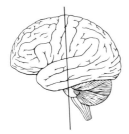

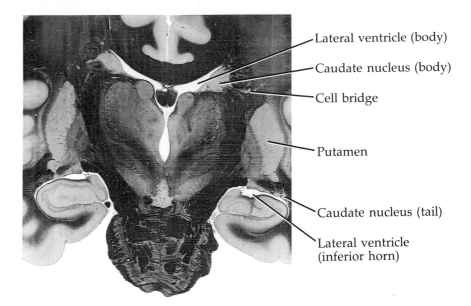

Lateral ventricle (body)

Caudate nucleus (body)

Cell bridge

Putamen

Caudate nucleus (tail)

Lateral ventricle
(inferior horn)

Figure 2.14 A coronal section (myelin-stained) through the cerebral hemisphere of the mature brain illustrates that portions of the caudate nucleus and lateral ventricle are located ventrally and dorsally. Inset shows plane of section.

poral horn of the lateral ventricle is seen in the temporal lobe. The caudate nucleus is also present in two locations: dorsally, in the wall of the body of the lateral ventricle, and ventrally, in the roof of the inferior horn. The partial separation of the caudate nucleus and putamen by the fibers of the internal capsule is reflected in the small cell bridges that link these two structures (Figure 2.14). The names of the different portions of the caudate nucleus will be considered in Chapter 11.

Summary

Nerve cells and glial cells are derived from a specialized portion of the ectoderm termed the *neural plate* (Figure 2.1). The edges of the neural plate fold, ultimately appose, and form the *neural tube* (Figure 2.1). The cerebral hemispheres and the brain stem develop from the rostral and intermediate portions of the neural tube, and the spinal cord develops from the caudal portions. The *neuroepithelium* (Figure 2.2) lines the neural tube and forms the cellular constituents of the central nervous system. Immature neurons arise from the neuroepithelium. The neural tube has two additional layers: the *mantle layer*, which becomes the gray matter of the central nervous system, and the *marginal layer*, which becomes the white matter (Figure 2.2). The cavity within the neural tube forms the ventricular system.

Three brain vesicles first form from the rostral neural tube (Figure 2.3): (1) *prosencephalon (forebrain)*, (2) *mesencephalon (midbrain)*, and (3) *rhombencephalon (hindbrain)*. The prosencephalon divides into the *telencephalon (cerebral cortex, hippocampal formation, basal ganglia, and amygdala)* and *diencephalon (thalamus and hypothalamus)*, and the rhombencephalon divides into the *metencephalon (pons and cerebellum)* and *myelencephalon (medulla)*. The spinal cord, like the mesencephalon, remains undivided throughout development. A persisting bend called the *cephalic flexure* occurs at the juncture of the mesencephalon and diencephalon (Figure 2.3).

Immature neurons in the developing brain stem and spinal cord organize into rostrocaudally oriented columns of cells (Figures 2.4, 2.6–2.9). There are two such columns in the spinal cord: the *alar plate* forms the *dorsal horn*, and the *basal plate* forms the *ventral horn* (Figure 2.4). In the brain stem, the alar and basal plates are divided into separate *somatic* and *visceral* columns, from which the cranial nerve nuclei derive (Figures 2.6–2.9). Other sensory and motor nuclei of the brain stem derive from immature neurons that migrate from the alar and basal plates. The cerebellum forms from a particular portion of the alar plate, the *rhombic lip* (Figure 2.10).

In contrast to the diencephalon (Figure 2.12), which remains roughly spherical in shape throughout development, structures of the cerebral hemispheres take on a C-shaped configuration (Figures 2.11–2.14). The cerebral cortex, a component of the cerebral hemisphere, has an overall C-shape (Figures 2.11 and 2.13); so too does the *caudate nucleus* (Figure 2.13). The *lateral ventricle*, which is located within the cerebral hemisphere, has a C-shape as well (Figure 2.13). C-shaped structures appear twice on transverse sections through the cerebral hemisphere (Figure 2.14): dorsal and ventral. ■

References

Heimer, L. 1983. The Human Brain and Spinal Cord. New York: Springer-Verlag.

Keibel, F., and Mall, F. P. (eds.). 1910–1912. Manual of Human Embryology. 2 vols. Philadelphia: Lippincott.

Pansky, B. 1982. Review of Medical Embryology. New York: Macmillan.

Patten, B. M. 1968. Human Embryology. New York: McGraw-Hill (Blackston Division).

Selected Readings

Cowan, W. M. 1979. The development of the brain. Sci. Am. 241:112–133.

Jacobson, M. 1978. Developmental Neurobiology, 2nd ed. New York: Plenum Press.

Jones, E. G., and Cowan, W. M. 1983. Nervous tissue. In Weiss, L. (ed.), Histology: Cell and Tissue Biology, 5th ed. New York: Elsevier Biomedical, pp. 283–370.

Langman, J. 1981. Medical Embryology. Baltimore: Williams & Wilkins.

Internal Organization of the Central Nervous System

3

Internal Organization of the Central Nervous System

In Chapter 2 we saw that the complex three-dimensional organization of the central nervous system is explained by its developmental plan. In the cerebral hemispheres, the enormous proliferation of cells forces many structures into a C-shaped configuration. By contrast, the brain stem and spinal cord remain relatively undifferentiated. In fact, the brain stem and spinal cord in the mature brain closely resemble their embryonic counterparts. In this chapter we begin to focus on the internal organization of the central nervous system by comparing the three-dimensional configuration of brain structures with their appearance in myelin-stained sections, which are two-dimensional slices.

Longitudinally Oriented Systems Have a Component at Each Level of the Neuraxis

Whereas the complex anatomy of the brain is difficult to learn, the task is simplified by focusing on components that are present at all levels of the neuraxis. As we saw in Chapters 1 and 2, the *ventricular system* (Figure 3.1A) has components in all six major divisions of the central nervous system. In addition to the ventricular system, certain functional systems are present at all levels of the neuraxis. The *dorsal column–medial lemniscal* system is a sensory pathway that has a longitudinal organization (Figure 3.1B). It is termed an *ascending system* because it brings information from sensory receptors in the periphery to lower levels of the central nervous system, such as the brain stem, and then to higher levels, such as the thalamus and cerebral cortex. The dorsal column–medial lemniscal system is the principal path for perception of tactile stimuli. The corticospinal tract (Figure 3.1C) is the principal pathway for voluntary movement. Because this system carries information from a higher level of the central nervous system, the cerebral cortex, to a lower level, the spinal cord, it is termed a *descending pathway* or *system*. Axons of the corticospinal tract actually travel along the ventral brain stem surface during their descending course. As a component of the sensory and motor systems and the ventricular system is present at all levels of the neuraxis, knowledge of their organization provides a frame of reference for remembering the locations of other structures. The overall organization of the ventricular system, the dorsal column–medial lemniscal system, and the corticospinal tract is surveyed here. In later sections of this chapter we will have the opportunity to synthesize an overall view of the organization of the central nervous system when we identify components of these three longitudinal systems in key sections through the spinal cord, brain stem, and cerebral hemisphere. The plan of this chapter is similar to that of the chapters on the functional systems (Chapters 5–15). The *overall organization* of a neural system is surveyed first and then the *various levels* of the neural system are examined in sequence on sections through the central nervous system.

The brain ventricles and the central canal of the spinal cord are illustrated in Figure 3.1A. There is a component of the ventricular system at each level of the neuraxis. The *lateral ventricles* and *third ventricle* are located within the cerebral hemisphere and diencephalon, respectively. They are connected by the interventricular foramina. The cerebral aqueduct, located in the midbrain, connects the third and the fourth ventricles. The fourth ventricle is located in the pons and medulla. The central

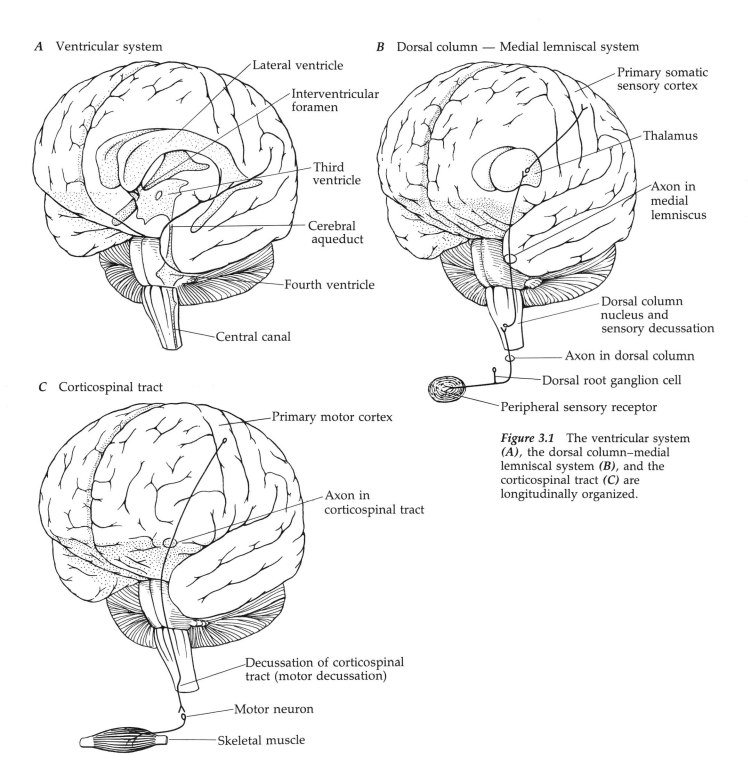

A Ventricular system

Lateral ventricle

Interventricular foramen

Third ventricle

Cerebral aqueduct

Fourth ventricle

Central canal

B Dorsal column — Medial lemniscal system

Primary somatic sensory cortex

Thalamus

Axon in medial lemniscus

Dorsal column nucleus and sensory decussation

Axon in dorsal column

Dorsal root ganglion cell

Peripheral sensory receptor

C Corticospinal tract

Primary motor cortex

Axon in corticospinal tract

Decussation of corticospinal tract (motor decussation)

Motor neuron

Skeletal muscle

Figure 3.1 The ventricular system *(A)*, the dorsal column–medial lemniscal system *(B)*, and the corticospinal tract *(C)* are longitudinally organized.

canal is the most caudal portion of the ventricular system, extending directly from the fourth ventricle into the spinal cord. In Chapter 2 it was shown that the complex three-dimensional shape of the ventricular system is a consequence of the developmental plan of the brain and spinal cord.

The dorsal column–medial lemniscal system (Figure 3.1B) is formed by a three-neuron circuit that links the periphery with the cerebral cortex, and in doing so traverses the six major divisions of the central nervous system. Its name derives from the names of two of its components: the axonal pathway in the spinal cord, called the *dorsal column*, and the pathway in the brain stem, the *medial lemniscus*. The first neurons in the circuit are the *dorsal root ganglion cells*, the class of neurons that innervate the peripheral sensory receptors. Dorsal root ganglion cells link the periphery, where the stimuli are received, with the spinal cord and brain stem. This component of the system is a fast transmission line that is visible on the dorsal surface of the spinal cord as the *dorsal column*. The first synapse is made in a *relay nucleus* in the medulla. A relay nucleus processes incoming signals and transmits this information to the next component of the circuit. Typically, the neural signal emerging from the relay nucleus is transformed from the incoming signal. Different relay nuclei transform neural signals in different ways, reflecting the particular feature of sensory processing the nucleus performs. The somatic sensory relay nucleus in the medulla is the *dorsal column nucleus*, and it contains the cell bodies of the second neurons in the pathway. The axons of these second-order neurons cross the midline, or *decussate* (termed the somatic sensory decussation). As a consequence of the decussation, sensory information from the right side of the body is processed by the left side of the brain. Most sensory (and motor) pathways decussate at some point along their course. This is a consistent neuroanatomical pattern whose functional significance is not known. The decussated axons ascend in the brain stem pathway, the *medial lemniscus*, to synapse in the *thalamus*. From here, third-order neurons send their axons to the primary somatic sensory cortex, which is located in the postcentral gyrus of the parietal lobe (Figure 3.1B).

The corticospinal tract originates from neurons in the cerebral cortex and terminates on motor neurons in the spinal cord. Many of the cells of the corticospinal tract that synapse directly on motor neurons are located in the primary motor cortex on the precentral gyrus of the frontal lobe (Figure 3.1C). The axons of these neurons leave the motor cortex and travel through the white matter underlying the cerebral cortex. As we will see later in the chapter, the corticospinal tract emerges from the cerebral hemisphere and courses along the ventral surface of the midbrain. The tract disappears below the ventral surface of the pons and reappears on the ventral surface of the medulla as the *medullary pyramid*. In the caudal medulla most of the axons in the corticospinal tract decussate (motor decussation). Once in the spinal cord, the descending cortical axons run along its lateral margin. This region is part of the white matter of the spinal cord because of the presence of myelinated axons. The axons terminate on motor neurons in the gray matter of the spinal cord. Since motor neurons innervate skeletal muscle, the motor cortex exerts a direct influence on movement.

The focus of the remaining sections of this chapter is on the internal structure of the central nervous system. We approach the problem of learning the individual nuclei and tracts of the brain and spinal cord by examining drawings and photographs of sections through key levels of the central nervous system. In addition, magnetic resonance scans of comparable sections of the living brain are examined. Because the central nervous system is so complex, the discussion in this chapter is limited to (1) those structures directly associated with the dorsal column–medial lemniscal system, the corticospinal tract, and the ventricular system, and (2) surface and internal landmarks that characterize the level of a particular slice. These landmarks are easily recognized by first-time viewers. Gradually, our neuroanatomy vocabulary will increase as we learn more of the functional organization of the brain in later chapters.

The Spinal Cord Has a Central Cellular Region Surrounded by a Region That Contains Myelinated Axons

Neurons of the dorsal root ganglia are sometimes termed primary sensory neurons because they provide the sensory input to the spinal cord (Figure 3.2), input that is used in perception, control of movement, and maintenance of arousal. The dorsal root ganglion cell receives sensory information from the periphery and transmits this information to the central nervous system. Each cell has two principal axon branches: (1) the peripheral branch projects to the peripheral tissue and provides the sensory innervation, and (2) the central branch enters the spinal cord through the *dorsal root*. The central branch has a complex branching pattern, with

Figure 3.2 A. Three-dimensional schematic view of a spinal cord segment, showing the branching pattern of dorsal root ganglion cells in the spinal cord. *B*. Circuit for the knee jerk reflex.

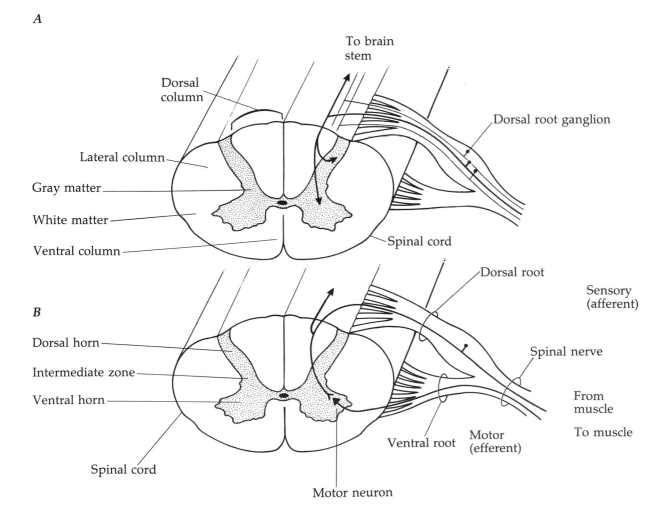

processes that terminate in the gray matter—the cellular region of the spinal cord—as well as ascend in the white matter—the axonal region of the spinal cord—to transmit sensory information to the brain stem (Figure 3.2A). The gray matter contains two functional regions, the *dorsal* and *ventral horns*, each of which contains columns of neurons oriented rostrocaudally. Recall that the dorsal horn develops from the alar plate and the ventral horn develops from the basal plate (see Chapter 2). Because neurons of the dorsal horn receive input from the dorsal root ganglion cells, they subserve sensory function. In contrast, neurons of the ventral horn subserve movement. Motor neurons are located here, and they send their axons out the ventral root.

There are monosynaptic connections between a certain type of dorsal root ganglion cell, stretch receptors called primary muscle spindle receptors, and motor neurons (Figure 2.2B). In certain segments of the lumbar spinal cord, this contact mediates a simple reflex, the *knee jerk reflex*. A tap to the patella tendon stretches the quadriceps muscle, thereby stretching primary spindle receptors in the muscle. A central branch of dorsal root ganglion cells that innervate these receptors synapse on quadriceps motor neurons. Because this synapse is excitatory, the quadriceps motor neurons are discharged and the muscle contracts. An understanding of this simple neural circuit helps one appreciate not only the functional organization of the spinal cord but also the information flow in the central nervous system. The sensory neuron is the *afferent* component of the reflex. An afferent path brings information into the central nervous system. The motor neuron is the *efferent* component of the reflex, relaying the neural command away from the central nervous system. The terms *afferent* and *efferent* also describe generally the direction of information flow within the central nervous system. An afferent pathway carries information toward structures in the central nervous system that process the information; an efferent pathway carries the processed information away.

Between the dorsal and ventral horns is the *intermediate zone*, which contains interneurons that link the sensory functions of the dorsal horn with the motor functions of the ventral horn. Whereas the knee jerk reflex is a monosynaptic reflex, other reflexes have numerous synapses interposed between the sensory and motor neurons, and many of these neurons are located in the intermediate zone. For example, touching a hot surface evokes a reflex withdrawal of the hand. This behavior is mediated by a polysynaptic reflex with interneurons located in the intermediate zone of the cervical spinal cord. In the thoracic and lumbar segments of the spinal cord, the intermediate zone mediates visceral motor function because autonomic preganglionic neurons are located there (Chapter 14).

Surrounding the gray matter of the spinal cord is the white matter (Figure 3.2). Unlike the gray matter, which contains rostrocaudally oriented columns of neuronal cell bodies, the white matter contains three rostrocaudally oriented columns in which axons ascend or descend. These are the *dorsal column*, in which a branch of the dorsal root ganglion cell ascends to the brain stem (Figure 3.2A), the *lateral column*, in which the corticospinal tract (and other tracts) descends, and the *ventral column*, in which both motor and sensory pathways travel.

The configuration of a slice through the spinal cord is shown in Figure 3.3. The section is stained for the presence of myelinated axons.

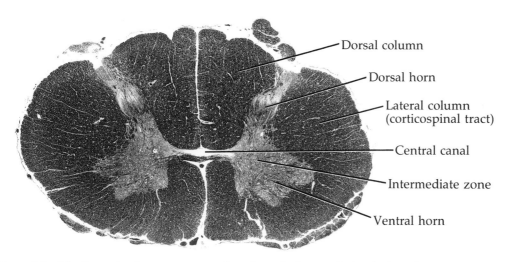

Dorsal column

Dorsal horn

Lateral column
(corticospinal tract)

Central canal

Intermediate zone

Ventral horn

Figure 3.3 Myelin-stained transverse section through the cervical spinal cord.

In myelin-stained sections (Chapter 1), the locations of the regions containing myelinated axons are stained dark and cellular regions are stained pale. Unfortunately, in myelin-stained material the white matter of the central nervous system stains black! Recall that the terms white matter and gray matter derive from the appearance of the nervous system in its *fresh state*. Between the intermediate zones on the two sides of the spinal cord is the *central canal*, a component of the ventricular system. (In the adult, the central canal is not usually patent for its entire rostral–caudal extent.)

Surface Features of the Brain Stem Correlate with Internal Structures

The rostral spinal cord merges with the brain stem. This can be seen in Figure 3.4, which illustrates the dorsal and ventral surfaces of the rostral spinal cord and brain stem. The cerebellum has been removed in Figure 3.4A to reveal the fourth ventricle. Whereas the surface features of the spinal cord do not change remarkably at different rostrocaudal levels, the surface anatomy of the brain stem is characterized by a series of important landmarks and nerve roots, and these landmarks and nerve roots are different for the three parts of the brain stem, the medulla, pons, and midbrain. Many of these surface features also can be seen on brain stem sections and therefore can help in recognizing the level of the brain through which a slice is obtained.

On the dorsal brain stem surface (Figure 3.4A) four important landmarks are easily recognized. At the juncture of the spinal cord and the brain stem, the *dorsal columns* (1) merge with swellings, *dorsal column tubercles* (2), that signify underlying nuclei. There are two tubercles on each side and two dorsal column nuclei: gracile, located medially, and cuneate, located laterally. The first neurons in the dorsal column–medial lemniscal system synapse on neurons in the dorsal column nuclei that form these tubercles. With the cerebellum removed the floor of the *fourth ventricle* (3) can be identified by its rhomboid shape. The key tubercles and sulci on the floor of the fourth ventricle will be examined in Chapter 12, where

A

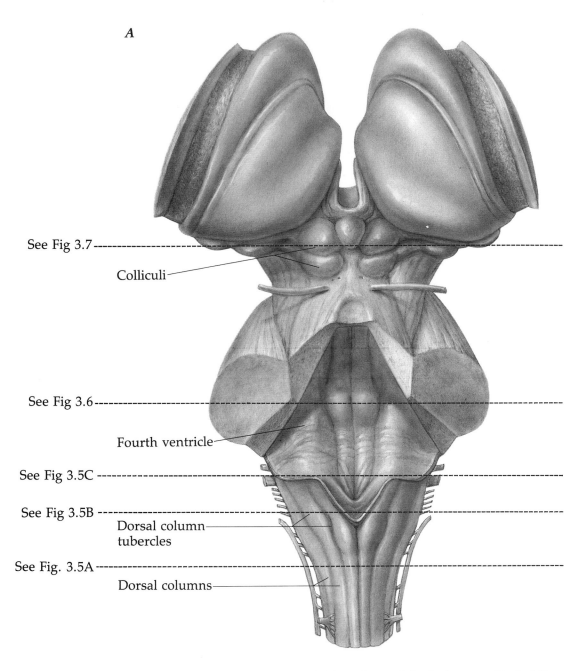

See Fig 3.7

Colliculi

See Fig 3.6

Fourth ventricle

See Fig 3.5C

See Fig 3.5B

Dorsal column
tubercles

See Fig. 3.5A

Dorsal columns

Figure 3.4 Dorsal *(A)* and ventral *(B)* surfaces of the brain stem. Dashed lines indicate the approximate levels through which sections in Figures 3.5–3.7 were obtained.

we will consider the cranial nerve nuclei in detail. The *colliculi* (4) are four bumps located on the dorsal surface of the midbrain. The rostral pair of bumps, termed the superior colliculi, are important visual reflex centers and the caudal pair of bumps, termed the inferior colliculi, process auditory information. There are also four important landmarks on the ven-

B

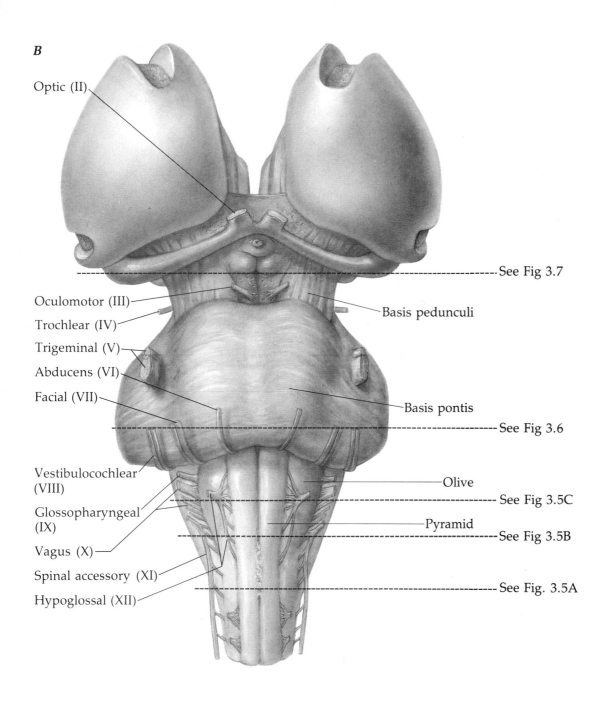

Optic (II)

- - - - - - See Fig 3.7

Oculomotor (III)

Basis pedunculi

Trochlear (IV)

Trigeminal (V)

Abducens (VI)

Facial (VII)

Basis pontis

- - - - - - See Fig 3.6

Vestibulocochlear (VIII)

Olive

- - - - - - See Fig 3.5C

Glossopharyngeal (IX)

Pyramid

Vagus (X)

- - - - - - See Fig 3.5B

Spinal accessory (XI)

Hypoglossal (XII)

- - - - - - See Fig. 3.5A

tral surface (Figure 3.4B) and, remarkably, all are key components of the motor system. The *medullary pyramids* (1) contain the axons of the corticospinal tract. The *olives* (2) are located lateral to the pyramids. The olives together with the *basis pontis* (3)—the large basal surface of the pons—provide the major source of afferent information to the cerebellum. Using this information, the cerebellum is thought to control the accuracy of movement. Finally, the *basis pedunculi* (4) are on the ventral surface of the midbrain. Many of the axons that are immediately beneath the ventral midbrain surface in the basis pedunculi course through the basis pontis and emerge on the medullary surface in the pyramid.

Another characteristic of the brain stem is the presence of the cranial nerves. Unlike the spinal cord, where the dorsal (sensory) and ventral (motor) roots have a segmented configuration, the cranial nerves in the mature nervous system appear to be regionally distributed (Figure 3.4). Thus, knowledge of their locations aids in development of a general understanding of brain stem anatomy. There are 12 pairs of *cranial nerves*, which, like the spinal nerves, mediate sensory and motor function, but of cranial structures. The first two cranial nerves, the *olfactory nerve* (*I*), which contains the sensory neurons that innervate the nasal mucosa, and the *optic nerve* (*II*), which relays visual information from the retina, enter the telencephalon and diencephalon, respectively. The optic nerve is actually a displaced central nervous system pathway, because the retina, from which optic nerve axons derive, develops from the central nervous system. The *oculomotor* (*III*) and the *trochlear* (*IV*) *nerves* are motor nerves, similar to the ventral roots, and innervate the extraocular muscles. They both exit from the midbrain. The *trigeminal nerve* (*V*) is located at the pons. It provides the somatic sensory innervation of the head, as well as the motor innervation of the jaw muscles. The next three cranial nerves enter and exit from the juncture of the pons and the medulla, a region termed the *pontomedullary junction*. The *abducens nerve* (*VI*), together with the oculomotor and trochlear nerves, controls eye movements. The *facial nerve* (*VII*) controls the muscles of facial expression and also mediates taste. The *vestibulocochlear nerve* (*VIII*) mediates audition and balance. The remaining four cranial nerves all enter or exit from the medulla. The *glossopharyngeal nerve* (*IX*) innervates a pharyngeal muscle and taste buds, and transmits visceral sensory information to the brain. The *vagus nerve* (*X*) has functions similar to those of the glossopharyngeal nerve and, in addition, innervates parts of the gut. The *spinal accessory nerve* (*XI*) innervates laryngeal muscles and two neck muscles. Finally, the *hypoglossal nerve* (*XII*) innervates tongue muscles.

The brain stem is extraordinarily complex. In this chapter we will approach the study of brain stem anatomy, as well as other parts of the nervous system, in stages. Here, we examine transverse sections through five key levels: (1) the spinal cord–medullary junction, (2) the caudal medulla, (3) the midmedulla, (4) the caudal pons, and (5) the rostral midbrain. We correlate the surface features that we observed earlier with internal structures of the brain stem. In later chapters, the detailed anatomy and connections of the various brain stem nuclei will be examined.

The Caudal Medulla and Spinal Cord Have a Similar Organization

The first of three key sections through the medulla that we will study is shown in Figure 3.5A. This section is at the transition between the spinal cord and medulla. The corticospinal tract is located in the ventral portion of the section, and at this level it decussates. The *pyramidal* (or

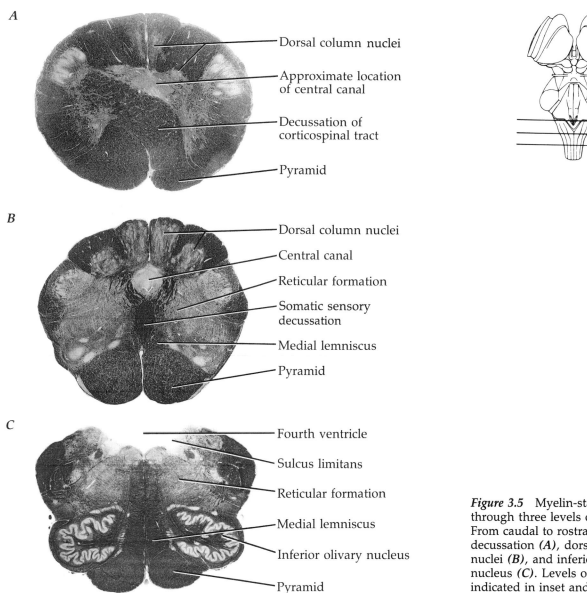

A

— Dorsal column nuclei

— Approximate location of central canal

— Decussation of corticospinal tract

— Pyramid

B

— Dorsal column nuclei

— Central canal

— Reticular formation

— Somatic sensory decussation

— Medial lemniscus

— Pyramid

C

— Fourth ventricle

— Sulcus limitans

— Reticular formation

— Medial lemniscus

— Inferior olivary nucleus

— Pyramid

Figure 3.5 Myelin-stained sections through three levels of the medulla. From caudal to rostral; pyramidal decussation *(A)*, dorsal column nuclei *(B)*, and inferior olivary nucleus *(C)*. Levels of sections are indicated in inset and in Figure 3.4.

corticospinal) decussation is actually visible on the ventral brain stem surface (Figure 3.4B). The significance of this decussation is that one side of the brain controls muscles of the opposite side of the body. Because this section is stained for myelin, the corticospinal tract appears dark, just as the lateral column of the spinal cord. The *dorsal column nuclei*, a collection of two nuclei (a pair on each side) along the dorsal portion of the medulla, are nested within the dorsal columns. The dorsal column nuclei (and the sensory relay nuclei of the trigeminal nerve, which innervates facial structures) constitute much of the dorsal medullary gray matter. This is similar to the gray matter of the spinal cord, where the dorsal horn subserves sensory function. Whereas the dorsal column nuclei are small in this section compared with the next (Figure 3.5B), their position within and at the base of the dorsal columns serves as an aid to understanding their afferent connections: the dorsal column nuclei receive their major input from the dorsal columns. There are three important similarities in the internal organization of the spinal cord and brain stem. First, the dorsal horn merges rostrally with the dorsal column nuclei and cranial nerve sensory nuclei. Second, the ventral horn merges with cranial nerve motor nuclei. Third, the intermediate zone of the spinal cord merges rostrally with the reticular formation. The reticular formation plays a role in sensory–motor integration, as does the intermediate zone, and, in addition, the reticular formation regulates arousal.

The Dorsal Column Nuclei Relay Somatic Sensory Information to the Thalamus

The dorsal column nuclei are large nuclei and therefore are located in transverse sections through wide regions of the medulla. The largest portion of the dorsal column nuclei is located rostral to the junction of the spinal cord and the medulla (Figure 3.5B) beneath the gracile and cuneate tubercles on the dorsal brain stem surface. Second-order neurons of the dorsal column–medial lemniscal system originate in these nuclei. Their axons decussate in the ventral portion of the medulla (somatic sensory decussation) and ascend to the thalamus in the *medial lemniscus*, which is located close to the midline. The significance of this decussation is that sensory information from one side of the body is processed by the other side of the brain. Because both the sensory and motor pathways decussate, the same side of the brain receives sensory input from and controls the muscles of the opposite side of the body. At this level the corticospinal tract is clearly separated from other regions of the medulla, in the medullary *pyramids* (Figure 3.4).

The Inferior Olivary Nucleus Sends Axons to the Cerebellum

The *olive* is a bulge located on the ventral medullary surface, lateral to the medullary pyramid, and it marks the position of the *inferior olivary nucleus*. The inferior olivary nucleus is also a prominent internal landmark, and like the surface structure, it is lateral to the pyramid (Figure 3.5C). As we saw in Chapter 2, developing neurons of the alar plate migrate from the ventricular surface to the ventral medulla to form the inferior olivary nucleus. In the mature brain, neurons in the inferior olivary nucleus project to the cerebellum where they form one of the strongest excitatory synapses in the entire central nervous system (see Chapter 10). The pyramid can be seen ventral to the medial lemniscus.

At this level the first view of the ventricular system of the brain becomes apparent. The central canal has "opened" to form the *fourth ventricle*. Recall the development of this brain stem region from Chapter 2 (Figure 2.6). The *sulcus limitans* separates the alar and basal plates in the embryonic central nervous system. In the mature nervous system, sensory and motor nuclei of the cranial nerves are separated by the sulcus limitans.

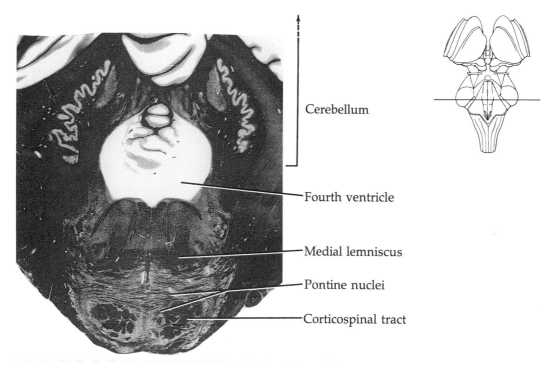

Cerebellum

Fourth ventricle

Medial lemniscus

Pontine nuclei

Corticospinal tract

Figure 3.6   Myelin-stained section through pons. Level of section is indicated in inset and in Figure 3.4.

The Pontine Nuclei Surround the Corticospinal Tract in the Base of the Pons

The dorsal surface of the pons is formed by the floor of the fourth ventricle (Figure 3.6). The medial lemniscus, which was located in the ventral portion of the medulla, is displaced dorsally at this level. This shift in the position of the medial lemniscus may be explained by the presence of the *pontine nuclei*, which, like the inferior olivary nucleus, are derived from immature neurons that migrate to this ventral pontine site from the ventricular floor. Neurons in the pontine nuclei transmit information from the cerebral cortex to the cerebellum, which lies dorsal to the pons, and may play an important role in the learning of motor skills. The pontine nuclei surround the fascicles of the corticospinal tract, and both of these components of the pons are located within the *basis pontis* (Figure 3.4).

The Dorsal Surface of the Midbrain Contains the Colliculi

The midbrain is traditionally divided into three regions, from the dorsal to the ventral surface (Figure 3.7): (1) the *tectum* (Latin for "roof"), (2) the *tegmentum*, and (3) the *basis pedunculi*.[1] The tectum contains the superior colliculi, at this level, and more caudally, the inferior colliculi.

---

[1] There is often confusion regarding terminology of midbrain regional anatomy. Strictly speaking, the cerebral peduncle refers to both the tegmentum and the basis pedunculi. Another term for basis pedunculi is crus cerebri.

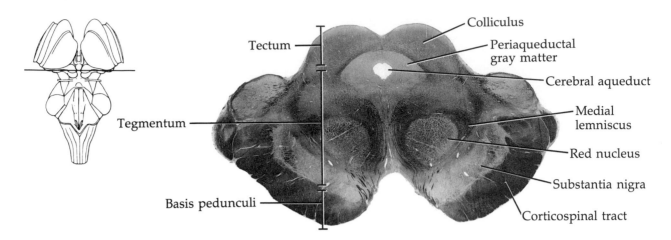

Figure 3.7 Myelin-stained section through the rostral midbrain, at the level of the superior colliculus. Level of section is indicated in inset and in Figure 3.4.

The superior colliculi play an important role in eye movement control and the inferior colliculi, in audition. The tectum and tegmentum are separated by the cerebral aqueduct, which connects the third and fourth ventricles. This ventricular conduit is surrounded by a nuclear region, termed the *periaqueductal gray*, which contains neurons that are part of the circuit for endogenous pain suppression: pain is perceived as less severe during intense emotional experiences, for example, during childbirth. The medial lemniscus is located within the tegmentum, whereas the *corticospinal tract* is located more ventral, in the basis pedunculi. The corticospinal tract is therefore seen on the ventral surfaces of both the midbrain (basis pedunculi) and the medulla (pyramid). A nucleus of major clinical significance, the substantia nigra, separates the corticospinal tract and the medial lemniscus. The substantia nigra functions closely with the basal ganglia in the control of movement. Neurons in this nucleus that use dopamine as a neurotransmitter are destroyed in patients with Parkinson's disease, and two major behavioral consequences are tremor and a paucity (and slowing) of voluntary movements. The red nucleus is another midbrain nucleus that participates in the control of movement. It is thought to play a key role in the recovery of motor function that may occur after damage to the corticospinal tract. Remarkably, these structures can be visualized on the magnetic resonance image shown in Figure 3.8. Recall that this is a noninvasive method for imaging brain anatomy.

The Thalamus Relays Information from Subcortical Structures to the Cerebral Cortex

The complex anatomy of the diencephalon and cerebral hemispheres is often difficult to understand. This is especially true when the most common way of representing these structures is with two-dimensional slices rather than diagrams of their overall three-dimensional shape. Here,

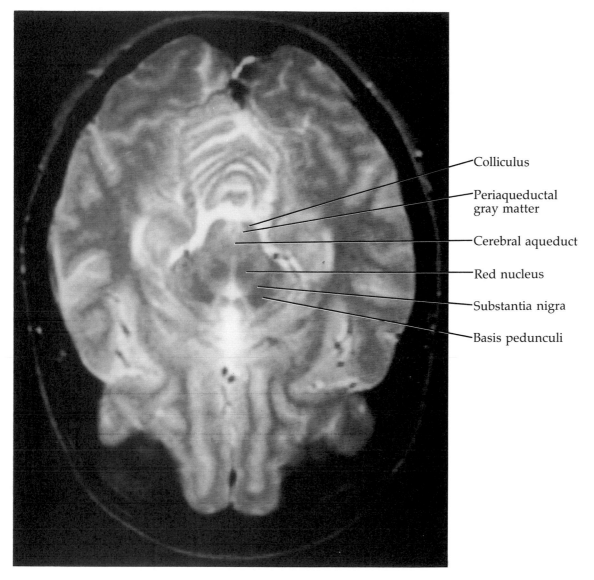

Figure 3.8 MRI scan through the cerebral hemisphere and midbrain. (Courtesy of Dr. Neal Rutledge, University of Texas at Austin.)

we expand our understanding of the general structure of the diencephalon and cerebral hemispheres by examining the thalamus and the cerebral cortex in relation to the connections of the dorsal column–medial lemniscal system and the corticospinal tract, and the location of the third and lateral ventricles. The thalamus and cerebral cortex are emphasized here because a general knowledge of these structures will aid in learning the organization of the sensory systems, the topic of Chapters 5–8. The other components of the diencephalon and cerebral hemispheres will be examined in later chapters when their connections and functions are discussed.

The shape of the thalamus and its position within the cerebral hemispheres are shown in Figure 3.9. The location of the thalamus, between the midbrain and cerebral hemispheres, reflects its major function, which is to receive information from subcortical structures and relay this information to the cerebral cortex. The thalamus is bilaterally paired, separated by the third ventricle. A small portion of each half of the thalamus adheres at the midline in most brains. This is termed the *thalamic adhesion* or massa intermedia. Neurons in each half of the thalamus project to the cerebral cortex on the same side (ipsilateral). Thalamic neurons are not distributed randomly, but rather are clustered and form anatomically and functionally separate nuclei. The organization of thalamic nuclei can be approached from a regional and a functional perspective.

On the basis of their locations, six separate nuclear groups can be identified in the thalamus (Figure 3.9). The names of the four major groups are determined by their locations with respect to bands of myelinated axons, called the *internal medullary laminae*: (1) anterior nuclei, (2) medial nuclei, (3) lateral nuclei, and (4) intralaminar nuclei, which lie

Figure 3.9 A three-dimensional view of the thalamus as well as its approximate location in cerebral hemispheres. The major nuclei are labeled. Nuclei of the lateral group of nuclei are numbered.

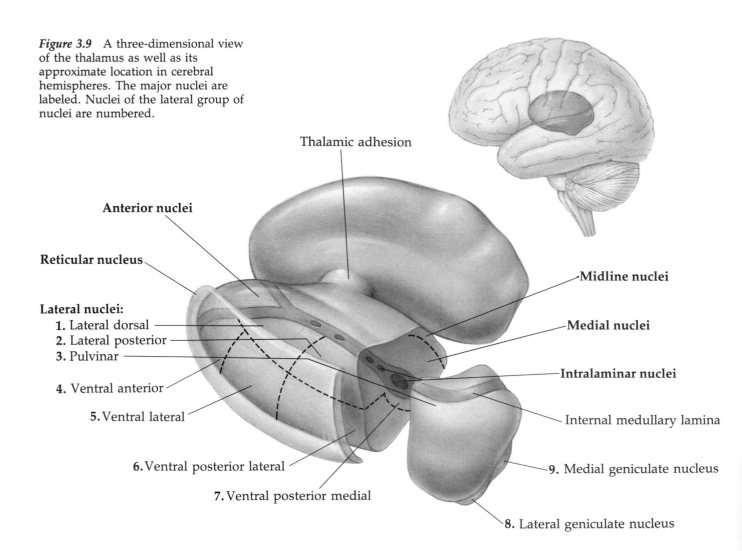

Thalamic adhesion

Anterior nuclei

Reticular nucleus

Lateral nuclei:
  1. Lateral dorsal
  2. Lateral posterior
  3. Pulvinar
  4. Ventral anterior
  5. Ventral lateral
  6. Ventral posterior lateral
  7. Ventral posterior medial

Midline nuclei

Medial nuclei

Intralaminar nuclei

Internal medullary lamina

9. Medial geniculate nucleus

8. Lateral geniculate nucleus

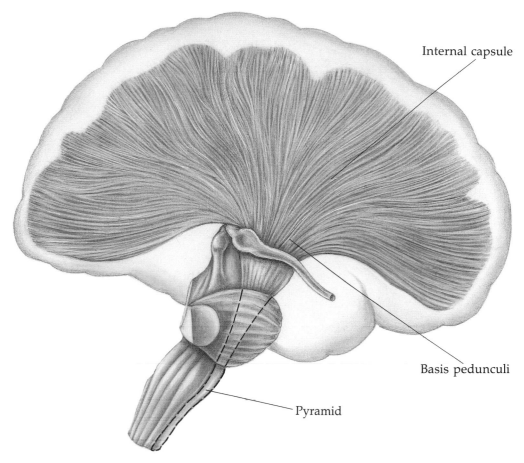

Internal capsule

Basis pedunculi

Pyramid

Figure 3.10   Three-dimensional view of the internal capsule. The descending cortical axons collect into a discrete tract in the brain stem. (Adapted from Carpenter, M. B., and Sutin, J. 1983. Human Neuroanatomy. Baltimore: Williams & Wilkins.)

within the laminae. The two other nuclei are the reticular nucleus (5) and the midline nuclei (6). The various thalamic nuclei are divided into two major functional classes: (1) relay nuclei and (2) diffuse-projecting nuclei.[2] *Relay nuclei* are involved in such functions as perception, control of voluntary movement, emotional responses, and language. They transmit information from particular subcortical inputs to a *restricted portion of the cerebral cortex*. The relay nuclei that mediate sensation and movement are located in the lateral portion of the thalamus. The *ventral posterior lateral nucleus*, the somatic sensory relay nucleus of the thalamus, receives its major input from the medial lemniscus. Other relay nuclei do not project to sensory or motor areas of the cerebral cortex, but rather to an *association*

---

[2] Relay nuclei are often referred to as *specific* relay nuclei because of the precise topography of their connections. Similarly, the diffuse-projecting nuclei were once considered *nonspecific* because of their widespread cortical connections. However, despite this more diffuse projection pattern, the connections are specific.

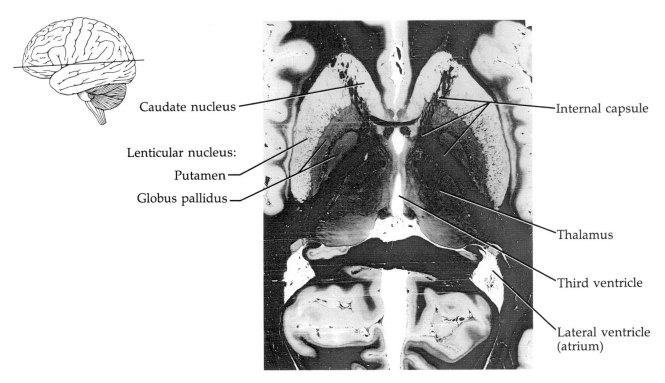

Caudate nucleus

Internal capsule

Lenticular nucleus:

Putamen

Globus pallidus

Thalamus

Third ventricle

Lateral ventricle
(atrium)

Figure 3.11 Myelin-stained horizontal section through the cerebral hemisphere, at the level of the thalamus. The level of this section is indicated in inset.

area. The anterior and medial thalamic nuclei, as well as some members of the lateral nuclei, are relay nuclei for association cortex. (Sometimes these nuclei are termed association nuclei.) *Diffuse-projecting nuclei* function in arousal. They receive input from many converging sources and in turn project widely to the cerebral cortex. The intralaminar nuclei are the principal nuclei in this class. The patterns of termination of neurons in diffuse-projecting nuclei are described as *regional* because they cross functional boundaries in the cortex. By contrast, the terminations of an individual relay nucleus are confined to a *single functional cortical area.*

Thalamic neurons project to the cerebral cortex via the *internal capsule.* The internal capsule is a two-way path, not only for transmission of information from the thalamus to the cerebral cortex, but also for transmission from the cerebral cortex to subcortical structures, such as the spinal cord. Whereas the ascending thalamocortical fibers are located entirely in the internal capsule, the descending cortical fibers course within and through the internal capsule and appear to condense to form the basis pedunculi. The three-dimensional configuration of the internal capsule is similar to that of a curved fan (Figure 3.10). When a slice is made through the cerebral hemispheres in the horizontal plane, the internal capsule resembles an arrowhead with the tip pointing medially (Figure 3.11). The magnetic resonance image shown in Figure 3.12 is in approximately the same plane as the myelin-stained section shown in Figure 3.11. The arrowhead-shaped configuration of the internal capsule is seen,

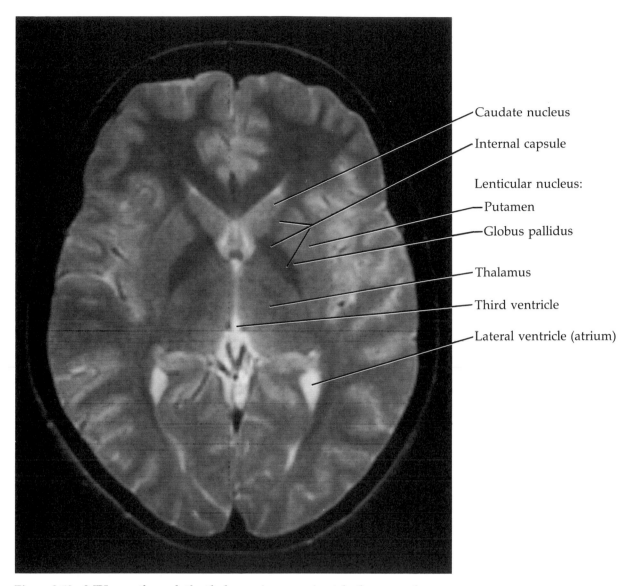

Caudate nucleus

Internal capsule

Lenticular nucleus:

Putamen

Globus pallidus

Thalamus

Third ventricle

Lateral ventricle (atrium)

Figure 3.12   MRI scan through the thalamus in approximately the same plane as shown in Figure 3.11. (Courtesy of Dr. Neal Rutledge.)

as are the thalamus and caudate nucleus, located medial to the internal capsule, and the putamen and globus pallidus, located lateral. The caudate nucleus, the putamen, and the globus pallidus are the three principal components of the basal ganglia. Collectively, the putamen and the globus pallidus are termed the *lenticular nucleus*, because they are shaped like a lens. The coronal slice (Figure 3.13) cuts through the thalamus, the lenticular nucleus, and the caudal part of the internal capsule. The axons from the ventral posterior lateral nucleus pass through this part of the internal capsule en route to the primary somatic sensory cortex. In addition, the axons of the corticospinal tract descend here. The magnetic

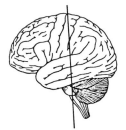

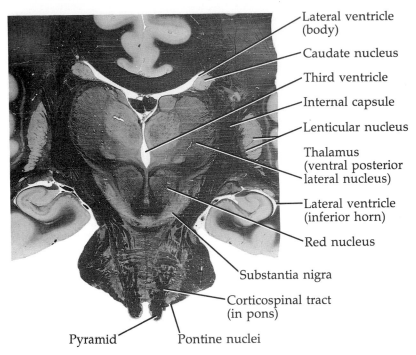

Lateral ventricle (body)

Caudate nucleus

Third ventricle

Internal capsule

Lenticular nucleus

Thalamus (ventral posterior lateral nucleus)

Lateral ventricle (inferior horn)

Red nucleus

Substantia nigra

Corticospinal tract (in pons)

Pyramid　　Pontine nuclei

Figure 3.13 Myelin-stained coronal section through the cerebral hemisphere, at the level of the thalamus. Inset shows plane of section.

resonance scan in Figure 3.14 is approximately in the same plane as the slice shown in Figure 3.13. The internal capsule and thalamus can be distinguished, as can the gray and white matter of the cerebral cortex.

In the various myelin-stained sections (Figures 3.11 and 3.13) and magnetic resonance images (Figures 3.12 and 3.14) two components of the ventricular system can be identified, the *lateral ventricles* and the *third ventricle*. Portions of the lateral ventricles can be identified in two locations in each of these figures. In the horizontal plane, the anterior horn of the lateral ventricle is located rostrally and the junction of the body, posterior horn, and inferior horn is located caudally (see Figure 3.1A). The junction of the body, posterior horn, and inferior horn of the lateral ventricle is termed the *atrium*. In the coronal plane, the body of the lateral ventricle is located dorsally and the inferior horn, ventrally (see also Chapter 2).

Neurons of the Cerebral Cortex Are Organized into Layers

The cerebral cortex is the structure to which the dorsal column–medial lemniscal system projects and the origin of the corticospinal tract. It has a characteristic structure: it contains neurons that are organized into discrete layers (Figure 3.15). Different cortical regions contain characteristically different numbers of cell layers. Most of the cerebral cortex contains at least six cell layers, and this cortex is termed *isocortex* (Figure 3.15A). Because isocortex dominates the cerebral cortex of phylogeneti-

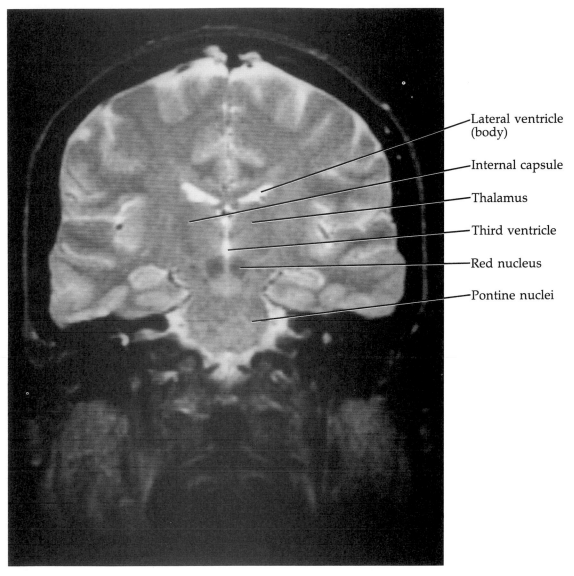

Lateral ventricle
(body)

Internal capsule

Thalamus

Third ventricle

Red nucleus

Pontine nuclei

Figure 3.14 MRI scan through the thalamus in approximately the same plane as shown in Figure 3.13. (Courtesy of Dr. Neal Rutledge.)

Figure 3.14

cally higher vertebrates, it is also termed *neocortex*. In contrast to isocortex, *allocortex* contains fewer than six layers (Figure 3.15B). Although present in higher vertebrates, allocortex dominates the cortex of phylogenetically more primitive vertebrates. The phylogenetically oldest type of allocortex, the *archicortex*, constitutes the hippocampal formation (Chapter 15). The example of allocortex shown in Figure 3.15 is archicortex. It contains three cell layers. *Paleocortex*, thought to be a somewhat more advanced allocortex, is associated with areas that mediate olfactory function (Chapters 8 and 15). Here, we consider further the neocortex because this is the type of cortex that comprises the major sensory, motor, and association areas.

A **Neocortex**

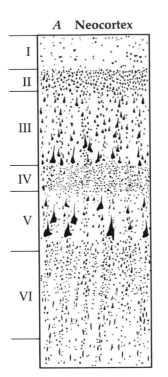

B **Allocortex**

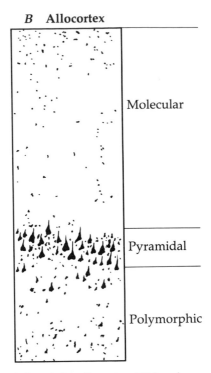

Molecular

Pyramidal

Polymorphic

Figure 3.15 The neocortex has six cell layers *(A)* and the allocortex *(B)* has fewer than six layers. The drawing of a Nissl-stained section through the neocortex of the human brain is semischematic. The section through allocortex is of a portion of the hippocampal formation. This is archicortex and it has three cell layers. (*A*, Adapted from Brodmann, K. 1909. Vergleichende Lokalisationslehre der Grosshirnrinde in ihren Prinzipien dargestellt auf Grund des Zellenbaues. Leipzig: Barth.)

Regions of neocortex that subserve different functions have a different microscopic anatomy: the thickness of the six neocortical cell layers varies. Areas that subserve sensation have a well-developed layer IV (Figure 3.16). This is the layer to which most thalamic neurons from the sensory relay nuclei project. The primary visual cortex has this morphology (Figure 3.16). In contrast, the primary motor cortex has a thin layer IV and a thick layer V (Figure 3.16). Layer V contains the neurons that project to the spinal cord, via the corticospinal tract. Association areas of the cerebral cortex, such as prefrontal and parietal association cortex, have a morphology that is intermediate between those of sensory cortex and motor cortex (Figure 3.16). Based primarily on differences in the thickness of cortical layers and on the sizes and shapes of neurons, the German

Figure 3.16 Different regions of the cerebral cortex have a different cytoarchitecture. (*Top*) Nissl-stained sections through various portions of the cerebral cortex. (Adapted from Campbell, 1905.) (*Bottom*) Brodmann's cytoarchitectonic areas of the cerebral cortex. (Adapted from Brodmann, K. 1909. Vergleichende Lokalisationslehre der Grosshirnrinde in ihren Prinzipien dargestellt auf Grund des Zellenbaues. Leipzig: Barth, and Campbell, A. W. 1905. Histological Studies on the Localization of Cerebral Function. New York: Cambridge University Press.) ▷

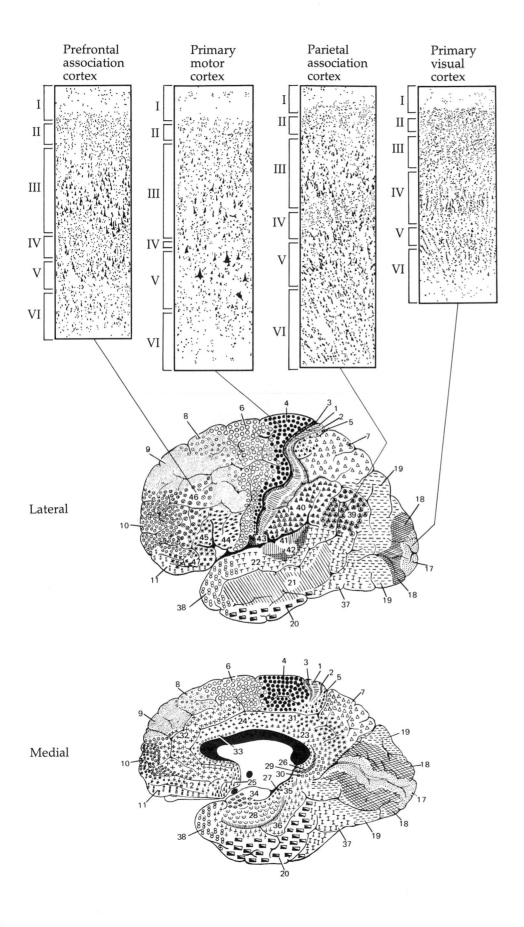

Prefrontal association cortex

Primary motor cortex

Parietal association cortex

Primary visual cortex

Lateral

Medial

anatomist Korbinian Brodmann identified more than 50 divisions (now termed *Brodmann's areas*, Figure 3.16 bottom). These *cytoarchitectonic* divisions are based on their constituent neuronal architecture and not on function. However, modern research on the cerebral cortex has shown that different functional areas of the cortex have different cytoarchitecture.

Summary

The spinal cord, the most caudal of the six major divisions of the central nervous system, has a central region that contains predominantly cell bodies of neurons (gray matter), surrounded by a region that contains mostly myelinated axons (white matter) (Figures 3.2 and 3.3). Both of these regions can be further subdivided. The *dorsal horn* of the gray matter subserves somatic sensation and the *ventral horn*, skeletal motor function. The *dorsal column* of the white matter carries somatic sensory information to the brain, the *lateral* and *ventral columns* carry both sensory and motor information (Figure 3.2).

Five key levels through the brain stem describe its essential features. The caudal medulla (Figure 3.5A) is similar in its organization to the spinal cord. At a more rostral level (Figure 3.5B) the medulla contains nuclei on its dorsal surface that subserve tactile sensation—the *dorsal column nuclei*—and a pathway on its ventral surface that subserves voluntary movement—the corticospinal tract, which is located in the medullary pyramid. The *medial lemniscus* is located dorsal to the pyramid. At the level of the *inferior olivary nucleus* (Figure 3.5C), the fourth ventricle forms the dorsal surface of the medulla. The pons (Figure 3.6) contains nuclei in its ventral portion, the *pontine nuclei*, that transfer information from the cerebral cortex to the cerebellum. The midbrain (Figure 3.7) contains the *colliculi* on its dorsal surface and the motor pathway on its ventral surface.

The *diencephalon* and the *cerebral hemisphere* have a more complex organization than that of the brain stem or spinal cord. The *thalamus*, which relays information from subcortical structures to the cerebral cortex, contains two different functional classes of nuclei: *relay* and *diffuse-projecting*. Three of the four main *anatomical* divisions of the thalamus (Figure 3.9) serve relay functions: (1) *anterior nuclei*, (2) *medial nuclei*, and (3) *lateral nuclei*. The fourth main anatomical division of the thalamus, *intralaminar nuclei*, contains diffuse-projecting nuclei. These anatomical divisions are based on the spatial location of nuclei with respect to the *internal medullary lamina*, bands of myelinated fibers in the thalamus. Thalamic neurons send their axons to the cerebral cortex via the *internal capsule* (Figure 3.10), as do cortical neurons that project to subcortical sites.

There are two types of cortex based on the presence or absence of six cell layers. *Neocortex* (or isocortex) has *six layers* (Figures 3.15A and 3.16), and the different layers have different thicknesses depending on the function of the particular cortical area. *Allocortex* (Figure 3.15B) has fewer than *six layers* and consists mainly of the *archicortex* of the *hippocampal formation* and the *paleocortex* of the *olfactory regions*. ■

References

Brodmann, K. 1909. Vergleichende Lokalisationslehre der Grosshirnrinde in ihren Prinzipien dargestellt auf Grund des Zellenbaues. Leipzig: Barth.

Campbell, A. W. 1905. Histological studies on the localisation of cerebral function. New York: Cambridge University Press.

Carpenter, M. B., and Sutin, J. 1983. Human Neuroanatomy. Baltimore: Williams & Wilkins.

Hassler, R. 1982. Architectonic Organization of the Thalamic Nuclei. In Shaltenbrand, G., and Warhen, W. W. (eds), Stereotaxy of the Human Brain. New York: G. Thieme Verlag, pp. 140–180.

Jones, E. G. 1984. Organization of the Thalamocortical Complex and Its Relation to Sensory Processes. In Darian-Smith, I. (ed.), Handbook of Physiology, Section 1: The Nervous System, Vol. III. Sensory Processes. Bethesda, Md.: American Physiological Society, pp. 149–212.

Nieuwenhuys, R., Voogd, J., van Huijzen, Chr. 1988. The Human Central Nervous System: A Synopsis and Atlas, 3rd edition. Berlin: Springer-Verlag.

Rexed, B. 1952. The cytoarchitectonic organization of the spinal cord in the cat. J. Comp. Neurol. 96:415–495.

Selected Readings

Brodal, A. 1981. Neurological Anatomy. New York: Oxford University Press.

Kandel, E. R., and Schwartz, J. H. 1985. Principles of Neural Science. New York: Elsevier.

Vasculature of the Central Nervous System

4

Vasculature of the Central Nervous System

Disorders of brain vasculature constitute one of the major classes of disease affecting the nervous system. One reason for this is that the principal source of nourishment for the central nervous system is glucose, and neither glucose nor oxygen is stored in appreciable amounts. Thus, the central nervous system is critically dependent on an adequate supply of blood and when this supply becomes interrupted, even for a brief period, brain functions become severely disrupted.

In this chapter we examine the blood supply of the central nervous system, in part by using images obtained from *cerebral angiography*, a method whereby the clinician can view the arterial and venous circulation radiologically. Not only is cerebral angiography an important clinical tool that permits localization of a vascular obstruction or other pathology, it also gives the student of neuroanatomy an opportunity to study the configuration of cerebral vasculature in the living brain.

The Vertebral and Carotid Arteries Supply Blood to the Central Nervous System

The arterial blood supply of the brain is provided by two arterial systems that receive blood from different systemic arteries: the *anterior circulation*, which is fed by the *internal carotid arteries*, and the *posterior circulation*, which receives blood from the *vertebral arteries* (Figure 4.1 inset). The vertebral arteries join at the juncture of the medulla and pons to form the *basilar artery*, an unpaired artery that lies along the midline (Figure 4.1).[1] The anterior circulation and posterior circulation are not independent; they are interconnected by a network of arteries on the cortical surface and communicating arteries on the ventral surface of the diencephalon. Whereas the cerebral hemispheres receive blood from both the anterior circulation and the posterior circulation, the brain stem receives its blood supply from the posterior circulation. The arterial supply of the spinal cord is provided by the systemic circulation and, to a lesser degree, by the vertebral arteries. In the following sections, first the arterial blood supply of the major divisions of the central nervous system is considered and then their venous drainage.

The Spinal and Radicular Arteries Supply Blood to the Spinal Cord

The spinal cord receives blood from branches of the vertebral arteries, the *anterior* and *posterior spinal arteries* (Figure 4.1), as well as from segmental vessels, the *radicular arteries* (Figure 4.2). The anterior and posterior spinal arteries typically do not form a single continuous vessel along their entire length, but rather form a network of communicating channels that are oriented along the rostral–caudal axis of the spinal cord. The vertebral arteries feed into this network of vessels rostrally, and the radicular arteries, caudally.

---

[1] The anterior circulation is also called the carotid circulation, and the posterior circulation, the vertebral–basilar circulation.

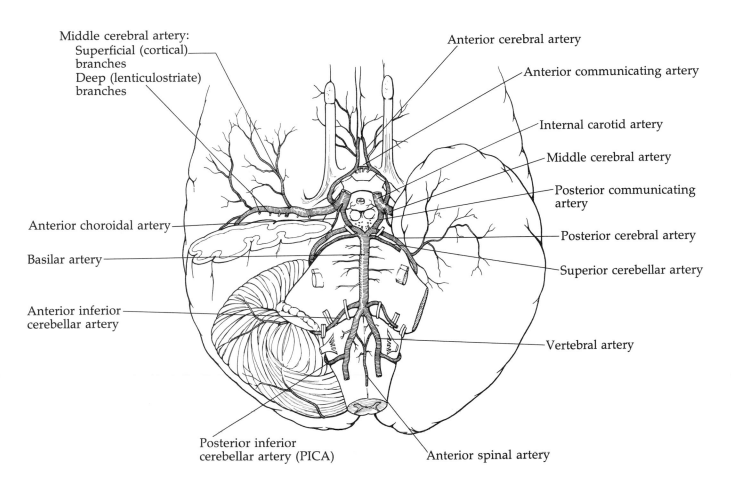

Middle cerebral artery:
Superficial (cortical) branches
Deep (lenticulostriate) branches

Anterior cerebral artery

Anterior communicating artery

Internal carotid artery

Middle cerebral artery

Posterior communicating artery

Anterior choroidal artery

Posterior cerebral artery

Basilar artery

Superior cerebellar artery

Anterior inferior cerebellar artery

Vertebral artery

Posterior inferior cerebellar artery (PICA)

Anterior spinal artery

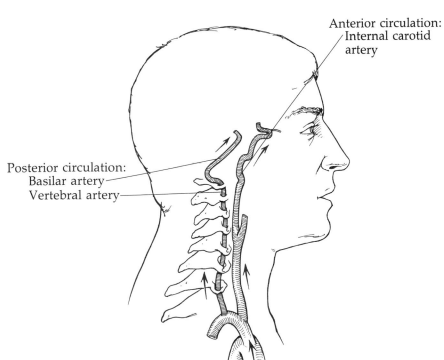

Anterior circulation:
Internal carotid artery

Posterior circulation:
Basilar artery
Vertebral artery

Figure 4.1 Diagram of the ventral surface of brain stem and cerebral hemispheres illustrating the key components of the anterior (carotid) circulation and the posterior (vertebral–basilar) circulation. The anterior portion of the temporal lobe is removed to illustrate the course of the middle cerebral artery through the lateral (Sylvian) fissure and the penetrating branches (lenticulostriate arteries). The circle of Willis is formed by the anterior communicating artery, the two posterior communicating arteries, and the three cerebral arteries. Inset **(below) shows the extracranial and cranial courses of the vertebral, basilar, and carotid arteries.**

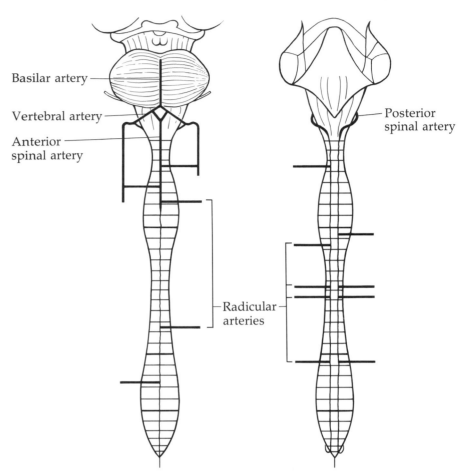

Basilar artery

Vertebral artery

Anterior spinal artery

Posterior spinal artery

Radicular arteries

Figure 4.2 Schematic ventral (left) and dorsal (right) views of the spinal cord and brain stem are illustrated with the atrerial circulation of the spinal cord. (Adapted from Carpenter, M. B., and Sutin, J. 1983. Human Neuroanatomy. Baltimore: Williams & Wilkins.)

Although both spinal and radicular arteries supply blood to the spinal cord, different spinal cord segments are preferentially supplied by one or the other system. The cervical spinal cord receives its blood supply primarily from vertebral and cervical arteries. In contrast, the principal source of blood to thoracic, lumbar, and sacral segments is the radicular arteries. The radicular artery that supplies the lumbosacral enlargement, which comprises those spinal cord segments that provide the innervation of the legs, is particularly prominent. It is termed the *artery of Adamkiewicz*.

Certain regions of the spinal cord are particularly susceptible to injury after arterial occlusion because of the lack of *collateral circulation*, which is the redundant supply of blood to a region. For example, individual rostral thoracic segments are supplied by fewer radicular arteries than more caudal segments. When a radicular artery that serves the rostral thoracic segments becomes occluded, damage may result because there is no backup system for perfusion. Collateral circulation is also an important concept in understanding perfusion of the cerebral hemispheres (see later).

The Brain Stem Receives Blood from the Vertebral and Basilar Arteries

Each of the three major divisions of the brain stem receives its arterial supply from the posterior circulation (Figure 4.3A). The medulla is supplied by the vertebral and spinal arteries. The pons and cerebellum are supplied by the basilar artery and its branches. The midbrain is supplied primarily by the posterior cerebral artery as well as the basilar artery. The major principle for understanding the regional distribution of arterial perfusion of the caudal brain stem is that different arteries perfuse regions of tissue that resemble wedge-shaped slices of a pie in transverse section (Figure 4.3B). Even though the spinal arteries primarily supply the spinal cord, they also supply the caudal medulla. The spinal arteries lie close to the dorsal and ventral midline and provide the blood for the most medial areas. More lateral areas are served by the vertebral arteries, or one of their major laterally emerging branches, the *posterior inferior cerebellar artery* (PICA). The vertebral arteries join to form the basilar artery at the junction of the medulla and pons.

The blood supply to the pons and cerebellum is provided by three sets of branches of the *basilar artery*: (1) paramedian, (2) short circumferential, and (3) long circumferential. The *paramedian branches* of the basilar artery supply regions of the pons that are located close to the midline. This supply is often bilateral. The *short circumferential branches* supply lateral wedge-shaped regions, and the *long circumferential branches* supply the dorsolateral portions of the pons and the cerebellum. The dorsolateral portion of the caudal pons is supplied by a long circumferential branch of the basilar artery, termed the *anterior inferior cerebellar artery (AICA)*. The region in the pons rostral to that supplied by the anterior inferior cerebellar artery is supplied by the *superior cerebellar artery*, another long circumferential branch of the basilar artery (Figure 4.3A). The cerebellum is supplied by distal branches of the posterior inferior cerebellar artery, the anterior inferior cerebellar artery, and the superior cerebellar artery (Figure 4.3A). Whereas the basilar artery supplies blood to the midbrain, the principal arterial supply to the midbrain is from the *posterior cerebral artery*. Proximal branches supply the base and tegmentum of the midbrain (see Figure 3.7), while the tectum is supplied by more distal branches as they course around the lateral midbrain surface.

The Anterior and Posterior Circulations Supply the Diencephalon and Cerebral Hemispheres

The three cerebral arteries supply blood to the cerebral cortex, basal ganglia, and thalamus (Figures 4.4 and 4.6). Two of them, the *anterior cerebral artery* and the *middle cerebral artery*, are part of the anterior circulation. The third cerebral artery, the *posterior cerebral artery*, is part of the posterior circulation even though it derives embryologically from the anterior system. These two arterial systems are interconnected at two locations: (1) at the terminal ends of the cerebral arteries, on the convexity of the cerebral cortex (Figure 4.4A), and (2) on the ventral surface of the diencephalon, where branches of the anterior and posterior circulations

A

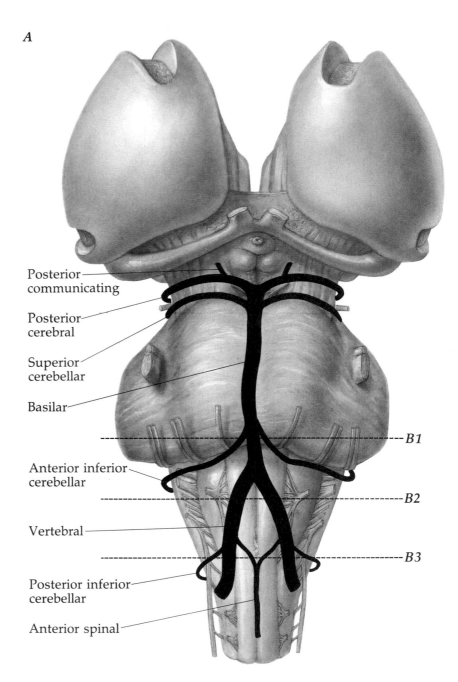

Posterior communicating

Posterior cerebral

Superior cerebellar

Basilar

------- *B1*

Anterior inferior cerebellar

------- *B2*

Vertebral

------- *B3*

Posterior inferior cerebellar

Anterior spinal

Figure 4.3 **A.** Arterial circulation of the brain stem is schematically illustrated on a view of the ventral surface of the brain stem. **B.** Three tranverse sections through the brain stem, illustrating wedge-shaped regions supplied by different arteries: (1) pons, (2) rostral medulla, (3) caudal medulla.

B1

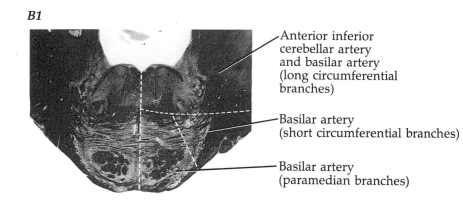

Anterior inferior
cerebellar artery
and basilar artery
(long circumferential
branches)

Basilar artery
(short circumferential branches)

Basilar artery
(paramedian branches)

B2

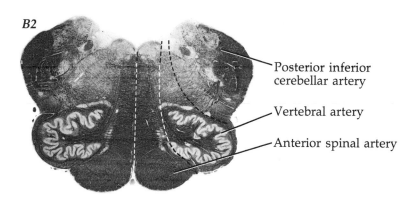

Posterior inferior
cerebellar artery

Vertebral artery

Anterior spinal artery

B3

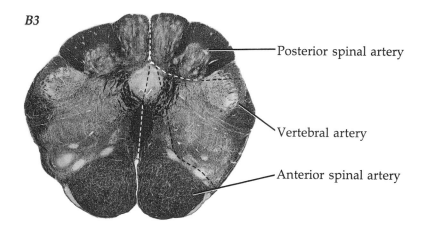

Posterior spinal artery

Vertebral artery

Anterior spinal artery

A

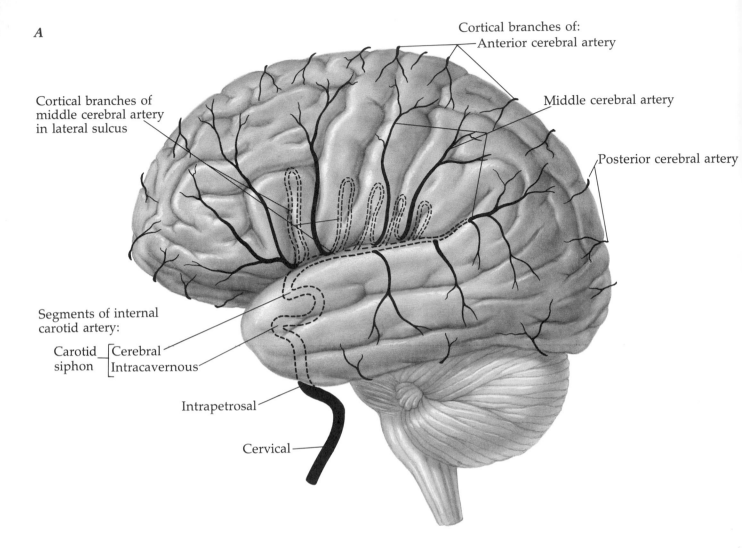

Cortical branches of:
Anterior cerebral artery

Cortical branches of
middle cerebral artery
in lateral sulcus

Middle cerebral artery

Posterior cerebral artery

Segments of internal
carotid artery:

Carotid   Cerebral
siphon   Intracavernous

Intrapetrosal

Cervical

Figure 4.4 The courses of the three cerebral arteries are illustrated in views of the lateral surface of the cerebral hemisphere *(A)* and the midsagittal surface *(B)*.

form an anastomotic network of arteries called the *circle of Willis* (Figure 4.1). The interconnection between the two arterial systems is important in compensation for reduced arterial perfusion when one system becomes nonfunctional (see later). In general, deep structures of the brain, for example, the diencephalon, receive blood directly from branches of the internal carotid artery and the proximal portions of the cerebral arteries (Figures 4.6 and 4.7). In contrast, the gray matter of the cerebral cortex and the underlying white matter are supplied by branches of more distal portions of the cerebral arteries. The internal carotid artery, which supplies the anterior system with blood, is discussed first. Then the circle of Willis, the proximal cerebral arteries, and the circulation to the thalamus, basal ganglia, and internal capsule are considered. Finally, the arterial supply of the cerebral cortex is examined.

B

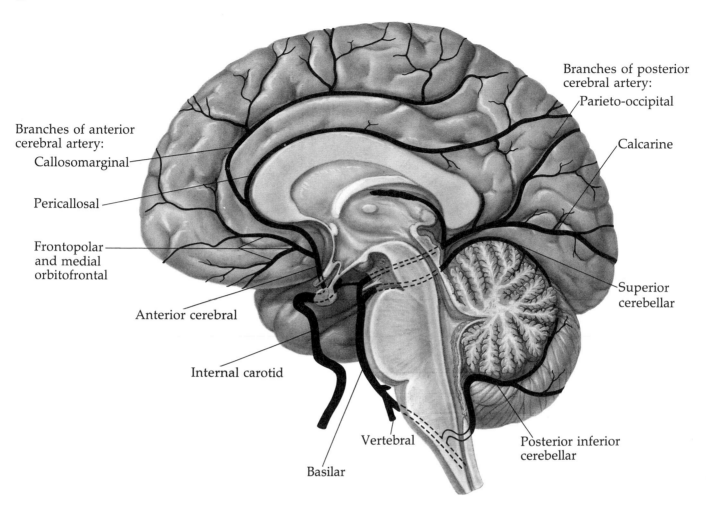

Branches of anterior cerebral artery:
  Callosomarginal
  Pericallosal
  Frontopolar and medial orbitofrontal
Anterior cerebral
Internal carotid
Basilar
Vertebral

Branches of posterior cerebral artery:
  Parieto-occipital
  Calcarine
Superior cerebellar
Posterior inferior cerebellar

The Internal Carotid Artery Has Four Principal Portions

The internal carotid artery consists of four segments (Figure 4.4B). The *cervical* segment (1) extends from the bifurcation of the common carotid (into the external and internal carotid arteries) to where it enters the carotid canal. The *intrapetrosal segment* (2) is surrounded by the petrous portion of the temporal bone. The *intracavernous segment* (3) courses through the cavernous sinus, a venous structure overlying the sphenoid bone (see Figure 4.10B). The *cerebral segment* (4) extends to the point at which the internal carotid artery bifurcates into the anterior and middle cerebral arteries. The intracavernous and cerebral portions are collectively termed the *carotid siphon*.

Figure 4.5 Cerebral angiographs of the anterior circulation are shown in a lateral projection *(A)* and a frontal projection *(B)*. (Courtesy of Dr. Neal Rutledge, University of Texas at Austin.)

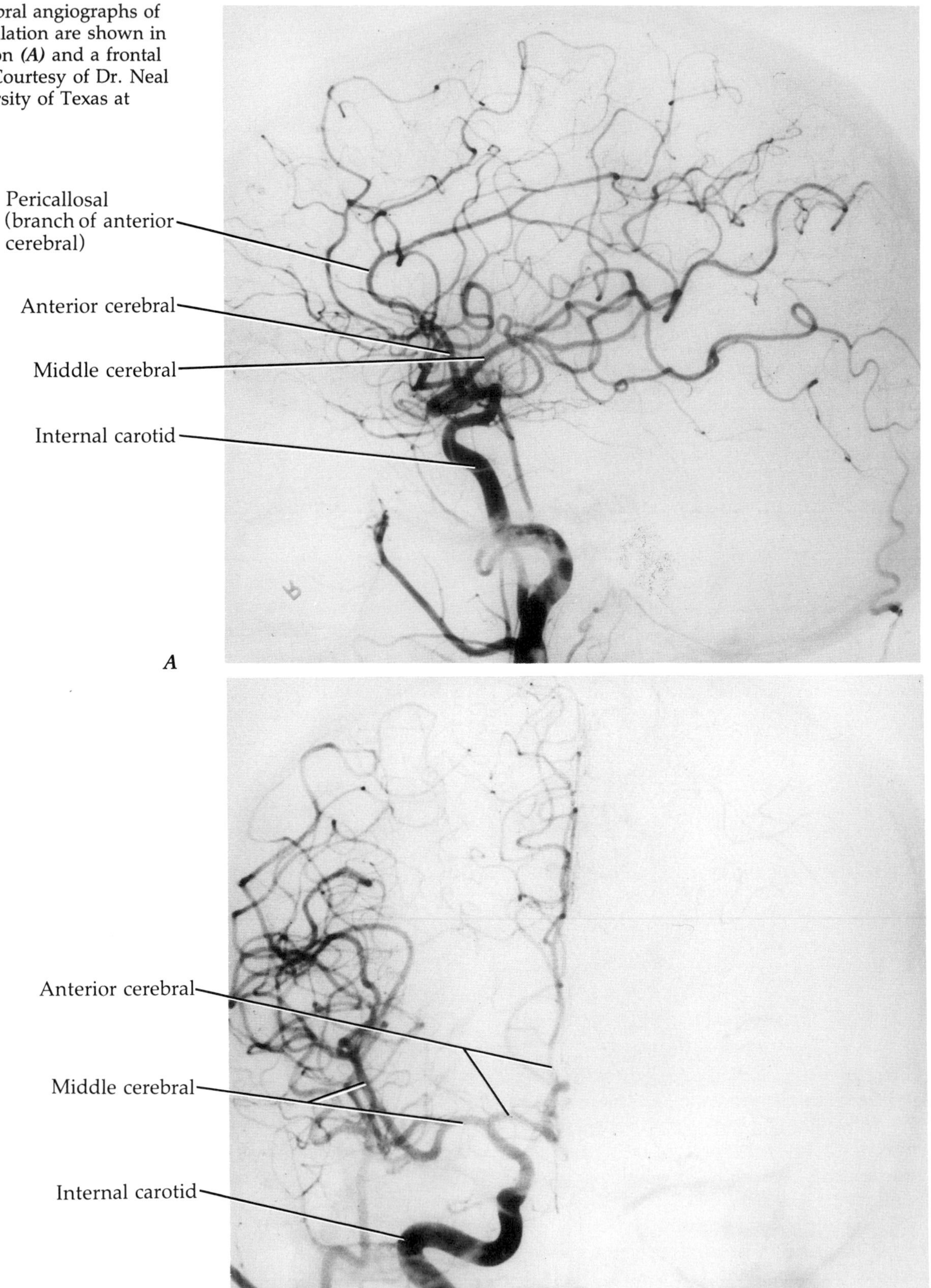

Pericallosal (branch of anterior cerebral)

Anterior cerebral

Middle cerebral

Internal carotid

A

Anterior cerebral

Middle cerebral

Internal carotid

B

Cerebral vessels can be visualized in vivo using the radiological technique of *cerebral angiography*. To obtain such an image, radiopaque material (termed *contrast medium*) is injected into either the anterior or the posterior arterial system, and a series of X-ray skull films are taken in rapid repetition as the contrast medium circulates. Films obtained while the contrast medium is within cerebral arteries are called arteriographs. Films obtained later, after the radiopaque substance has reached the cerebral veins or the dural sinuses, are called venographs. Images may be obtained from different angles with respect to the cranium. Two views are common—from the side (lateral projection) and from the front (frontal projection). The internal carotid artery is well visualized in cerebral angiographs (Figure 4.5). Indeed, with the exception of the intrapetrosal portion, which is surrounded by very dense bone, the entire course of the internal carotid artery can be identified.

The internal carotid artery also has branches that supply cerebral and other cranial structures. The major branches of the internal carotid artery, in order of emergence, are (1) the ophthalmic artery, (2) the posterior communicating artery, which forms part of the circle of Willis, and (3) the anterior choroidal artery (Figures 4.1, 4.3B, and 4.5).

The Circle of Willis Is Formed by the Communicating and Cerebral Arteries

The internal carotid artery divides near the basal surface of the cerebral hemisphere to form the *anterior cerebral artery* and the *middle cerebral artery* (Figures 4.1 and 4.4B). The *posterior cerebral artery* is part of the vertebral–basilar system and originates at the bifurcation of the basilar artery at the midbrain (Figures 4.1 and 4.3A). These three cerebral arteries are interconnected by two communicating arteries and collectively form the *circle of Willis*. The *posterior communicating artery* (1) links the middle and posterior cerebral arteries, and the *anterior communicating artery* (2), which is the only artery of the circle of Willis that is not paired, links the anterior cerebral arteries on both sides of the cerebral hemispheres (Figure 4.1B). When occlusion of either the posterior or anterior arterial circulation occurs, collateral circulation may occur through the circle of Willis to rescue the region deprived of blood. Because the anatomy of the circle of Willis is variable, and a functional "circle" is often not achieved, perfusion by the surviving system may not be complete.

Branches of the internal carotid artery and the proximal portions of the three cerebral arteries supply the diencephalon, basal ganglia, and internal capsule (Figures 4.6 and 4.7). The internal capsule, the structure through which axons pass to and from the cerebral cortex, is supplied by the *lenticulostriate arteries*, which are branches of the middle cerebral artery, and the *anterior choroidal artery*. The basal ganglia receive their arterial blood supply from two principal sources, the *anterior choroidal artery*—a branch of the internal carotid artery—and the lenticulostriate arteries (Figure 4.7). The anterior choroidal artery also supplies the choroid plexus of the lateral ventricle. The thalamus, together with the caudal hypothalamus, is fed by branches of the *posterior cerebral artery*, whereas the anterior hypothalamus and preoptic area—a region of the diencephalon and telencephalon that is located rostral to the optic chiasm (see Chapter 14)—are fed by branches of the *anterior cerebral artery*.

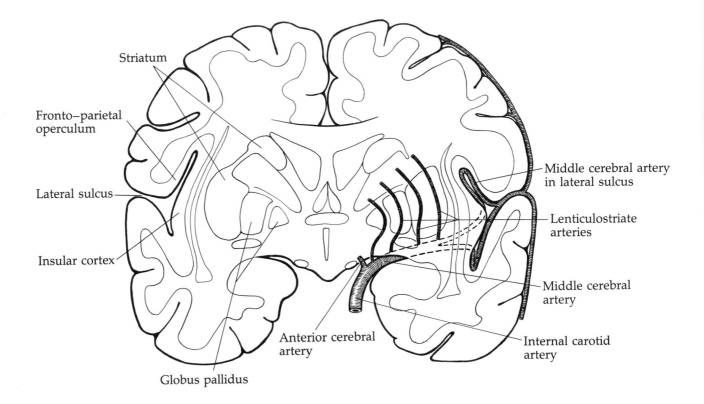

Striatum

Fronto–parietal
operculum

Lateral sulcus

Insular cortex

Globus pallidus

Anterior cerebral
artery

Middle cerebral artery
in lateral sulcus

Lenticulostriate
arteries

Middle cerebral
artery

Internal carotid
artery

Figure 4.6 The course of the middle cerebral artery through the lateral sulcus and along the insular and opercular surfaces of the cerebral cortex is shown in a schematic coronal section. (Adapted from DeArmond, S. J., Fusco, M. M., and Dewey, M. M. 1976. Structure of the Human Brain. New York: Oxford University Press.)

Different Functional Areas of the Cerebral Cortex Are Supplied by Different Cerebral Arteries

The arterial supply of the cerebral cortex is provided by the distal branches of the anterior, middle, and posterior cerebral arteries. These branches are often termed "cortical" branches. The *anterior cerebral artery* has a C-shaped configuration, like many components of the cerebral hemispheres. It originates at the bifurcation of the internal carotid artery, and courses within the interhemispheric fissure and around the rostral and dorsal surfaces of the corpus callosum (Figure 4.4B). It is important to become familiar with the approximate boundaries of the cortical regions that are supplied by the different cerebral arteries because this knowledge provides insight into the functional disturbances that follow vascular obstruction, or other pathology, of the cerebral vessels. As its gross distribution would suggest, the anterior artery supplies the dorsal and medial portions of the frontal and parietal lobes (Figure 4.4A, B). The angiographs in Figure 4.5 illustrate the course of the anterior cerebral artery in the living brain. Its C-shaped trajectory can be seen in the lateral view (A), and its position with respect to the midline is shown in the frontal view (B).

The *middle cerebral artery*, which originates at the bifurcation of the internal carotid artery, courses through the lateral sulcus (Sylvian fissure) en route to the lateral convexity of the cerebral hemisphere, to which it supplies blood. The course of the middle cerebral artery through the lateral sulcus is indirect (Figure 4.6). It courses along the surface of the insular cortex, over the inner opercular surface of the frontal, temporal, and parietal lobes, and finally emerges on the lateral convexity. The complex configuration of the middle cerebral artery can be seen in the an-

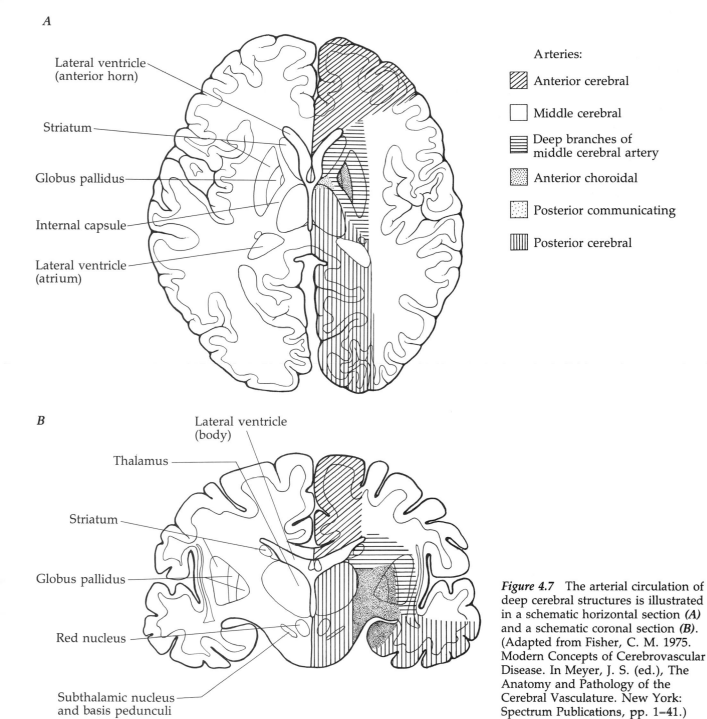

A

Lateral ventricle
(anterior horn)

Striatum

Globus pallidus

Internal capsule

Lateral ventricle
(atrium)

Arteries:

Anterior cerebral

Middle cerebral

Deep branches of
middle cerebral artery

Anterior choroidal

Posterior communicating

Posterior cerebral

B

Lateral ventricle
(body)

Thalamus

Striatum

Globus pallidus

Red nucleus

Subthalamic nucleus
and basis pedunculi

Figure 4.7 The arterial circulation of deep cerebral structures is illustrated in a schematic horizontal section *(A)* and a schematic coronal section *(B)*. (Adapted from Fisher, C. M. 1975. Modern Concepts of Cerebrovascular Disease. In Meyer, J. S. (ed.), The Anatomy and Pathology of the Cerebral Vasculature. New York: Spectrum Publications, pp. 1–41.)

giographs in Figure 4.5. The rostro–caudal course of the middle cerebral artery, from where it enters the lateral sulcus to where it emerges and distributes over the lateral surface of the cerebral cortex, is revealed in Figure 4.5A. In Figure 4.5B, its course can be followed from medial to lateral. The middle cerebral artery forms loops at the juncture of the insular cortex and the opercular surface of the frontal and parietal lobes.

Figure 4.8 Cerebral angiograph of the posterior circulation (lateral projection). (Courtesy of Dr. Neal Rutledge, University of Texas at Austin.)

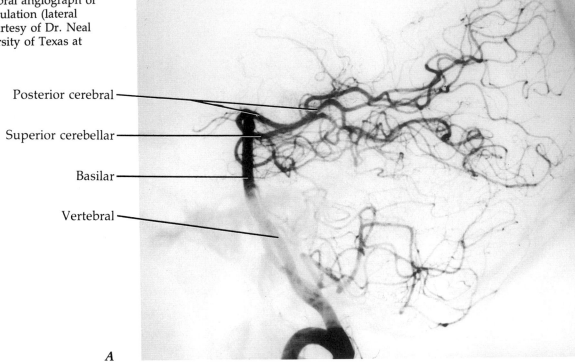

Posterior cerebral

Superior cerebellar

Basilar

Vertebral

A

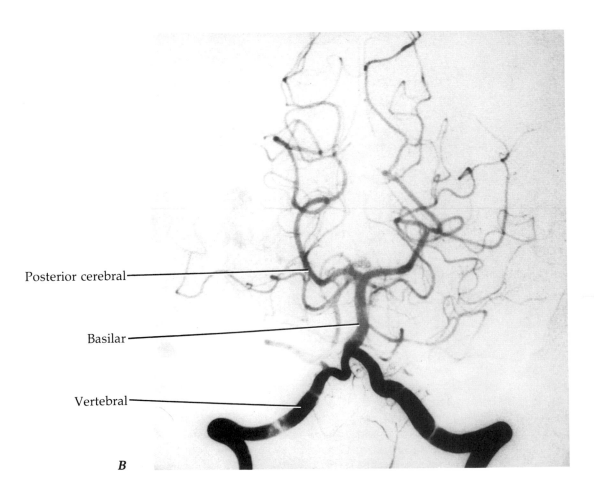

Posterior cerebral

Basilar

Vertebral

B

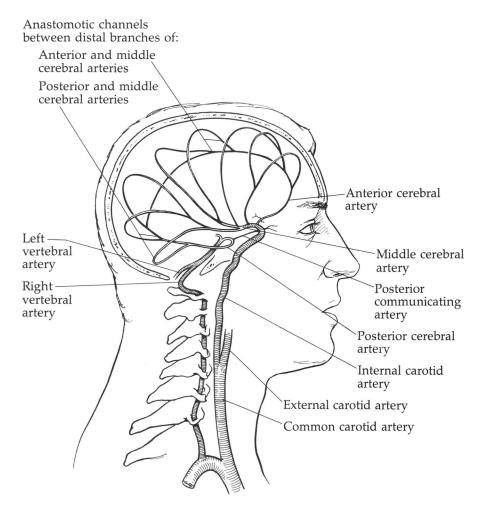

Anastomotic channels
between distal branches of:

Anterior and middle
cerebral arteries

Posterior and middle
cerebral arteries

Left
vertebral
artery

Right
vertebral
artery

Anterior cerebral
artery

Middle cerebral
artery

Posterior
communicating
artery

Posterior cerebral
artery

Internal carotid
artery

External carotid artery

Common carotid artery

Figure 4.9 Course of the major
cerebral arteries over the lateral and
medial cortical surfaces. Anastomotic
channels between the middle and
anterior cerebral arteries, which is
one site for collateral circulation, are
depicted. (Adapted from Fisher,
C. M. 1975. Modern Concepts of
Cerebrovascular Disease. In Meyer,
J. S. (ed.), The Anatomy and
Pathology of the Cerebral
Vasculature. New York: Spectrum
Publications, pp. 1–41.

The positions of these loops are radiological landmarks that aid in esti-
mating the position of the brain in relation to the skull. When a space-
occupying lesion is present, such as a tumor or a large blood clot, the
position of the brain in the skull is changed. The clinician can recognize
this displacement by noting the change in the position of the middle
cerebral artery.

The *posterior cerebral arteries* originate at the bifurcation of the basilar
artery (Figures 4.1 and 4.4B), and each one courses around the lateral
margin of the midbrain. The posterior cerebral artery supplies the occipital
lobe and portions of the medial and inferior temporal lobe. A lateral view
of an arteriograph of the posterior circulation is shown in Figure 4.8.

On the lateral convexity of the cerebral hemisphere, the terminal
ends of the different cerebral arteries form anastomoses with each other
(Figure 4.9). These anastomoses occur between surface branches only,
not when the artery has penetrated the surface. When major arteries
become occluded, these anastomoses limit the extent of damage. For example, if a branch of a cerebral artery becomes occluded, the ischemic
tissue may be rescued by collateral circulation from another cerebral artery
with which the occluded vessel is anastomotically connected. This cola-
teral circulation can best rescue the gray matter of the cerebral cortex. In
contrast, there is little collateral circulation between the regions perfused

by the cerebral arteries in the white matter. Although collateral circulation provides the cerebral cortex with a margin of safety during arterial occlusion, the anastomotic network that permits collateral circulation creates a different kind of vulnerability. When the systemic blood pressure is reduced, the region served by this anastomotic network is particularly susceptible to ischemia because such anastomoses occur at the terminal ends of the arteries, regions where perfusion pressure is lowest. The peripheral borders of the territory supplied by major vessels are termed *border zones* and an infarction occurring in these regions is termed a *border zone infarct*.[2]

Venous Drainage of the Central Nervous System

The venous drainage of the central nervous system is achieved through either of two routes. In one case venous blood returns directly to the systemic circulation. The blood supply to the spinal cord and caudal medulla drains by this direct path. A network of spinal veins and plexes empty into the systemic venous return. By contrast, most cerebral structures are drained by veins that empty into the *dural sinuses* (Figures 4.10 and 4.11; see also Figure 1.10). The dural sinuses are a collection of large channels located between layers of the *dura* (Figure 4.10A). The dural sinuses function as low-pressure channels for the flow of venous blood back to the systemic circulation.

The *superior sagittal sinus* runs along the midline of the cranial cavity, at the superior margin of the falx cerebri (Figure 4.10A). The *inferior sagittal sinus* runs along the inferior margin of the falx cerebri just superior to the corpus callosum. The inferior sagittal sinus together with the *great cerebral vein* (*of Galen*) return venous blood to the *straight* (sometimes called *rectus*) *sinus* (Figure 4.10B). At the occipital pole, the superior sagittal sinus and the straight sinus join to form the two *transverse sinuses*. The *confluence of the sinuses* is located here, although rarely is the confluence formed from the juncture of all four dural sinuses. Finally, the transverse sinus drains into the sigmoid sinus, which, in turn, drains into the internal jugular vein. The cavernous and petrosal sinuses are also illustrated in Figure 4.10B.

Venous drainage of the cerebral hemispheres is provided by superficial and deep cerebral veins. The superficial cerebral veins arise from the cerebral cortex and underlying white matter. The veins anastomose in the pia mater and drain into the sagittal and straight sinuses. The superficial cerebral veins are quite variable in their course.[3] The *deep cerebral veins* drain the deeper portions of the white matter, the basal ganglia, and parts of the diencephalon. The *great cerebral vein* (of Galen) (Figure 4.10B) collects venous blood from many deep cerebral veins and, in turn, drains into the straight sinus. The venous drainage of the brain stem, like that of the cerebral hemispheres, is into the dural sinuses. Veins of the caudal brain stem drain into the sigmoid or petrosal sinuses (Figure 4.10B). The cerebellar veins drain into the great cerebral vein, which in turn drains into the *straight sinus*, or they drain directly into the straight

---

[2] Another term used to describe a border zone infarction is *watershed infarct*.

[3] Two cerebral veins are often distinguishable: the superior anastomotic vein (of Trolard) lying across the parietal lobe and the inferior anastomotic vein (of Labbé) on the surface of the temporal lobe.

A

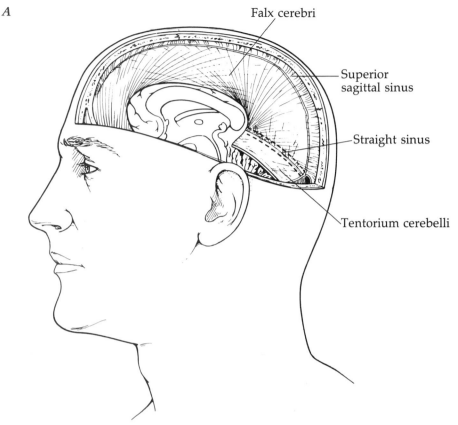

Falx cerebri

Superior
sagittal sinus

Straight sinus

Tentorium cerebelli

Figure 4.10 *A.* Falx cerebri and
superior sagittal sinus from a lateral
perspective. *B.* View of the ventral
surface of the anterior and middle
cranial fossae, and the sinuses on the
dorsal surface of the tentorium
cerebelli and the ventral cranium.

B

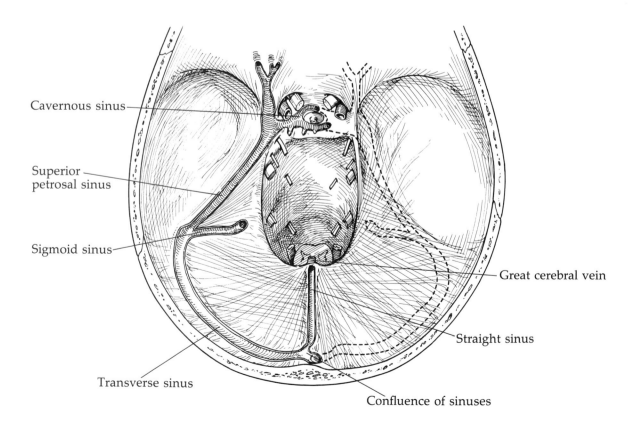

Cavernous sinus

Superior
petrosal sinus

Sigmoid sinus

Great cerebral vein

Straight sinus

Transverse sinus

Confluence of sinuses

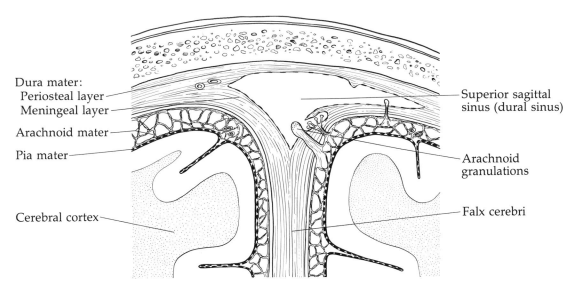

Dura mater:
  Periosteal layer
  Meningeal layer
Arachnoid mater
Pia mater

Superior sagittal sinus (dural sinus)

Arachnoid granulations

Cerebral cortex

Falx cerebri

Figure 4.11   The flow of cerebrospinal fluid is shown on a view of the midsagittal surface of the central nervous system. (Adapted from Davson, H., Keasley, W., and Segal, M. B. 1987. Physiology and Pathophysiology of the Cerebrospinal Fluid. Edinburgh: Churchill Livingstone.)

sinus and the *transverse sinus*. The venous drainage of the midbrain is via the great cerebral vein or the deep cerebral veins, and then to the straight sinus.

The Dural Sinuses Provide the Return Path for Cerebrospinal Fluid

In addition to their role in draining cerebral veins, the dural sinuses also are the sites for reabsorption of cerebrospinal fluid. Here, the production and flow of cerebrospinal fluid is surveyed, and absorption of cerebrospinal fluid into the vascular system is considered. The ventricles and subarachnoid space contain approximately 125 ml of cerebrospinal fluid (25 ml in the ventricles and 100 ml in the subarachnoid space). Approximately two-thirds of the cerebrospinal fluid is secreted by the *choroid plexus*, which is located in the ventricles (Figure 4.11; see also Figure 1.11). The additional one-third of cerebrospinal fluid production is secreted by brain capillaries. The total amount of cerebrospinal fluid production is approximately 500 ml per day. Cerebrospinal fluid is returned to the systemic circulation through valves in the dural sinuses (see later). Cerebrospinal fluid produced by the choroid plexus in the lateral ventricles (Figure 4.11, dashed line) flows through the interventricular foramen and mixes with cerebrospinal fluid produced in the third ventricle. From here, it flows through the cerebral aqueduct and into the fourth ventricle, which is another site for cerebrospinal fluid production because choroid plexus is also located there. Three apertures in the roof of the fourth ventricle are the sites for drainage of cerebrospinal fluid from the ventricular system into the subarachnoid space: the *foramen of Magendie*, which is located on the midline, and the two *foramina of Luschka*, which are located at the lateral margins of the fourth ventricle. The subarachnoid space is dilated in certain locations, termed *cisterns*. Five prom-

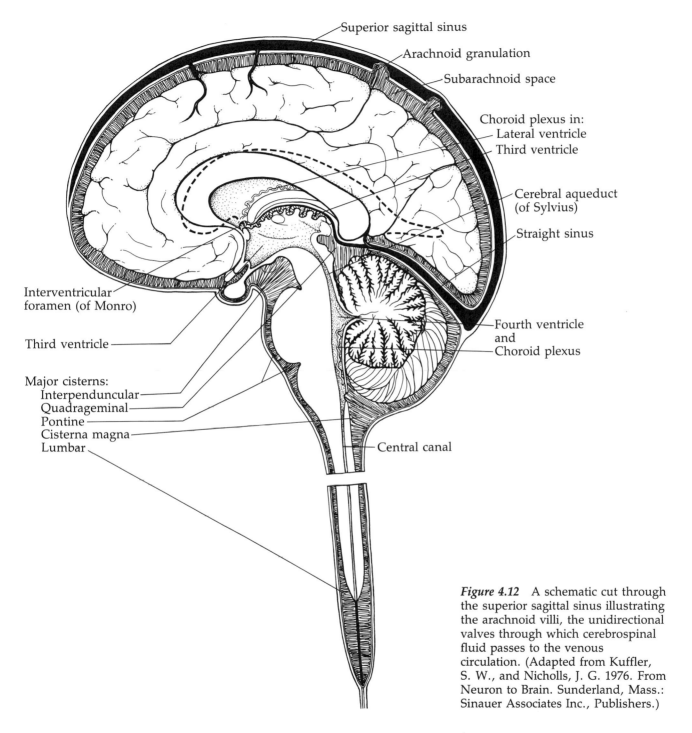

Superior sagittal sinus

Arachnoid granulation

Subarachnoid space

Choroid plexus in:
Lateral ventricle
Third ventricle

Cerebral aqueduct
(of Sylvius)

Straight sinus

Interventricular
foramen (of Monro)

Third ventricle

Major cisterns:
Interpenduncular
Quadrageminal
Pontine
Cisterna magna
Lumbar

Fourth ventricle
and
Choroid plexus

Central canal

Figure 4.12 A schematic cut through the superior sagittal sinus illustrating the arachnoid villi, the unidirectional valves through which cerebrospinal fluid passes to the venous circulation. (Adapted from Kuffler, S. W., and Nicholls, J. G. 1976. From Neuron to Brain. Sunderland, Mass.: Sinauer Associates Inc., Publishers.)

inent cisterns are located on the midline: the (1) *interpeduncular* and (2) *quadrageminal*[4] cisterns are both located at the level of the midbrain, (3) the *pontine cistern* is located ventral to the pons, (4) the *cisterna magna* is located dorsal to the medulla, and (5) the *lumbar cistern* is located in the caudal vertebral canal (Figure 4.11).

---

[4] The quadrageminal cistern is located dorsal to the superior and inferior colliculi. This cistern derives its name from the quadrageminal bodies—in total, the four colliculi.

Cerebrospinal fluid passes from the subarachnoid space to the venous blood through small unidirectional valves, termed *arachnoid villi*, which are located in the walls of the dural sinuses (Figure 4.12). Arachnoid villi are microscopic evaginations of the arachnoid mater. Numerous clusters of arachnoid villi are especially prominent over the dorsal (superior) convexity of the cerebral hemispheres in the superior sagittal sinus, where they form a macroscopic structure called the *arachnoid granulations*.

Summary

The arterial supply of the spinal cord is provided by the *vertebral arteries* and the *radicular arteries* (Figures 4.1 and 4.2). The brain is supplied by the *internal carotid arteries (the anterior circulation)* and the *vertebral arteries*, which join at the pontomedullary junction to form the *basilar artery* (collectively termed the *posterior circulation*) (Figure 4.1). The brain stem is supplied by the posterior system (Figure 4.3A). The medulla receives blood directly from small branches of the *vertebral arteries* as well as from the *spinal arteries* and the *posterior inferior cerebellar artery (PICA)* (Figure 4.3A, B). The pons is supplied by *paramedian* and *short circumferential branches* of the *basilar artery*. Two major long circumferential branches are the *anterior inferior cerebellar artery (AICA)* and the *superior cerebellar artery* (Figure 4.3C). The midbrain receives its arterial supply primarily from the *posterior cerebral artery* as well as from the basilar artery (Figure 4.3A).

The cerebral hemispheres and diencephalon are supplied by both the *anterior* and the *posterior circulations*. The cerebral cortex receives its blood supply from the three cerebral arteries: the *anterior* and *middle cerebral arteries*, which are part of the anterior circulation, and the *posterior cerebral artery*, which is part of the posterior circulation (Figures 4.1, 4.4, 4.6, and 4.7). The diencephalon, basal ganglia, and internal capsule receive blood from branches of the *internal carotid artery*, the three *cerebral arteries*, and the *posterior communicating artery* (Figures 4.1, 4.6, and 4.7).

The anterior and posterior systems are interconnected by two networks of arteries: (1) the *circle of Willis*, which is formed by the three *cerebral arteries*, the *posterior communicating artery*, and the *anterior communicating artery* (Figure 4.1), and (2) terminal branches of the cerebral arteries, which anastomose on the superior convexity of the cerebral cortex (Figures 4.4 and 4.9).

The venous drainage of the spinal cord is direct to the systemic circulation. By contrast, veins draining the cerebral hemispheres and brain stem drain into the *dural sinuses* (Figure 4.10). Cerebrospinal fluid also drains into the dural sinuses (Figure 4.11) through unidirectional valves termed *arachnoid villi* (Figure 4.12). ■

References

Carpenter, M. B., and Sutin, J. 1983. Human Neuroanatomy. Baltimore: Williams & Wilkins.

DeArmond, S. J., Fusco, M. M., and Dewey, M. M. 1976. Structure of the Human Brain. New York: Oxford University Press.

Ferner, H., and Staubestand, J. (eds.) 1983. Sobotta: Atlas of Human Anatomy. Vol. 1. Head, neck, upper extremities. Baltimore: Urban and Schwarzenberg.

Kuffler, S. W., and Nicholls, J. G. 1976. From Neuron to Brain. Sunderland, Mass.: Sinauer Associates Inc., Publishers.

Selected Readings

Davson, H., Keasley, W., and Segal, M. B. 1987. Physiology and Pathophysiology of the Cerebrospinal Fluid. Edinburgh: Churchill Livingstone.

Fisher, C. M. 1975. Modern Concepts of Cerebrovascular Disease. In Meyer, J. S. (ed.), The Anatomy and Pathology of the Cerebral Vasculature. New York: Spectrum Publications, pp. 1–41.

Fishman, R. A. 1980. Cerebrospinal Fluid in Diseases of the Nervous System. Philadelphia: Saunders.

Kistler, J. P., Ropper, A. H., and Martin, J. B. 1987. Cerebrovascular diseases. In Braunwald, E., Isselbacher, F. J., Peterdorf, R. G., et al. (eds.) Harrison's Principles of Internal Medicine, 11th edition. New York: McGraw-Hill, pp. 1930–1960.

The Somatic
Sensory System

5

The Somatic Sensory System

The sensory systems of the brain are the focus of this and the next three chapters. Here we consider the anatomical organization of the somatic sensory system, which processes stimuli that impinge on the body surface or originate from within the body—from the muscles, joints, and viscera. The somatic sensory system functions in perception of tactile stimuli, limb position sense, pain, and temperature. In addition, the somatic sensory system is critically involved in the maintenance of arousal and in the sensory control of movement. The anatomical systems that process information from the limbs and trunk are separate from those that process information from facial structures, although the general features of their organization are similar. In this chapter, the anatomical systems that subserve somatic sensation from the limbs and trunk are discussed. These systems, which receive afferent information from the spinal nerves, constitute the ascending spinal cord pathways. Somatic sensation from the head, which is carried by the cranial nerves, will be considered in Chapter 12 where the general organization of the cranial nerves and cranial nerve nuclei are examined.

In approaching the study of the anatomical organization of different functional components of the somatic sensory system, we first survey their general organization, an organization that parallels the longitudinal axis of the central nervous system. This will be accomplished in the next section of this chapter. During this initial examination, we focus on concepts to gain an overall view rather than focus on anatomical details. In the latter sections of the chapter the anatomical organization of the specific components is examined at various levels through the nervous system.

The Dorsal Column–Medial Lemniscal System and the Anterolateral System Differ in Anatomical Organization

Somatic sensation of the limbs and trunk is mediated principally by two ascending neural systems: (1) the *dorsal column–medial lemniscal system* (Figures 5.1B and 5.2A), which is important for discriminative tactile sensations, vibration, and upper limb position sense, and (2) the *anterolateral system* (Figures 5.1C and 5.2B), which subserves pain and temperature sense and a less discriminative—or crude—form of tactile sense.[1] The organization of the dorsal column–medial lemniscal system was considered briefly in Chapter 3 in our initial exposure to the internal organization of the central nervous system. Here, its organization will be compared with that of the anterolateral system. There are four key differences in the organization of these pathways.

1. In Chapter 3 we saw that the dorsal root ganglion cell is a primary sensory neuron, providing sensory information to the somatic sensory system. Afferent input from different functional classes

---

[1] The spinocervical tract is an important somatic sensory ascending pathway in carnivores. It exists in primates but it is not as well developed. It may play a role in the recovery of somatic sensory function after dorsal column lesion. Lower limb position sense is subserved by axons that course in the lateral column.

of dorsal root ganglion cells contribute information to the two systems. The dorsal column–medial lemniscal system receives input from sensory receptors that are sensitive to *mechanical* stimuli. In contrast, sensory receptors sensitive to *noxious* (i.e., painful) and *thermal* stimuli provide the major afferent input to the anterolateral system. Although the segregation of the different types of afferent input into the two ascending systems is not absolute, it is sufficiently complete to have important clinical consequences. After a lesion of the dorsal column–medial lemniscal system, only a less discriminative—or crude—form of touch remains. Although simple tactile thresholds may not be elevated, discriminative capabilities are reduced. Individuals suffering from such a lesion, using only residual somatic sensory capabilities, may not be able to distinguish different gradations of rough and smooth, or the shapes of objects without the aid of vision; nor would they be capable of telling an examiner arm position. By contrast, a lesion of the anterolateral system leaves tactile and limb position senses unaffected but pain thresholds are elevated.

2. The first major relay in the dorsal column–medial lemniscal system is in the *dorsal column nuclei,* in the medulla. This is where the first-order neurons in the pathway—the primary sensory neurons—synapse on second-order neurons. In contrast, the anterolateral system first relays in the *dorsal horn* of the spinal cord. The general aspects of the anatomy of these two systems are presented in Figure 5.1B and C. Schematic sections through the spinal cord, brain stem, and cerebral hemisphere are illustrated along with the patterns of connections between anatomical structures on the various sections. Figure 5.2A and B presents a comparison of the anatomical organization of the two systems. The course of the dorsal column–medial lemniscal system is illustrated in part A and the course of the anterolateral system is shown in part B.

3. The dorsal column–medial lemniscal system decussates (crosses the midline) in the medulla (Figure 5.2A) and the anterolateral system decussates in the spinal cord (Figure 5.2B). The two systems are similar to the extent that in each system it is the axon of the second neuron in the circuit that decussates. Knowledge of the level at which neurons in a system decussate is important in identifying the location of a lesion.

4. The dorsal column–medial lemniscal system represents a relatively homogenous and anatomically discrete pathway that processes somatic sensory information and transmits this information to the ventral posterior lateral nucleus of the thalamus and then to the primary somatic sensory cortex in the parietal lobe (Figure 5.1A). On the other hand, the anterolateral system contains three separate pathways that ascend in parallel: the *spi-*

A

Central sulcus

Primary somatic
sensory cortex

Secondary somatic
sensory cortex

B

Cerebral cortex
and thalamus

Primary somatic
sensory cortex

Internal capsule
(posterior limb)

Ventral posterior
lateral nucleus

Midbrain

Pons

Medial lemniscus

Medulla

Dorsal column nuclei:
Gracile nucleus
Cuneate nucleus

Internal arcuate fibers

Medulla

Gracile fascicle

Cuneate fascicle

Spinal
cord

Large diameter fiber

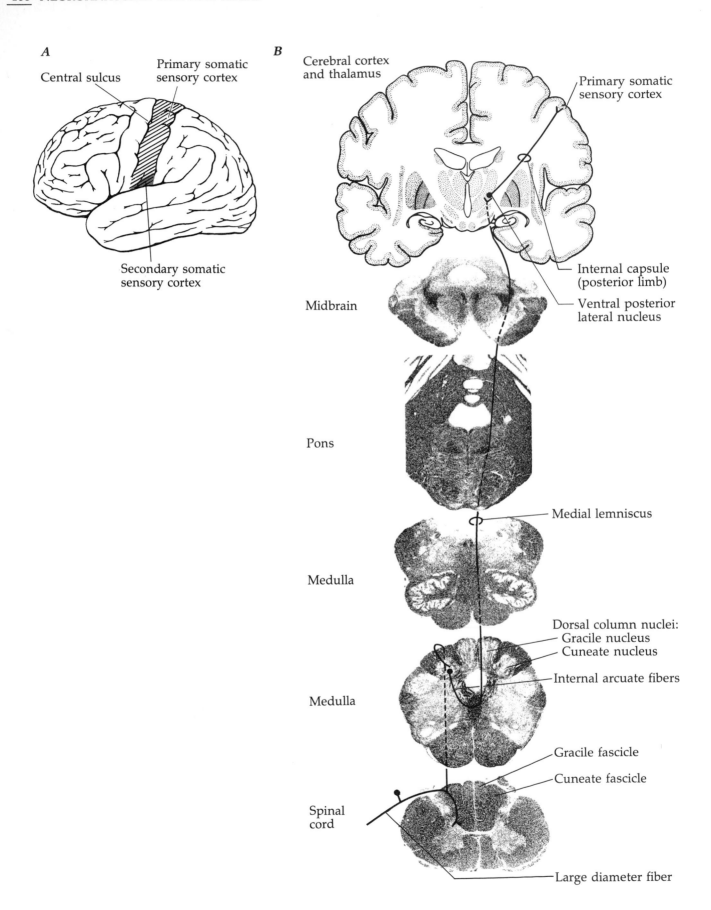

C

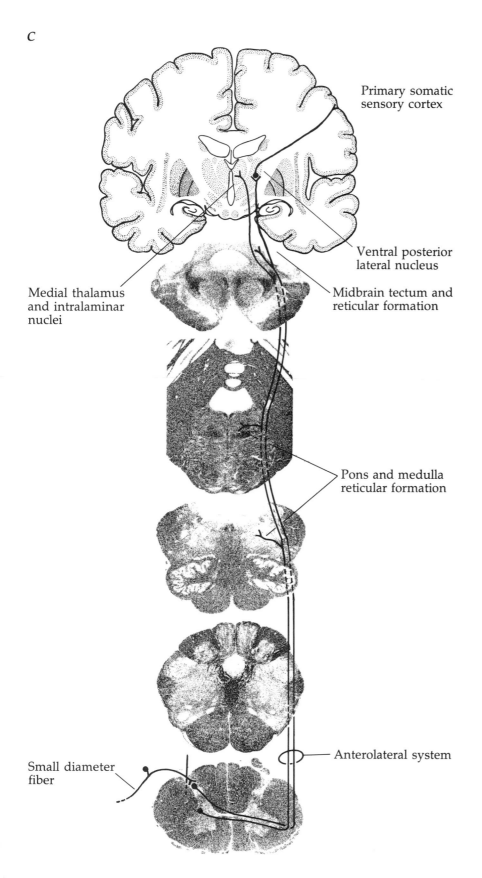

Primary somatic sensory cortex

Ventral posterior lateral nucleus

Medial thalamus and intralaminar nuclei

Midbrain tectum and reticular formation

Pons and medulla reticular formation

Anterolateral system

Small diameter fiber

Figure 5.1 The general organization of the ascending somatic sensory pathways. *A.* View of lateral surface of the cerebral cortex and the primary and secondary somatic sensory cortex. *B.* Dorsal column–medial lemniscal system. *C.* Anterolateral system.

A

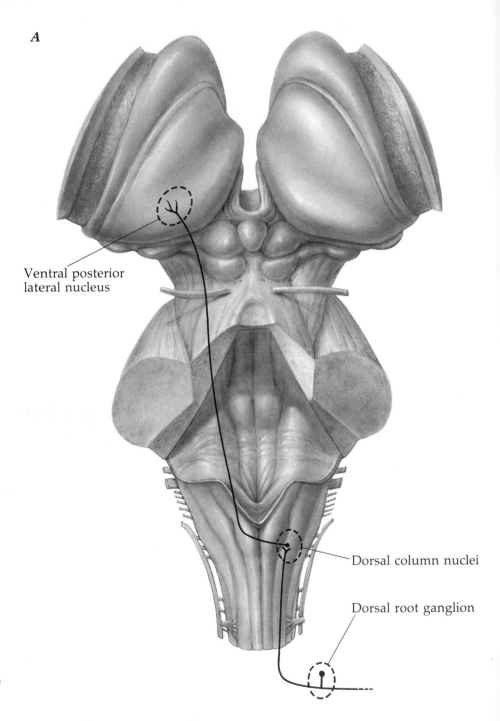

Ventral posterior
lateral nucleus

Dorsal column nuclei

Dorsal root ganglion

Figure 5.2 Dorsal view of the brain
stem without the cerebellum
illustrating the course of the dorsal
column–medial lemniscal system *(A)*
and the anterolateral system *(B)*.

nothalamic tract, the *spinoreticular tract*, and the *spinotectal tract*.[2]
These three pathways intermingle in the spinal cord and brain
stem. The spinothalamic tract parallels the anatomy and function
of the dorsal column–medial lemniscal system more closely than

---

[2] Based on phylogenetic considerations, the spinothalamic tract is also termed the
neospinothalamic tract, and the spinoreticular tract is called the *paleospinothalamic tract*.

B

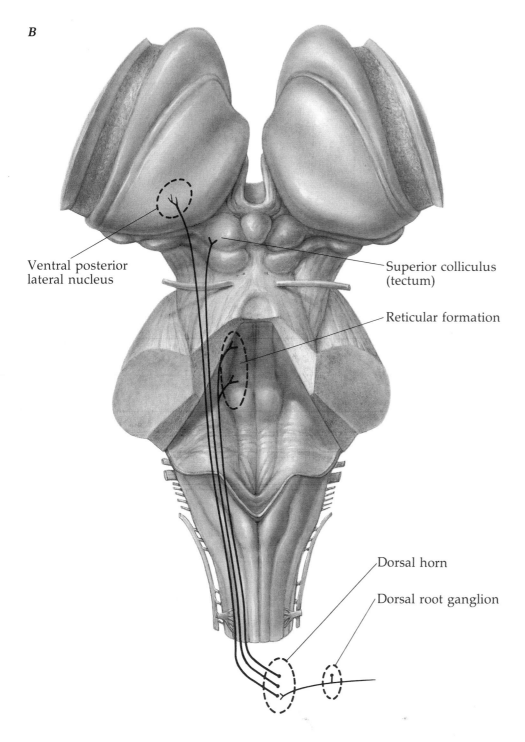

Ventral posterior lateral nucleus

Superior colliculus (tectum)

Reticular formation

Dorsal horn

Dorsal root ganglion

the other contingents of the anterolateral system. It carries information to the ventral posterior lateral nucleus and then to the primary somatic sensory cortex. The projection of both the spinothalamic tract and the medial lemniscus to the ventral posterior lateral nucleus is thought to be important in the discriminative aspects of somatic sensations, for example, the precise spatial localization of a tactile stimulus or pin prick. In addition, a portion of the spinothalamic tract terminates more medially in the thalamus, in the intralaminar nuclei. This projection and the one to the reticular formation via the spinoreticular tract are thought to be important in the motivational and affective aspects of somatic sensation and in maintaining arousal. The spinotectal tract terminates in the midbrain tectum (primarily in the superior colliculus). This path may participate in integrating visual and somatic sensory information for orienting the head and body to salient stimuli (Chapter 6).

In the remaining sections of this chapter the different regions of the nervous system that function in somatic sensation are examined. The various components of the dorsal column–medial lemniscal system and anterolateral system and their spatial locations are compared at different levels, progressing in sequence from the periphery to the cerebral cortex. An understanding of the *regional organization* is important because when a discrete portion of the central nervous system is injured, components of different functional systems are often affected indiscriminately. In later chapters, similar levels through the neuraxis will be reexamined, but from the perspective of the different functional systems. Gradually, we will build a complete picture of the anatomical and functional organization of a region.

The First Neuron in the Somatic Sensory Pathway Is the Dorsal Root Ganglion Cell

The *dorsal root ganglion cells* (Figure 5.3) transduce sensory information into neural signals, and transmit these signals to the central nervous system. These neurons derive their name from the *dorsal root ganglia*, in which their cell bodies are located. Ganglia are collections of neuronal cell bodies that are located outside the central nervous system. The dorsal root ganglia are located in the intervertebral foramina. Dorsal root ganglion cells are *pseudounipolar neurons*[3], each with two axonal branches: one directed toward the periphery and the other, centrally. The *peripheral* branch innervates the tissue (for example, skin and muscle). The distal terminal of the peripheral branch is the only portion of the neuron that is sensitive to stimulus energy. This portion is the *sensory receptor*, which is where stimulus transduction occurs. The *primary afferent fiber*, a term commonly used to describe the peripheral branch of the dorsal root ganglion cell, transmits the sensory information to the central nervous system. There is a relationship between the diameter of the primary afferent fiber, important features of its physiology, and the connections it makes with structures in the central nervous system. Large-diameter primary afferent fibers are myelinated and their peripheral receptive portion is sensitive to *mechanical* stimuli. The peripheral receptive portions of the majority of small-diameter myelinated fibers and unmyelinated primary fibers are sensitive to *noxious* and *thermal* stimuli. Table 5.1 lists the func-

---

[3] Early in development dorsal root ganglion cells have a bipolar morphology, with a peripheral and a central branch emerging from the two poles of the cell body. Later, the proximal portions of the two axonal processes fuse.

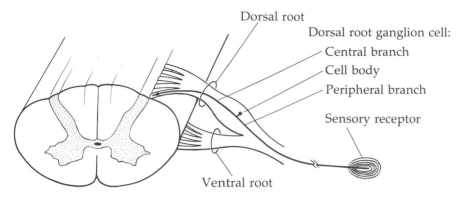

Figure 5.3   The dorsal root ganglion cell and the organization of the primary afferent fiber. The sensory receptor illustrated is a mechanoreceptor, a Pacinian corpuscle.

tional categories of primary afferent fibers, including the afferent fiber nomenclature based on axonal diameter. Alternate schemes exist for classifying afferent fibers: A-α, A-β, A-δ, and C fibers compared with I, II, III, and IV respectively. Mechanoreceptors have a morphologically specialized ending (for example, the morphologically specialized mechanoreceptor in Figure 5.3 is a Pacinian corpuscle) whereas nociceptors and thermoreceptors have bare nerve endings. The dorsal column–medial lemniscal system receives afferent input principally from the large-diameter fibers, whereas the anterolateral system receives afferent input mostly from the smaller diameter myelinated and unmyelinated fibers.

The *central branches* of dorsal root ganglion cells collect into the *dorsal roots* and enter the spinal cord (Figure 5.3). As the dorsal roots approach the spinal cord, they branch into numerous rootlets that enter along the dorsolateral margin of a single spinal segment (Figure 5.3 see also, Figure 1.4). The area of skin innervated by the axons in a single dorsal root is termed a *dermatome*. The key feature of their organization is that the dermatomes of adjacent dorsal roots overlap extensively with those of their neighbors. This feature has important clinical consequences. When a cli-

Table 5.1

Fiber Diameter (μm)	Class		Myelination[a]	Receptor Type
13–20	A-α	I	Myelinated	Mechanoreceptors (muscle and tendon)
6–12	A-β	II	Myelinated	Mechanoreceptors (skin, muscle, and deep tissue)
1–5	A-δ	III	Myelinated	Nociceptors, thermoreceptors[a]
0.2–1.5	C	IV	Unmyelinated	Nociceptors, thermoreceptors

[a] A small number of thinly myelinated and unmyelinated fibers are sensitive to mechanical stimuli. These mechanoreceptors are present in the hairy skin.

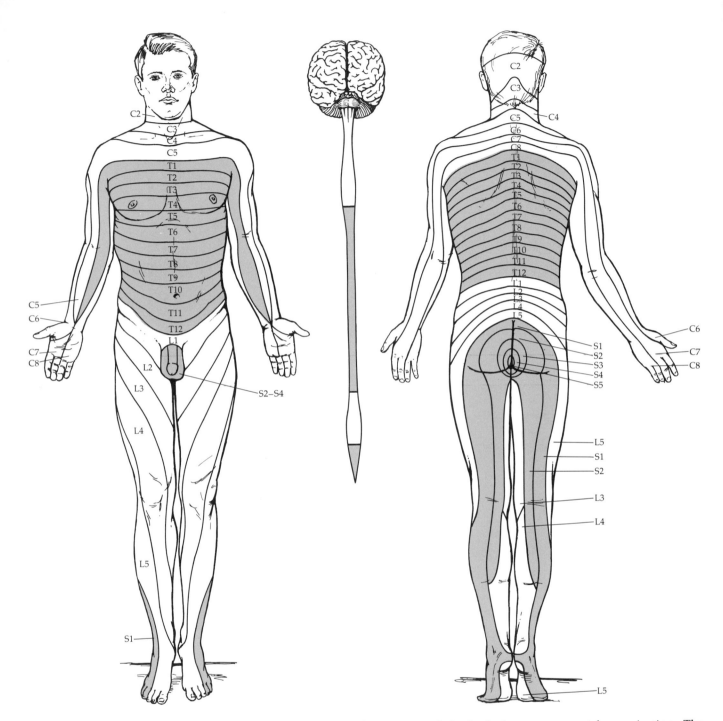

Figure 5.4 The dermatomes of the body have a segmental organization. The correspondence between the spinal cord divisions (shown on a ventral view of the central nervous system) and dermatome locations is shown. The brain and spinal cord are enlarged for clarity.

nician probes sensory capacity after injury to a single dorsal root, typically no anesthetic area is observed. This is because the adjacent dorsal roots, which are intact, also innervate the peripheral area that was innervated by the damaged root. Rather than produce a clear sensory deficit (patients

THE SOMATIC SENSORY SYSTEM

are sometimes aware of tingling or even a diminished sensory capacity), dorsal root injury commonly produces *radicular pain*, which is localized to the dermatome of the injured root. The different portions of the body that are innervated by the different spinal cord segments are shown in Figure 5.4, which illustrates the dermatomes of the body. By comparing the location of a sensory disturbance, for example radicular pain, with a dermatomal map, the clinician can localize the site of the central nervous system damage.

Dorsal Root Axons with Different Diameters Terminate in Different Central Nervous System Locations

The central branch of a dorsal root ganglion cell enters the spinal cord at its dorsolateral margin (Figures 5.3 and 5.5). Even at the entrance to the spinal cord, axons that serve different sensory functions are segregated. Large-diameter axons, which mediate tactile, vibration, and limb position senses, enter medial to the small-diameter axons, which mediate pain and temperature sense (Figure 5.5B and C). The locations of entry can be distinguished (Figure 5.5A): the *large diameter fiber entry zone* and the *zone of Lissauer*, which is where small diameter myelinated fibers and unmyelinated fibers enter. Once in the spinal cord, dorsal root ganglion cells branch extensively. As we saw in Chapter 3 (Figure 3.2A), a general pattern of branching persists in which three broad classes of termination can be recognized: segmental, ascending, and descending (Figure 5.5B). *Segmental* branches (1) enter the gray matter of the spinal cord and synapse on a variety of neuron types, such as interneurons and motor neurons that are part of reflex circuits, and neurons that project to the brain (see later). The *ascending branch* (2) carries sensory information to the brain. The *descending branch* (3) synapses on spinal cord interneurons located caudal to the level of entry and contributes sensory information for intersegmental reflexes.

Ascending and descending branches of *large-diameter* dorsal root ganglion cells course within a circumscribed region of the white matter, the *dorsal column* (Figure 5.5). The two other regions of the spinal cord white matter, the lateral and ventral columns, contain axons of central nervous system neurons and not branches of dorsal root ganglion cells. A large diameter fiber, on entering the spinal cord, skirts around the cap of the gray matter to enter the dorsal column (Figure 5.5B). The main function of the ascending branch is to relay information to the medulla for perception. Large-diameter fibers also terminate in specific locations in the gray matter (Figure 5.5B). To understand the pattern of termination of the afferent fibers in the gray matter of the spinal cord, we must first briefly consider the cytoarchitecture of the three divisions of the gray matter: dorsal horn, intermediate zone, and ventral horn (Figure 5.5A). As other areas of the central nervous system, spinal cord neurons are clustered into nuclei (Table 5.2). The Swedish neuroanatomist Bror Rexed further recognized that the nuclei in the dorsal horn are arranged in the form of sheets of neurons that run parallel to the long axis of the central nervous system. The individual sheets, termed *Rexed's laminae*, contain neurons that have different anatomical connections and functions. Neurons of the intermediate zone and the ventral horn are also parceled into

A

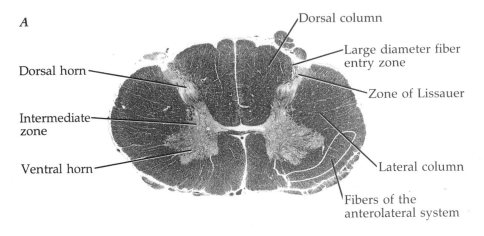

Dorsal column

Large diameter fiber entry zone

Dorsal horn

Zone of Lissauer

Intermediate zone

Ventral horn

Lateral column

Fibers of the anterolateral system

B

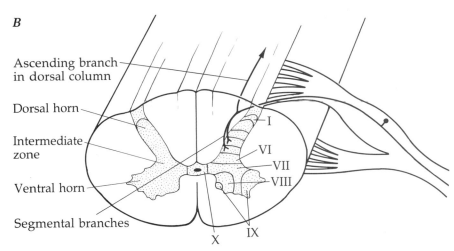

Ascending branch in dorsal column

Dorsal horn

I

Intermediate zone

VI

VII

VIII

Ventral horn

Segmental branches

X   IX

C

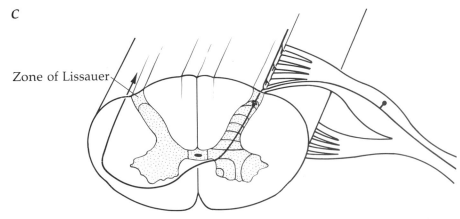

Zone of Lissauer

Figure 5.5   *A*. Myelin-stained section through the cervical spinal cord. *B, C*. Schematic drawings based on the section in A and illustrating the pattern of termination of large-diameter fibers *(B)* and small-diameter fibers *(C)*. Note that small diameter fibers also terminate in lamina II.

Table 5.2

Region	Rexed's Lamina	Nuclei
Dorsal horn	I	Marginal zone
Dorsal horn	II	Substantia gelatinosa
Dorsal horn	III, IV	Nucleus proprius
Intermediate zone	VII	Clarke's nucleus
Intermediate zone	VII	Intermediolateral nucleus
Ventral horn	IX	Motor nuclei

laminae; however, rather than forming clear sheets, these laminae are actually shaped like rods or columns. There are ten Rexed's laminae. The dorsal horn is formed by laminae I through VI, the intermediate zone corresponds to lamina VII,[4] and the ventral horn is composed of laminae VIII and IX. Lamina X is the gray matter surrounding the central canal. Some laminae also correspond to spinal cord nuclei and a comparison between the laminar organization and spinal cord nuclei is presented in Table 5.2. The nuclear nomenclature is simply an alternate scheme for categorizing the locations of spinal cord neurons. The laminar nomenclature is more commonly used because there is a relationship between individual laminae, the pattern of termination of afferent fibers, and the location of neurons that send their axons to the brain stem or thalamus (see later). Large-diameter fibers do not terminate in the superficial laminae of the dorsal horn, but rather in *laminae III through VI.* Large-diameter fibers also terminate in the *intermediate zone* and *ventral horn.*

The pattern by which small-diameter axons that subserve pain and temperature senses enter and terminate in the spinal cord (Figure 5.5C) is quite different from that of the large-diameter axons. Once a small diameter fiber enters the spinal cord, it branches and ascends and descends within the *zone of Lissauer*, the white matter region that caps the dorsal horn (Figure 5.5). The zone of Lissauer appears pale on myelin-stained sections because it contains many unmyelinated fibers. The segmental branches that enter the dorsal horn derive directly from the ascending and descending branches of the small-diameter fibers. Whereas large-diameter axons terminate in laminae III through VI of the dorsal horn, small-diameter myelinated and unmyelinated axons terminate in *laminae I and II.*

The Dorsal Columns Have Two Separate Components That Mediate Tactile Sense from the Upper and Lower Extremities

The dorsal column transmits sensory information from the *ipsilateral side of the body* to the medulla. The majority of dorsal column axons are ascending branches of dorsal root ganglion cells. A significant minority are axons of dorsal horn neurons and therefore are postsynaptic to the primary afferent fibers. These neurons, which are located in the *deeper laminae of the dorsal horn*, receive afferent input from segmental branches of afferent fibers (Figure 5.5B).

---

[4] Some investigators place lamina VI in the intermediate zone; however, the function of neurons in this layer is more like that of neurons of the dorsal horn.

There is a systematic relationship between the position of an axon in the dorsal column and the body location from which it receives input. Input from the leg is carried by axons in the most medial portion of the dorsal column, a region termed the *gracile fascicle* (Figure 5.6). Afferent input from the lower trunk is transmitted rostrally by axons located lateral to the leg input, but still within the gracile fascicle. Sensory information from the rostral trunk, arm, neck, and back of the head ascends in the *cuneate fascicle*. The cuneate fascicle begins approximately at the level of the sixth thoracic segment. The gracile and cuneate fascicles are separated by the *dorsal intermediate septum*, whereas the dorsal columns of the two halves of the spinal cord are separated by the *dorsal median septum* (Figure 5.6). This organization of sensory input, which in the spinal cord is determined by the sequential ordering of the dorsal roots, is characteristic of how sensory information from the body surface is represented in the central nervous system. This is the *somatotopic organization*: there is an orderly representation of the various body parts within central nervous system structures that process somatic sensory information such that *neighborhood relations in the periphery are preserved in the central nervous system*. For example, from medial to lateral in the dorsal columns, axons transmit sensory information from the leg, trunk, arm, neck, and occiput (Figure 5.6). Thus, sensory information from adjacent structures in the periphery is transmitted by axons in adjacent parts of the dorsal column. Somatotopy is a major determinant of the organization of the other components of the somatic sensory system. Similar principles apply to the organization of the visual system (retinotopy) and the auditory system (tonotopy).

The somatotopic organization of the dorsal columns also can be appreciated by examining post mortem tissue from individuals who sustained trauma to the spinal cord during their lifetime. The sections shown in Figure 5.7A were taken from a patient whose lumbar spinal cord had

Figure 5.6 The dorsal columns and the ascending axons of the anterolateral system are somatotopically organized.

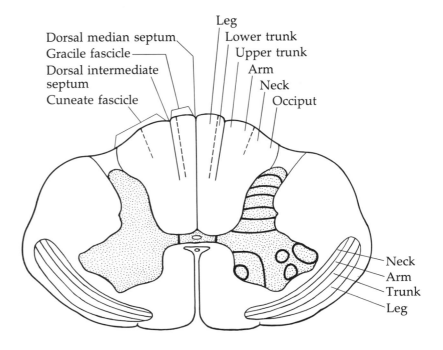

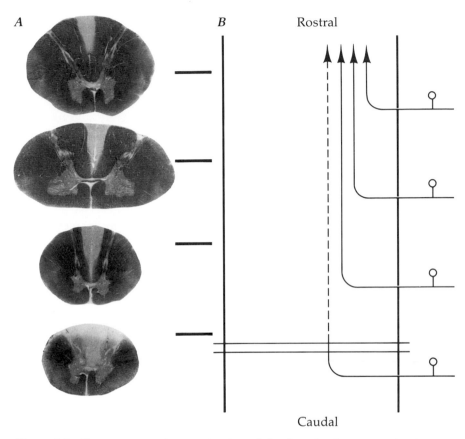

Figure 5.7 The somatotopic organization of the dorsal columns can be demonstrated by examining spinal cord sections from a patient that sustained damage to the lumbar spinal cord. *A*. Four levels through the spinal cord, rostrocaudally from top to bottom, a section rostral to the cervical enlargement, through the cervical enlargement and two thoracic sections. *B*. The course taken by the central branches of the dorsal root fibers as they enter the spinal cord and ascend in the dorsal columns. Dashed line depicts course of degenerated axon.

been crushed. The sections are stained for myelin. Axons that have degenerated have lost their myelin sheath, and as a consequence, are not stained (i.e., demyelination; see Chapter 1 for discussion of methodology). The bottom segment in Figure 5.7A is from the caudal thoracic spinal cord, close to the crushed portion. Nearly the entire gracile fascicle is demyelinated. Demyelination of the dorsal columns is restricted to a region close to the midline in the higher thoracic segments (Figure 5.7A, middle) because contingents of healthy axons continue to enter the spinal cord rostrally and are added on lateral to the degenerated axons from the lumbar spinal cord. In the cervical enlargement (Figure 5.7A, top), the degenerated region is confined to a small wedge along the midline. The pattern by which axons enter and ascend in the dorsal columns is shown schematically in Figure 5.7B.

Examination of the configuration of the spinal cord sections in Figure 5.7A reveals that there are variations in the shape of the gray matter and white matter. Two general morphological differences characterize these variations. First, the white matter of the spinal cord increases in size from caudal to rostral, because at successively more rostral levels, the white matter must accommodate a greater number of both ascending and descending axons. Thus, in Figure 5.7A there is a progressive increase in the size of the white matter from the most caudal section (bottom section in part A) to the most rostral section (top). Second, the gray matter is enlarged in certain locations (the fifth cervical to the first thoracic segments—*cervical enlargement*—and the first lumbar to the second sacral segments—*lumbosacral enlargement*) because neurons in these levels provide the sensory and motor innervation of the limbs. For example, compare the area of gray matter in the second section in Figure 5.7A, which is through the cervical enlargement, with the other three sections. (These differences also can be appreciated by examining the transverse sections through five levels of the spinal cord in Appendix II.)

Axons of the Anterolateral System Originate in the Dorsal Horn

In contrast to the dorsal columns, virtually all the axons of the anterolateral system originate in the gray matter of the spinal cord. These neurons, called *ascending projection neurons*, are widely scattered in the dorsal horn, the intermediate zone, and the ventral horn. There is a specific relationship between the lamina in which a projection neuron is located and the termination site of its axon in the brain. The pathway to the ventral posterior lateral nucleus of the thalamus originates from neurons in laminae I and V. The spinal cord neurons whose axons project to the intralaminar nuclei and reticular formation of the pons and medulla are more scattered in the gray matter, in laminae I, V, and VI through VIII. The projection to the tectum and reticular formation of the midbrain originates from neurons in laminae I and V, similar to the projection to the ventral posterior lateral nucleus.

The axons of the neurons that project to the thalamus decussate in the spinal cord before ascending. The group of neurons that project to the pontine and medullary reticular formation has two contingents, one whose axons decussate and a second, whose axons remain on the side ipsilateral to the cell body. The trajectory of the decussating axons is a complex one: they cross the midline over a rostral–caudal length of approximately three spinal cord segments (see Figure 5.8). The clinical significance of this pattern of decussation is that sensory deficits associated with damage to the anterolateral system are actually present on body parts that are innervated by one or two segments caudal to the level of the lesion. The site at which the actual decussation occurs is in the region of the white matter that is ventral to the central canal, the *ventral (anterior) commissure* (see Figure 5.9A). Commissures are white matter sites in the central nervous system where axons cross from one side to the other. The *corpus callosum*, for example, is the principal commissure of the cerebral hemispheres. Axons of the anterolateral system ascend in the anterior portion of the lateral column, hence the name *anterolateral system* (Figures 5.5 and 5.6). The general region of the spinal cord white matter in which the anterolateral system is located can be seen by examining the degenerated area in the lateral column in Figure 5.7A. Demyelination in the lateral column is attributed largely to degeneration of anterolateral fibers. Axons of the anterolateral system are somatotopically organized: axons from more caudal segments are located lateral to those from more rostral segments (Figure 5.6). However, the somatotopic organization in the anterolateral system is not as precise as that for the dorsal columns, which is why a systematic trend is not readily apparent when viewing the sections in Figure 5.7A. Ascending spinocerebellar axons also course in this region of the white matter (Chapter 10).

Three Key Sensory Deficits That Follow Spinal Cord Injury Permit Localization of Trauma

Spinal cord injury results in deficits in somatic sensation and in the control of body musculature caudal to the level of the lesion. Motor deficits that follow spinal cord injury will be considered in Chapter 9. Here, sensory deficits are considered. Sensory deficits have three major attributes: (1) the sensory *modality* that is affected, for example, whether pain, temperature, or tactile sensation is impaired, (2) the side of the body (*laterality*) where deficits are observed, and (3) the body regions that are affected (*somatotopy*). We consider the sensory consequences of spinal cord *hemisection* because this injury illustrates deficits in all three attributes. The clinical condition resulting from the combined sensory and motor deficits that follow spinal cord hemisection is known as the *Brown–Sequard syndrome* (Figure 5.8).

The two principal ascending pathways mediate different somatic sensory modalities and these two pathways cross the midline in different locations in the central nervous system. These two facts provide the basis for unambiguous identification of the side of injury. Because the axons in the dorsal columns relay sensory information from the ipsilateral side of the body, *deficits in tactile sensation, vibration sense, and limb position sense are present ipsilateral to the spinal cord lesion* (Figure 5.8). In contrast, the axons of the anterolateral system decussate in the spinal cord. Therefore,

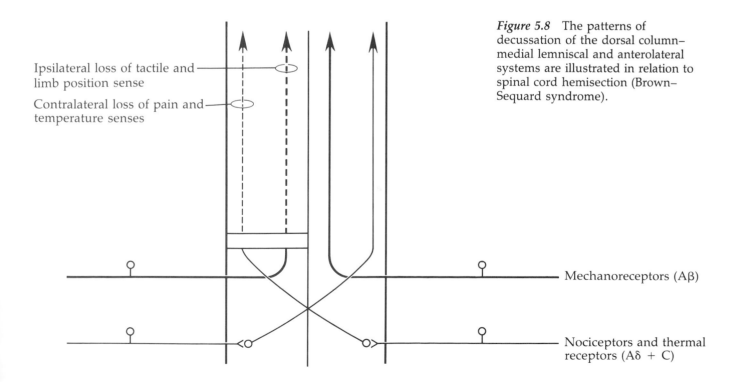

Ipsilateral loss of tactile and limb position sense

Contralateral loss of pain and temperature senses

Mechanoreceptors (Aβ)

Nociceptors and thermal receptors (Aδ + C)

Figure 5.8 The patterns of decussation of the dorsal column–medial lemniscal and anterolateral systems are illustrated in relation to spinal cord hemisection (Brown–Sequard syndrome).

A

Large-diameter fiber
(tactile, vibration, and
position senses)

Small-diameter fiber
(pain and temperature
senses)

Decussating axons
in ventral commissure

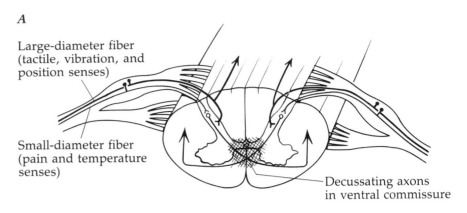

Figure 5.9 Syringomyelia disrupts the decussating fibers of the anterolateral system but usually not the ascending fibers of the dorsal column–medial lemniscal system. *A*. Spinal cord cross section showing the patterns of terminations of small- and large-diameter axons and how the components of the anterolateral system decussate and ascend. The dorsal column–medial lemniscal system ascends ipsilaterally in the spinal cord. The cross-hatching indicates the region that is affected by the formation of a syrinx (cavity). *B*. Distribution of loss of pain and temperature sense over body. (Adapted from Kandel, E. R., and Schwartz, J. H. 1985. Principles of Neural Science. New York: Elsevier.)

B

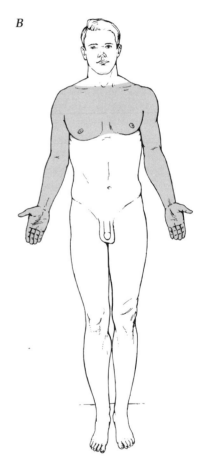

pain and temperature senses are impaired on the side of the body that is contralateral to the lesion. This pattern of ipsilateral loss of tactile sense and limb position sense and contralateral loss of pain and temperature sense is the hallmark of spinal cord hemisection. The spinal cord level at which injury occurs is determined by first mapping the distribution of sensory loss and then comparing the pattern of this loss with dermatomal maps (see Figure 5.4). The injured spinal cord level is about two segments higher than the most rostral dermatome in which pain and temperature senses are not intact.

Two pathological processes distinguish between the dorsal column–medial lemniscal and the anterolateral systems. First, in *tabes dorsalis*, an advanced stage of neurosyphilis, dorsal root ganglion cells with large-diameter axons are lost. As a consequence, patients suffering from this disease lose tactile sensation, vibration sense, and limb position sense. Fortunately, tabes dorsalis is rarely seen in present times. Patients with dorsal column symptoms more commonly have sustained spinal cord trauma. Second, in *syringomyelia*, a cavity forms in the central portion of the spinal cord (Figure 5.9A). In the early stages of this condition the decussating axons of the anterolateral system are damaged selectively. Because this condition interrupts decussating axons from both sides of the body, a symmetrical loss of pain and temperature sense is usually observed, typically in a capelike distribution on the arms, shoulder, and upper trunk, sparing the axons of the dorsal columns, which mediate tactile, vibration, and limb position senses (Figure 5.9B).

The spatial separation of the anterolateral and dorsal column–medial lemniscal systems in the spinal cord is clinically relevant. Although rarely performed at present, a surgical procedure for the relief of intractable pain, termed *anterolateral cordotomy*, is transection of the portion of the spinal cord in which axons carrying pain information project to the brain. With time, recovery of pain and temperature senses (partial or even complete) may occur. This recovery process can be explained by the presence of an intact *ipsilateral* ascending projection and other ascending pathways that become more important for function after destruction of the contralateral projection. This is a clear example of the plastic capabilities of the mature human central nervous system.

The Somatic Sensory Decussation in the Medulla Is Located Rostral to the Pyramidal Decussation

The dorsal column axons synapse on neurons in the *dorsal column nuclei* (Figures 5.10A and B), the first major relay in the ascending pathway for tactile, vibration, and limb position senses. These nuclei, as well as other relay nuclei, do not simply transmit information to the next level in the sequence—or *hierarchy*—of the pathway. Rather, somatic sensory information is transformed in the dorsal column nuclei. Local inhibitory synaptic interactions in the dorsal column nuclei function to enhance contrast so that when adjacent portions of the skin are stimulated, the stimulus configuration can be identified more accurately. Axons of the gracile fascicle synapse in the *gracile nucleus*, whereas those from the cuneate fascicle synapse in the *cuneate nucleus*. The section shown in Figure 5.10A is at the level of the motor decussation (or pyramidal decussation). The gracile nucleus is located in the gracile fascicle and the cuneate nucleus is located at the base of the cuneate fascicle. At this level, the cuneate nucleus can be seen "emerging" from the deeper portion of the dorsal horn. These nuclei are larger in the more rostral level shown in Figure 5.10B. From the dorsal column nuclei, the axons sweep ventrally through the medulla and decussate. These axons are called the *internal arcuate fibers* (Figure 5.10B). Next, the fibers ascend to the thalamus in the *medial lemniscus*. Axons from the gracile nucleus decussate ventral to axons from the cuneate nucleus and ascend in the ventral part of the medial lem-

A

B

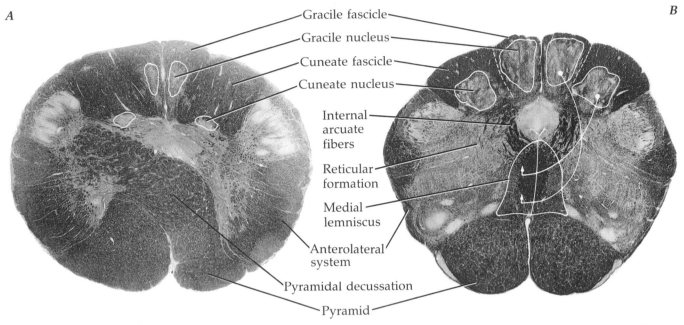

Gracile fascicle
Gracile nucleus
Cuneate fascicle
Cuneate nucleus
Internal arcuate fibers
Reticular formation
Medial lemniscus
Anterolateral system
Pyramidal decussation
Pyramid

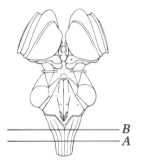

— B
— A

Figure 5.10 Myelin-stained transverse sections through two levels of the medulla. *A*. Level of the motor decussation. *B*. Dorsal column nuclei. Inset indicates the approximate planes of section. Trajectories of internal arcuate fibers from the gracile and cuneate nuclei are shown to the right.

niscus, compared with axons from the cuneate nucleus (Figure 5.10B). Because of this pattern, the somatotopic organization of the medial lemniscus in the medulla approximates a *person standing upright*: legs ventral, followed by the trunk and arms proceeding dorsally. Input from the face and intraoral structures, which reaches the brain stem via the trigeminal nerve, is relayed in the most dorsal position of the medial lemniscus thereby completing the image of the upright person. The organization of the trigeminal system will be discussed in Chapter 12. Note that the decussation of the dorsal column–medial lemniscal system—the sensory decussation (Figure 5.10B)—occurs at a more rostral level than the pyramidal decussation—the motor decussation (Figure 5.10A).

Figure 5.11 illustrates a sagittal section cut a few millimeters from the midline. Because of the proximity of the section to the midline, the gracile fascicle and nucleus are present. The arrow indicates the approximate level of the section shown in Figure 5.10B. Compare the dorsoventral sequence of structures located close to the midline in Figure 5.10B and at the level of the arrow in Figure 5.11. In both sections, three regions can be identified: (1) the gracile fascicle and nucleus, (2) gray matter in the central medulla (corresponding to cranial nerve and other nuclei), and (3) a large expanse of white matter in the ventral medulla corresponding to the medial lemniscus and the pyramid. The medial lemniscus and pyramid can be followed rostrally to the pons where they separate.

In contrast to the dorsal column–medial lemniscal system which ascends in the medial medulla, the anterolateral system ascends along its ventrolateral margin (Figure 5.10). For the spinothalamic and spinotectal tracts, the medulla is simply a conduit through which axons must pass

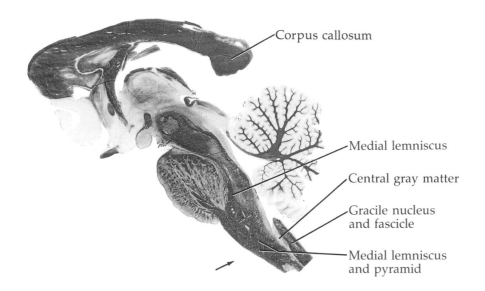

Corpus callosum

Medial lemniscus

Central gray matter

Gracile nucleus
and fascicle

Medial lemniscus
and pyramid

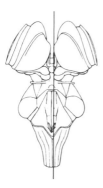

Figure 5.11 A myelin-stained sagittal section through the brain stem. The arrow marks the approximate level of the section shown in Figure 5.10B.

to reach more rostral locations. In contrast, some fibers of the spinoreticular tract terminate in the *medullary reticular formation*.

Vascular Lesions of the Caudal Brain Stem Differentially Affect the Somatic Sensory Pathways

As we saw in Chapter 4, the caudal brain stem receives blood from the *vertebral–basilar*, or the *posterior*, circulation. Small perforating branches of this arterial system supply blood to pie-shaped slices (each with the apex pointed dorsal and medial) of the medulla and pons (see Figure 4.3). The areas served by the posterior inferior cerebellar artery, vertebral artery, and anterior spinal artery are illustrated in Figure 5.12. Occlusion of the *posterior inferior cerebellar artery*, which supplies lateral portions of the medulla and pons, interrupts the ascending anterolateral system fibers and, as a consequence, produces a deficit in pain and temperature sensation. The side of the deficit is contralateral to the lesion

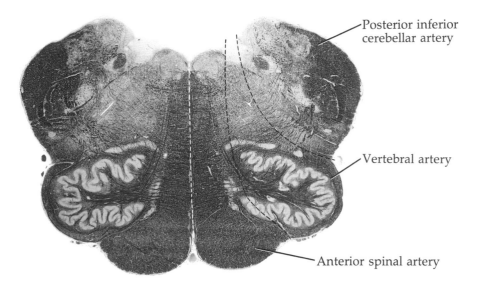

Posterior inferior
cerebellar artery

Vertebral artery

Anterior spinal artery

Figure 5.12 The pattern of arterial perfusion of the rostral medulla.

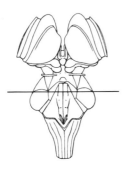

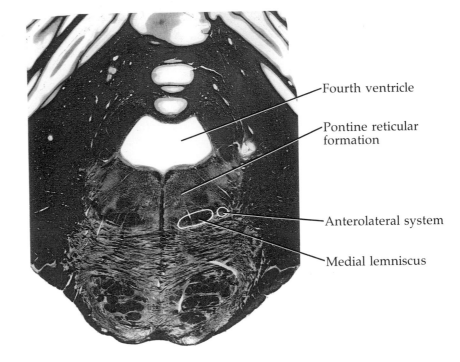

Fourth ventricle

Pontine reticular
formation

Anterolateral system

Medial lemniscus

Figure 5.13 A myelin-stained
transverse section through the pons.
Inset shows approximate plane of
section.

because the axons of the anterolateral system decussated in the spinal
cord (see Figure 5.8). Other sensory and motor deficits are associated
with occlusion of the posterior inferior cerebellar artery. These other deficits will be discussed when the different functional systems are considered. The complex set of deficits constitutes the *lateral medullary syndrome*
or *Wallenberg's syndrome.*

The Medial Lemniscus and the Anterolateral System
Remain Segregated in the Pons

In the pons the medial lemniscus is located more dorsally and is
oriented from medial to lateral rather than dorsoventral as it is in the
medulla. Many of the axons of the spinoreticular tract terminate at this
level, in the *pontine reticular formation.* The position of the anterolateral
system in Figure 5.13 is difficult to determine precisely because neighboring structures are similarly myelinated. This problem calls attention
to how we identify structures in normal myelin-stained sections. Many
structures are distinguished clearly from their neighbors because of morphological changes at boundaries; for example, a tract is clearly identifiable when it is surrounded by a region containing neurons. For example,
in Figure 5.10, the heavily myelinated (and darkly stained) medial lemniscus is distinguishable from neighboring structures in the reticular formation which contain mostly neuronal cell bodies and therefore are lightly
stained. Unfortunately, a more common occurrence is that functionally
different structures that have similar staining properties are intermingled.
Thus, the anterolateral system is localizable to only a general region because it is surrounded by other myelinated axons. In these cases, precise
identification cannot be made without additional information. Histori-

cally, this information was obtained by comparing normal and lesioned material. This method is used to identify the boundaries of the gracile fascicle in Figure 5.7A. More recently, axon tracing methods have been used in experimental animals as an important tool for precisely localizing a structure.

The Medial Lemniscus and the Anterolateral System Lie Adjacent to One Another in the Midbrain

The midbrain contains two levels with different morphologies: the caudal midbrain, at the level of the *inferior colliculus*, and the rostral midbrain, at the level of the *superior colliculus*. From the perspective of the ascending somatic sensory systems, the rostral and caudal levels of the midbrain are organized similarly. We therefore consider only the level of the superior colliculus here (Figure 5.14). The level of the inferior colliculus will be considered in Chapter 7. For the dorsal column–medial lemniscal system, the midbrain is simply a conduit for the axons of the medial lemniscus which synapse in the thalamus. The medial lemniscus lies in a horn-shaped collection of myelinated axons adjacent to the red nucleus, a motor control nucleus (Figure 5.14). Fibers of the anterolateral system are located dorsal and lateral to the medial lemniscus. The *spinothalamic tract* is like the medial lemniscus in that it only courses through the midbrain en route to the thalamus. The *spinotectal tract* projects to the superior colliculus (Figure 5.14) (see Chapter 6) and there is a projection to the midbrain reticular formation from the *spinoreticular tract*.

Neurons in the gray matter surrounding the cerebral aqueduct in the midbrain and beneath the floor of the fourth ventricle in the pons play a key role in the modulation of the perception of pain. A *descending pain inhibitory system* originates from this region. Receiving complex patterns of input from diencephalic and telencephalic structures involved in emotions (Chapters 14 and 15), the *periaqueductal gray matter* projects to the *raphe nuclei* in the medulla. These medullary neurons, which use *serotonin* as their neurotransmitter, project to the dorsal horn of the spinal cord to inhibit dorsal horn ascending projection neurons that transmit information about painful stimuli to the brain.

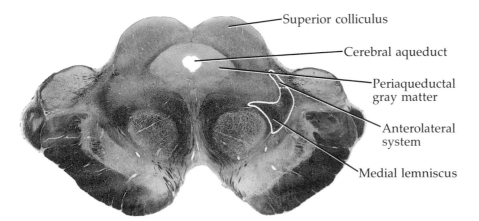

Superior colliculus

Cerebral aqueduct

Periaqueductal gray matter

Anterolateral system

Medial lemniscus

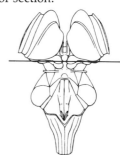

Figure 5.14 A myelin-stained transverse section through the midbrain. Inset shows approximate plane of section.

The Ventral Posterior Nucleus Is the Somatic Sensory Relay Nucleus of the Thalamus

The thalamus (Figure 5.15) is a nodal point for the dorsal column–medial lemniscal and anterolateral systems and their subsequent projections to the cerebral cortex. Indeed, with the exception of olfaction, all sensory systems relay in the thalamus en route to the cerebral cortex. There are two major thalamic regions that receive somatic sensory input. One, located laterally, is the *ventral posterior nucleus* (Figures 5.15 and 5.16). This is the somatic sensory relay nucleus. The second region is located medially in the thalamus, the *intralaminar nuclei*, and includes primarily the central lateral nucleus. Intralaminar nuclei are diffuse-projecting nuclei located within the internal medullary laminae (Figure 5.15). The terminations of the spinothalamic tract and the medial lemniscus in these thalamic regions are somewhat different. Both the medial lemniscus and the spinothalamic tract project to the ventral posterior nucleus, whereas the spinothalamic tract also projects to the intralaminar nuclei. Even though both systems terminate in the ventral posterior nucleus, their terminal fields do not overlap.

The ventral posterior nucleus has two divisions that separately mediate somatic sensations of the face and perioral structures and the limbs and trunk. The *ventral posterior medial nucleus* (1) (Figures 5.15 and 5.16B)

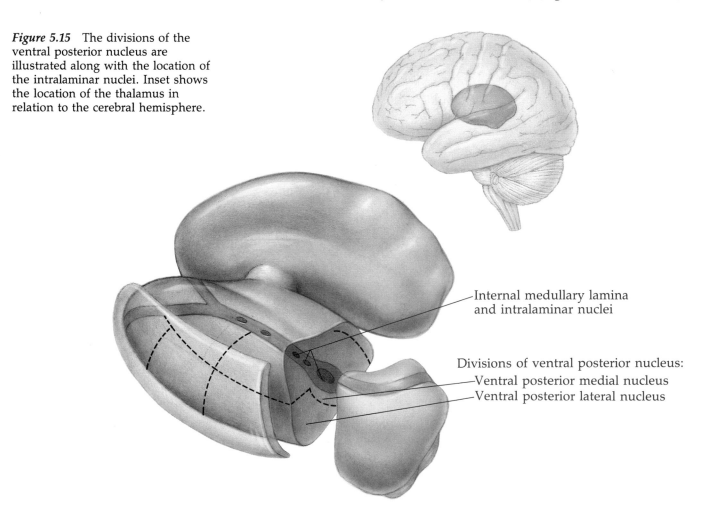

Figure 5.15 The divisions of the ventral posterior nucleus are illustrated along with the location of the intralaminar nuclei. Inset shows the location of the thalamus in relation to the cerebral hemisphere.

Internal medullary lamina and intralaminar nuclei

Divisions of ventral posterior nucleus:
Ventral posterior medial nucleus
Ventral posterior lateral nucleus

A

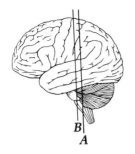

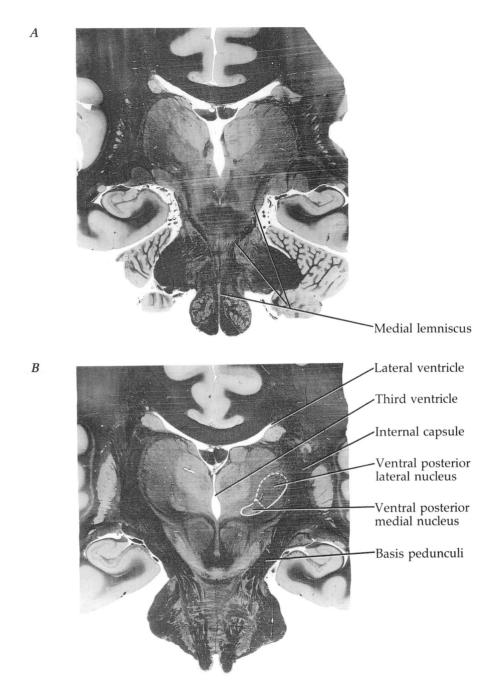

Medial lemniscus

B

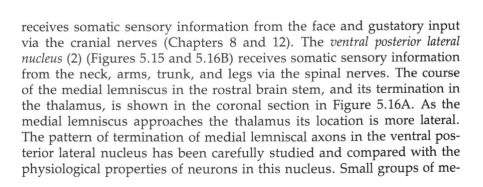

Lateral ventricle

Third ventricle

Internal capsule

Ventral posterior
lateral nucleus

Ventral posterior
medial nucleus

Basis pedunculi

Figure 5.16 Myelin-stained
transverse sections through the
diencephalon. The section illustrated
in *A* is located caudal to the section
shown in *B*. Inset shows
approximate planes of section.

receives somatic sensory information from the face and gustatory input
via the cranial nerves (Chapters 8 and 12). The *ventral posterior lateral
nucleus* (2) (Figures 5.15 and 5.16B) receives somatic sensory information
from the neck, arms, trunk, and legs via the spinal nerves. The course
of the medial lemniscus in the rostral brain stem, and its termination in
the thalamus, is shown in the coronal section in Figure 5.16A. As the
medial lemniscus approaches the thalamus its location is more lateral.
The pattern of termination of medial lemniscal axons in the ventral posterior lateral nucleus has been carefully studied and compared with the
physiological properties of neurons in this nucleus. Small groups of me-

dial lemniscal axons terminate in elongated rod-shaped fields that are oriented along the rostral–caudal axis. The neurons within a given rod-shaped region form a functional unit; they all process information about a single somesthetic modality and from a similar body location. Neurons in a rod-shaped field, in turn, project to a small group of cortical neurons that also constitute a functional unit, the *cortical column*. Neurons in a cortical column, spanning layers II through VI (layer I is largely devoid of neurons), all receive input from the same somatic sensory modality and a similar peripheral location (see later). The cortical column is the fundamental processing unit of the cerebral cortex, not only in the somatic sensory cortex but in other sensory cortical areas, as well as association and motor areas.

The *posterior nuclear group*, a collection of nuclei located at the junction of the midbrain and diencephalon, has long been thought to participate in pain sensation. This nuclear group, which includes the suprageniculate and limitans nuclei, the magnocellular nucleus of the medial geniculate complex, and the posterior nucleus, receives input from diverse sources and is likely to be part of a variety of *functional circuits* including the processing of somatic sensory information. The suprageniculate and limitans nuclei receive input from the midbrain tectum and may participate in visuomotor function. The magnocellular nucleus of the medial geniculate complex is a diffuse-projecting nucleus with a regional pattern of termination. Only a portion of the *posterior nucleus* receives a major input from the ascending somatic sensory pathways and it projects to a cortical region within the lateral sulcus (see later).

The Primary Somatic Sensory Cortex Is Located in the Postcentral Gyrus

The *primary somatic sensory cortex*, which is located in the postcentral gyrus of the parietal lobe, is the principal region of the cerebral cortex to which the ventral posterior nucleus projects. The axons from the ventral posterior nucleus travel to the cerebral cortex through the *posterior limb of the internal capsule* (see Figure 11.6), which is bounded by the thalamus and caudate nucleus medially and the globus pallidus and putamen laterally (Figure 5.16). The thalamic axons terminate predominantly in the deep part of layer III and layer IV. There is a precise topographic relationship between the locations of projection neurons in the ventral posterior nucleus and the region of the primary somatic sensory cortex to which their axons project (Figure 5.17). The lateral portion of the ventral posterior lateral nucleus receives somatic sensory input from the leg and lower trunk and projects to the medial portion of the postcentral gyrus. Much of the lower limb representation is on the medial surface of the parietal lobe, in the sagittal (or interhemispheric) fissure. The medial part of the ventral posterior lateral nucleus receives input from the neck, arm, and upper trunk and projects to the postcentral gyrus on the lateral hemisphere surface. The ventral posterior medial nucleus, the thalamic relay nucleus for facial somatic sensory information, projects to the most lateral part of the post-central gyrus, adjacent to and within the lateral sulcus (see Chapter 12).

We have seen that a key feature of all levels of the somatic sensory system is its somatotopic organization. In the somatic sensory cortex, the

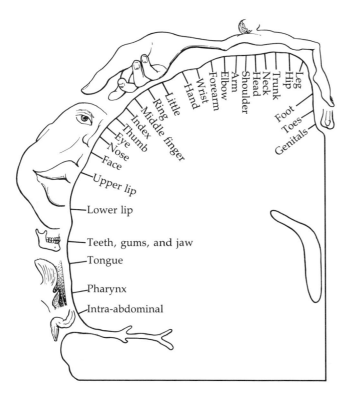

Figure 5.17   The primary somatic cortex is somatotopically organized. This figure illustrates a schematic coronal section through the postcentral gyrus. (Adapted from Penfield, W. and Rasmussen, T. 1950. The Cerebral Cortex of Man: A Clinical Study of Localization Function. New York: Macmillan.)

somatotopic organization is remarkably similar to a map of the surface of the body, a configuration termed the *sensory homunculus*. However, this map is not isomorphic with body form. Rather, the portions of the body used as discriminative tactile organs, such as the fingers, have a disproportionately greater representation on the map than areas that are not as important for tactile discrimination, such as the leg (Figure 5.17). It was once thought that these areal differences were fixed and simply reflected the density of peripheral receptors. It is now known that the body map is not static, but dynamically controlled by the pattern of use of different body parts in tactile exploration. If one body part is prevented from use in tactile discrimination (for example, after peripheral nerve injury), its cortical representation shrinks. In contrast, if one part is used more extensively (for example, by selectively reinforcing the use of one finger for tactile exploration in an experimental animal), its representation expands.

The Primary Somatic Sensory Cortex Has a Modality-Specific Organization

In the primary somatic sensory cortex, as in other cortical areas, regions with different cytoarchitecture subserve different functions. The primary somatic sensory cortex consists of four cytoarchitectonic divisions, or *Brodmann's areas* (Figure 3.16). These divisions are numbered 1,

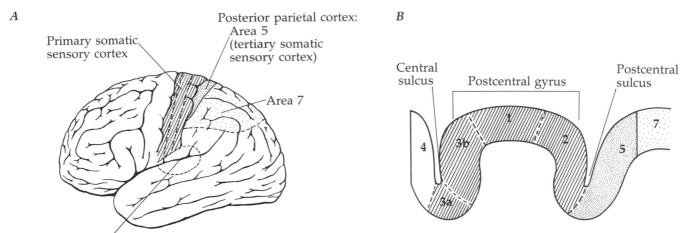

Figure 5.18 *A.* The locations of the primary and secondary somatic sensory areas are indicated on a lateral view of cerebral cortex. *B.* A schematic section cut perpendicular to the mediolateral axis of the postcentral gyrus. (Adapted from Kandel, E. R., and Schwartz, J. H. 1985. Principles of Neural Science. New York: Elsevier.)

2, 3a, and 3b (Figure 5.18). These areas receive projections from the ventral posterior nucleus that differ in at least two ways: (1) the specific modality of somatic sensory information they receive, and (2) the density of thalamic terminations. Areas 3a and 2 receive information from receptors located in deep structures, for example, the muscles and joints, and areas 3b and 1 receive information from mechanoreceptors of the skin. Area 3b receives the densest thalamic projections and area 2, the sparsest. These differences in input modality and density of thalamic terminations provide important insights into the functions subserved by the four primary somatic sensory cortical areas. The differences in the modality of the inputs indicate that the different somatic sensory modalities are each processed separately in the cortex, with areas 3a and 2 playing an important role in limb position sense and areas 3b and 1, a major role in tactile sensation. The functional importance of the differences in the density of thalamic projections is more subtle. Area 2 receives the fewest thalamic projections but is the recipient of a cascade of intracortical projections, from area 3b to 1 and then to area 2. Both studies with experimental animals and clinical examinations of patients who have sustained circumscribed parietal lobe infarcts indicate that when area 3b is damaged, the functions of the four cytoarchitectonic divisions are disrupted. In contrast, the functional consequences of damage restricted to area 2 are more limited.

Higher Order Somatic Sensory Cortical Areas Are Located in the Banks of the Lateral Sulcus and the Insular Cortex

The primary somatic sensory cortex is not the only area of the parietal lobe that is involved in somatic sensory function. Indeed, multiple regions of the parietal lobe and insular cortex process somatic sensory information. There are three major additional areas: (1) secondary somatic sensory cortex, (2) posterior insular cortex, and (3) posterior parietal lobe.

The *secondary somatic sensory cortex*, located largely on the parietal operculum receives its major source of input from the primary somatic sensory
cortex (see next section). Like the primary somatic sensory cortex, the
secondary area contains a representation of the body surface. However,
the body representation is of the contralateral surface in the primary somatic sensory cortex whereas there is a bilateral representation of the
body surface in the secondary somatic sensory cortex.

The *posterior insular cortex* receives its major somatic sensory input
from the secondary somatic sensory cortex. Because this portion of the
insular cortex projects to parts of the limbic system (Chapter 15) that are
important for memory and learning, it appears that a pathway from the
primary somatic sensory cortex to the secondary somatic sensory cortex
and then to the insular cortex may mediate *object recognition by touch*.
Similar pathways exist for vision and audition. The *posterior parietal cortex*,
which includes Brodmann's areas 5 and 7, receives somatic sensory input
from the somatic sensory cortical areas. Area 5 is considered by some
investigators to be the *tertiary somatic sensory cortex* because, like the primary and secondary areas, it contains a representation of the body surface. We will see in Chapter 6 that the visual system also contains multiple
representations of the retina in the cerebral cortex. This is a general principle of organization of sensory systems.

Efferent Projections Arise from the Primary Somatic Sensory Cortex

The somatic sensory cortical areas, as well as other functional regions
of cortex, contain three kinds of efferent projections mediated by three
separate classes of neurons: corticocortical association, callosal, and descending projection. The various classes of efferent projection neurons
have a laminar distribution. *Corticocortical association neurons* give rise to
projections that can be considered "ascending," in much the same sense
as the ascending somatic sensory pathways of the spinal cord and brain
stem are considered. This is because they are directed to higher order
sensory cortical areas, association areas, and motor areas, which collectively further process the somatic sensory information for perception and
planning and controlling a behavioral response. Corticocortical association neurons are predominantly located in layers II and III. *Callosal neurons*
make the second type of projection, which is to the contralateral somatic
sensory cortical areas via the *corpus callosum* (Figure 5.11). It is thought
that one function of callosal connections in sensory systems is to "stitch
together" the representations of the body in the primary somatic sensory
cortex of each hemisphere. In accord with this hypothesis, only neurons
located in the representation of proximal body parts, and not the hand
and foot areas, are connected with the contralateral hemisphere. Like the
association neurons, the callosal neurons are also located in layers II and
III. The third type of cortical projection neuron is termed a *descending
projection neuron*. The axons of these neurons descend to either (1) the
striatum (the caudate nucleus and putamen), (2) the ventral posterior
nucleus of the thalamus, (3) the brain stem, especially the dorsal column
nuclei, or (4) the dorsal horn of the spinal cord. The descending projection
neurons are located in layers V and VI. Those located in layer V terminate

in the striatum, brain stem, and spinal cord, whereas those neurons that project to the thalamus are located in layer VI. Except for the projection to the striatum, whose function is poorly understood, the descending projections from the somatic sensory cortex are thought to serve a feedback function by regulating the quantity of somatic sensory information that ascends through the central nervous system.

Summary

There are two major somatic sensory pathways (Figures 5.1 and 5.2): the *dorsal column–medial lemniscal system*, which mediates *tactile, vibration sense, and limb position sense*, and the *anterolateral system*, which mediates *pain and temperature sense* and a less discriminative form of tactile sense. These systems differ in four major ways: (1) modality sensitivity of input from dorsal root ganglion cells, (2) location of first relay site, (3) level of decussation, and (4) functional and anatomical homogeneity of the pathway.

Dorsal root ganglion cells receive somatic sensory information and transmit this information from the periphery to the spinal cord (Figure 5.3). Dorsal root ganglion cells with large-diameter axons are sensitive to mechanical stimuli (A-β), and those with small-diameter axons are sensitive to noxious and thermal stimuli (Aδ, C) (Table 5.1). The axons of dorsal root ganglion cells enter the spinal cord via the *dorsal root*. A *dermatome* is the area of skin innervated by a single dorsal root (Figures 5.3 and 5.4). The afferent information carried by adjacent dorsal roots overlaps nearly completely on the body surface. Once in the spinal cord, dorsal root ganglion cells have three branches: *segmental, ascending*, and *descending* (Figure 5.5). The principal branching pattern of large-diameter fibers is to ascend to the brain stem in the dorsal columns. Whereas small-diameter fibers ascend and descend in the *zone of Lissauer*, they eventually terminate in the gray matter of the spinal cord.

The ascending somatic sensory pathways course in two locations in the spinal cord. The dorsal column–medial lemniscal system ascends in the *dorsal columns*. The dorsal columns have two fascicles (Figures 5.6 and 5.7). The *gracile fascicle* carries axons from the leg and lower trunk, and the *cuneate fascicle* carries axons from the upper trunk, arm, neck, and back of the head. The majority of the axons in the dorsal columns are central branches of dorsal root ganglion cells. The axons of the anterolateral system derive from dorsal horn neurons, and decussate in the *ventral commissure* (Figure 5.9). The anterolateral system ascends in the lateral column (Figures 5.5 and 5.6).

Dorsal column axons terminate in the *dorsal column nuclei* in the caudal medulla (Figures 5.10 and 5.11). Axons of neurons in the dorsal column nuclei decussate and ascend in the *medial lemniscus* (Figures 5.13, 5.14, and 5.16A) and terminate in the lateral division of the ventral posterior nucleus of the thalamus (*ventral posterior lateral nucleus*) (Figures 5.15 and 5.16B). Fibers of the anterolateral system terminate in the *reticular formation* (Figures 5.10 and 5.13) (*spinoreticular tract*), *midbrain tectum* (Figure 5.14) (*spinotectal tract*), and *thalamus* (*spinothalamic tract*) (Figures 5.15 and 5.16). The major spinothalamic tract terminations include the *ventral posterior lateral nucleus* and the *intralaminar nuclei*. The major projection of the ventral posterior lateral nucleus is to the *primary somatic sensory cortex* (Figure 5.18).

There are three other major somatic sensory cortical areas (Figure 5.18). The *secondary somatic sensory cortex* (1) and the *posterior parietal cortex* (sometimes termed the tertiary somatic sensory cortex) (2) receive their input primarily from the primary somatic sensory cortex. The *posterior insular cortex* (3) receives its input primarily from the secondary somatic sensory cortex. The primary (Figure 5.17), secondary, and tertiary somatic sensory cortical areas are somatotopically organized. Efferent projections from the somatic sensory cortical areas arise from specific cortical layers. *Corticocortical association* connections (with other cortical areas on the same side of the cerebral cortex) are made by neurons in layers II and III. *Callosal* connections (with the other side of the cerebral cortex) are also made by neurons in layers II and III. *Descending projections* to the striatum, brain stem, and spinal cord originate from neurons located in layer V, whereas the projection to the thalamus originates from neurons located in layer VI. ∎

References

Appelberg, A. E., Leonard, R. B., Kenshalo Jr, D. R., et al. 1979. Nuclei in which functionally identified spinothalamic tract neurons terminate. J. Comp. Neurol. 188:575–586.

Burton, H., and Jones, E. G. 1976. The posterior thalamic region and its cortical projection in new world and old world monkeys. J. Comp. Neurol. 168:249–302.

Collins, R. D. 1962. Illustrated Manual of Neurologic Diagnosis. Philadelphia: Lippincott.

Craig, A. D., Jr., and Burton, H. 1981. Spinal and medullary laminal projection to nucleus submedius in medial thalamus: A possible pain center. J. Neurophysiol. 45:443–466.

Gobel, S. 1979. Neural circuitry in the substantia gelatinosa of Rolando: Anatomical insights. In Bonica, J. J. (ed.), Advances in Pain Research and Therapy, Vol. 3. New York: Raven Press, pp. 175–195.

Jones, E. G. 1984. Organization of the thalamocortical complex and its relation to sensory processes. In Darian-Smith, I. (ed.), Handbook of Physiology, Section 1: The Nervous System, Vol. III. Sensory Processes. Bethesda, Md.: American Physiological Society, pp. 149–212.

Jones, E. G., and Friedman, D. P. 1982. Projection pattern of functional components of thalamic ventrobasal complex on monkey somatosensory cortex. J. Neurophysiol. 48:521–544.

Jones, E. G., and Leavitt, R. Y. 1974. Retrograde axonal transport and the demonstration of non-specific projections to the cerebral cortex and striatum from thalamic intralaminar nuclei in the rat, cat and monkey. J. Comp. Neurol. 154:349–378.

Jones, E. G., and Powell, T. P. S. 1971. An analysis of the posterior group of thalamic nuclei on the basis of its afferent connections. J. Comp. Neurol. 143:185–216.

Mantyh, P. W. 1983. The spinothalamic tract in the primate: A reexamination using wheat germ agglutinin conjugated to horseradish peroxidase. Neurosci. 9:847–862.

Martin, J. H. 1985. Anatomical substrates for somatic sensation. In Kandel, E. R., and Schwartz, J. H., Principles of Neural Science. New York: Elsevier, pp. 301–315.

Ralston III, H. J., and Ralston, D. D. 1982. The distribution of dorsal root axons to laminae IV, V, and VI of the Macaque spinal cord: A quantitative electron microscopic study. J. Comp. Neurol. 212:435–448.

Willis, W. D., Kenshalo, D. R., Jr., and Leonard, R. B. 1979. The cells of origin of the primate spinothalamic tract. J. Comp. Neurol. 188:543–574.

Selected Readings

Brown, A. G. 1981. The terminations of cutaneous nerve fibers in the spinal cord. Trends in Neuroscience 4:64–67.

Dubner, R., and Bennett, G. J. 1983. Spinal and trigeminal mechanisms of nociception. Ann. Rev. Neurosci. 6:381–418.

Kandel, E. R. 1985. Central representation of touch. In Kandel, E. R., and Schwartz, J. H., Principles of Neural Science. New York: Elsevier, pp. 316–330.

Kelly, D. D. 1985. Central representation of pain and analgesia. In Kandel, E. R., and Schwartz, J. H., Principles of Neural Science. New York: Elsevier, pp. 331–343.

Martin, J. H. 1985. Receptor physiology and submodality coding in the somatic sensory system. In Kandel, E. R., and Schwartz, J. H., Principles of Neural Science. New York: Elsevier, pp. 286–300.

Mountcastle, V. B. 1984. Central Nervous Mechanisms in Mechanoreceptive Sensibility. In Darian-Smith, I. (ed.), Handbook of Physiology, Section 1: The Nervous System, Vol. III. Sensory Processes. Bethesda, Md.: American Physiological Society, pp. 789–878.

Willis, W. D. 1985. Nociceptive pathways: Anatomy and physiology of nociceptive ascending pathways. Phil. Trans. Soc. Lond. B 308:253–268.

Willis, W. D., and Coggeshall, R. E. 1978. Sensory Mechanisms of the Spinal Cord. New York: Plenum.

The Visual System

6

The Visual System

Visual perception, like perception of other sensory modalities, is not a passive process whereby the eyes simply receive visual stimulation. Rather, the position of the eyes is precisely controlled in order to scan the environment and to attend selectively and orient to specific visual stimuli. There are two anatomically separate visual pathways. Oculomotor control is principally mediated by one visual pathway. This component of the visual system concomitantly controls the orientation of the head and body to visual stimuli. Visual perception is mediated largely by the second pathway. We begin this chapter with an overview of these two visual pathways; then the structure and anatomical connections of their components are considered. Finally, we examine how the physician can use knowledge of the organization of the visual system to localize disturbances of brain function with precision.

Anatomically Separate Visual Pathways Mediate Perception and Reflex Function

The different sensory systems share many organizing principles. Similar to the somatic sensory system (Chapter 5) where the topography of connections is determined by the organization of the receptive sheet, the somatotopic organization, connections in the visual system are determined largely by the *retinotopic organization*. This is another example of the systematic and precise projection of sensory receptors on central nervous system structures. Another similarity is the *hierarchical* and *parallel* organization of sensory systems. A hierarchically organized system is one in which components can be assigned to *distinct functional levels with respect to one another* and such levels have clear anatomical substrates. The two separate visual pathways each have a hierarchical organization. The dorsal column–medial lemniscal and anterolateral systems are two examples of parallel somatic sensory pathways, each of which have a hierarchical organization.

The Pathway to the Primary Visual Cortex Mediates the Perception of Visual Form, Color, and Movement

All visual pathways originate in the retina, where the photoreceptors, which transduce visual stimuli, are located (inset to Figure 6.1A). The photoreceptors synapse on retinal interneurons which, in turn, synapse on ganglion cells. *Ganglion cells* are the retinal neurons that project to the thalamus and their axons travel in the *optic nerve*. The axons of certain ganglion cells decussate in the *optic chiasm* (Figure 6.1A; see later) and, together with the fibers from the ipsilateral side, course in the *optic tract*. The principal thalamic target for the ganglion cells is the *lateral geniculate nucleus*. This thalamic nucleus, in turn, projects to the *primary visual cortex* via a pathway called the *optic radiations*. The primary visual cortex is located in the occipital lobe, along the banks and within the depths of the *calcarine fissure* (Figure 6.10B). The structure and function of the primary visual cortex were considered briefly in Chapter 1. Efferent projections from the primary visual cortex follow one of three principal paths. One contingent "ascends" to *secondary* and *higher order visual cortical*

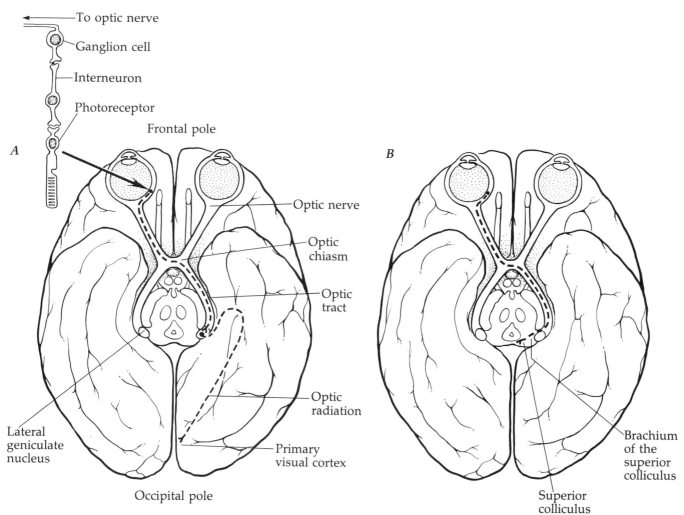

Figure 6.1 Organization of the two visual pathways, the retinal–geniculate–calcarine pathway **(A)** and the pathway to the midbrain **(B).** Inset shows the general organization of the retina. The photoreceptor transduces visual stimuli and relays the sensory information, encoded in the form of nonpropagated potentials, to retinal interneurons. The interneurons transmit the visual information to the ganglion cells. Ganglion cell axons form the optic nerve once they exit the eyeball.

areas in the occipital and temporal lobes and may mediate spatial vision and object recognition respectively. Visuomotor centers in the midbrain and the pons receive a "descending" projection from a second contingent. Finally, the axons of a third contingent of neurons "decussate" in the corpus callosum and terminate in the contralateral primary visual cortex.

The Pathway to the Midbrain Is Important in Oculomotor Reflexes and the Orientation of the Head and Body to Visual Stimuli

Certain ganglion cells project to the midbrain, principally to two structures (Figure 6.1B): (1) the *superior colliculus* and (2) the *pretectal nuclei*. The superior colliculus is located in the *tectum* of the midbrain, which is the portion located *dorsal to the cerebral aqueduct* (Figure 6.1B; see Figure 3.7). The pretectal nuclei are located rostral to the tectum, at the midbrain–diencephalic juncture, and participate in pupillary as well as other visual reflexes. These are topics that will be covered in Chapter 13. The superior colliculus is a key structure for form vision in lower vertebrates; however, in mammals, and especially humans, the superior colliculus has a minimal role in perception but an important role in coordination of eye and head movements.

The pathways for visual perception and visuomotor function do not remain completely separate. Rather, at certain sites in the cerebral cortex and in the superior colliculus the two systems converge. Certain superior colliculus neurons have an axon that ascends to the thalamus, to nuclei that project to the *association areas of the parietal, temporal, and occipital lobes*. Here in the cerebral cortex, the visuomotor pathway converges with the visual perception pathway. These cortical association areas are involved in complex aspects of perception and the planning of eye movement. Examples of their function in visual perception include the analysis of visual information during eye movements and the ability to direct attention selectively to specific visual stimuli. The other site for convergence of the two visual pathways is the superior colliculus because it receives a descending projection from the primary visual cortex.

The next six sections of this chapter examine the anatomy of the visual system from a regional perspective. First, the structure of the retina and the optical properties of the eye are considered, followed in sequence by the anatomy of the superior colliculus, lateral geniculate nucleus, primary visual cortex, and higher-order visual cortical areas. Finally, we consider some clinical applications of visual system anatomy.

The Retina Contains Five Major Layers

The retina is part of the peripheral component of the visual system, the portion where the photoreceptors are located (Figure 6.2). However, unlike the somatic sensory system where the dorsal root ganglion cells are part of the peripheral nervous system (they develop from the neural crest; see Chapter 2), the retina is actually a displaced portion of the central nervous system (it develops from the diencephalon). The location of the retina in relation to the eyeball is illustrated in Figure 6.2A. A section through the retina, oriented at a right angle to its surface, is shown in Figure 6.2B. At this peripheral level of the visual system the neurons are ordered into discrete layers, in a nearly geometrical arrangement. At subsequent levels in the visual system, the organization is also laminated. Lamination is one way the nervous system packs together neurons with similar functional attributes and patterns of connections.

The anatomical organization of the retina is somewhat paradoxical: light must travel through retinal layers that contain projection neurons and interneurons to reach the photoreceptors. However, in the region of the *fovea*—a specialized high-resolution portion of the retina—the retinal interneurons and ganglion cells are displaced, thereby exposing the photoreceptors directly to visual stimuli and optimizing the optical quality of the image. The fovea is the central portion of a morphologically distinct part of the retina, termed the *macula lutea*, where photoreceptors, especially cones, are most dense. The position of the eyes is precisely controlled to ensure that the principal portion of an image we view falls on the fovea of each eye. Indeed, the midbrain visual structures are devoted largely to positioning of the eyes to accomplish this purpose.

The retina contains five principal layers, three contain neuronal cell bodies and two are regions of synaptic contacts (Figure 6.2C): (1) outer nuclear layer, (2) outer synaptic (or plexiform) layer, (3) inner nuclear layer, (4) inner synaptic (or plexiform) layer, and (5) ganglion cell layer. In addition to the five principal layers, there are numerous strata that contain processes of particular retinal cells. The nomenclature describing the locations of the different layers has, as its spatial reference point, the *three-dimensional center* of the eye. The inner, or proximal, layers are located close to the *center of the eye*, whereas the *outer*, or distal, layers are located *farther from the center* (Figure 6.2A).[1] The *outer nuclear layer* (1) contains the cell bodies of photoreceptors. There are two classes of photoreceptors—*rods* and *cones*—each with different visual pigments. The discriminative aspects of human visual perception occur during daylight hours when light intensities are high. This is when the cones are activated. Cones contain pigments for color vision, and there are three different classes of cones each of which has different absorption spectra: red, green, and blue. In contrast, rods are optimally suited to low levels of illumination, such as during dusk or night time. In fact, a single photon may activate a rod cell. Connections between photoreceptors and retinal interneurons are made in the *outer synaptic (or plexiform) layer* (2). The *inner nuclear layer* (3) contains the cell bodies and proximal processes of interneurons: bipolar cells, horizontal cells, amacrine cells, and interplexiform cells. *Bipolar cells* link the photoreceptors directly with ganglion cells. There are two principal classes of bipolar cells: cone bipolar cells and rod bipolar cells. The *cone bipolar cells* receive synaptic input from a small number of cone cells, thereby setting the stage for a component of the visual system that has *high visual acuity*. By contrast, *rod bipolar cells* receive convergent input from many rods. Acuity is lost but sensitivity to *low levels of illumination* is gained. *Horizontal cells* and *amacrine cells*, mediate interactions between laterally located photoreceptors and bipolar cells and subserve physiological mechanisms for enhancing the contrast of visual images. Horizontal cells are located in the outer portion of the inner nuclear layer, whereas amacrine cells are located in the inner portion. The fourth retinal interneuron is the *interplexiform cell* (not illustrated in Figure 6.2C). As the name implies, these retinal interneurons connect the inner and outer synaptic layers (which are also termed inner and outer plexiform layers). They receive their input in the inner synaptic layer, and while they also synapse on retinal cells in this layer, their major synaptic connections are made in the outer synaptic layer. Connections between the bipolar cells and the ganglion cells are made in the *inner synaptic (or plexiform) layer* (4). The innermost retinal layer is the *ganglion cell layer* (5) named after the retinal output cells.

Ganglion cell axons collect along the inner retinal surface (Figures 6.2C and 6.3A) and leave the eye at a single, morphologically distinct

---

[1] It is interesting to note that the arterial supply of the inner and outer portions of the retina is different. The inner retina is supplied by branches of the ophthalmic artery—a branch of the internal carotid. The outer retina is devoid of blood vessels. Its nourishment derives from the choroidal circulation.

A

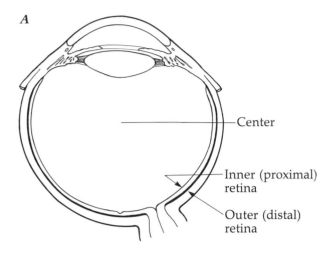

Center

Inner (proximal) retina

Outer (distal) retina

B

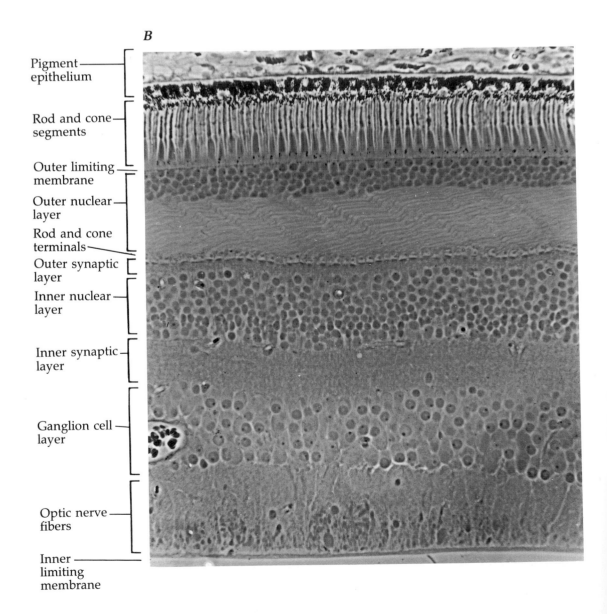

Pigment epithelium

Rod and cone segments

Outer limiting membrane

Outer nuclear layer

Rod and cone terminals

Outer synaptic layer

Inner nuclear layer

Inner synaptic layer

Ganglion cell layer

Optic nerve fibers

Inner limiting membrane

location on the retina called the *optic disk* (Figure 6.3A). There are no photoreceptors or interneurons here, only ganglion cell axons en route to form the optic nerve. Consequently, there is a blind spot in the retina of each eye that corresponds to the location of the optic disk. Interestingly, we are not aware of the presence of the blind spot until it is demonstrated (see later). Ganglion cell axons do not become myelinated until they exit from the retina (Figure 6.3A). A single optic nerve contains all the axons of ganglion cells in the ipsilateral retina. The optic nerve is called the

Figure 6.2   Anatomy of the retina. *A.* Schematic diagram of eyeball indicating the inner and outer portions of the retina. *B.* A transverse section of the retina. *C.* Wiring diagram of the generalized vertebrate retina. It should be noted that in mammalian retinae, horizontal cells do not synapse on cones. (*A,* Courtesy of Dr. John E. Dowling, Harvard University; adapted from Boycott, B. B., and Dowling, J. E. 1969. Organization of the primate retina: Light microscopy. Proc. Trans. R. Soc. Lond. B 255:109–184; *C,* Adapted from Dowling, J. E., and Boycott, B. B. 1966. Organization of the primate retina: Electron microscopy. Proc. R. Soc. Lond. B 166:80–111.)

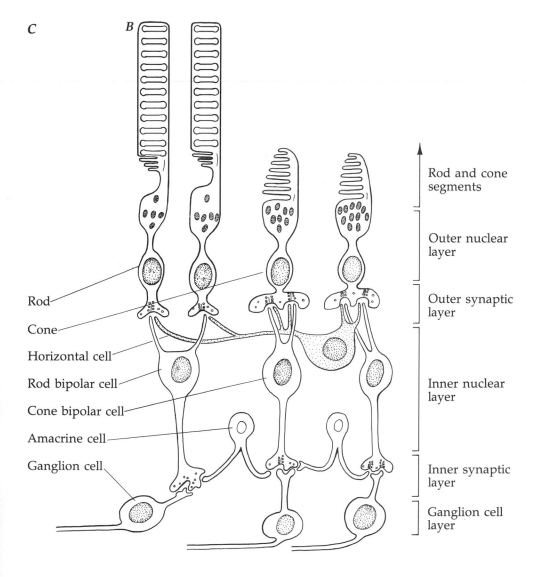

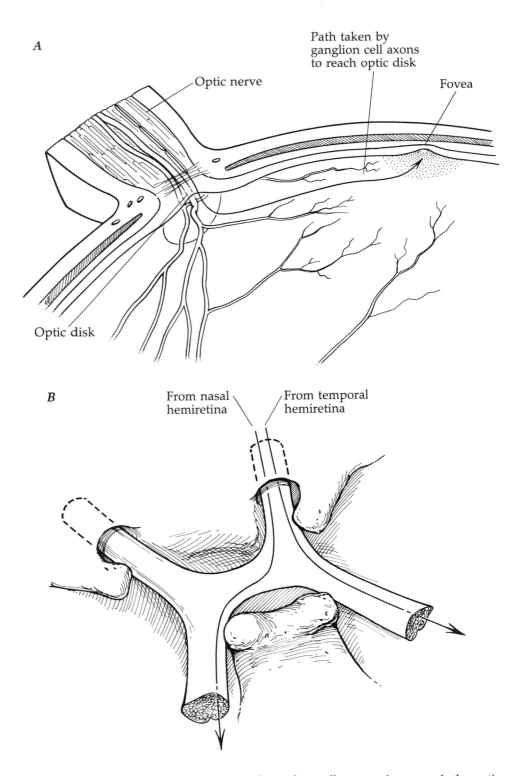

Figure 6.3 The path that the retinal ganglion cell axons take to reach the optic tract. *A.* Course of ganglion cell axons along the surface of the retina and into the optic nerve at the optic disk. *B.* Regional anatomy of the optic chiasm. Direction of arrows indicate axon trajectory toward lateral geniculate nucleus and midbrain. (Adapted from Patten, H. 1977. Neurological Differential Diagnosis. New York: Springer-Verlag.)

second cranial nerve, but it is actually a central nervous system pathway displaced to the periphery rather than part of the peripheral nervous system. The other sensory cranial nerves are components of the peripheral nervous system. The optic nerves from the two eyes converge at the *optic chiasm* (Figures 6.1 and 6.3B). Here the axons from certain ganglion cells decussate and enter the *contralateral optic tract*, whereas others do not decussate, but pass directly to the *ipsilateral optic tract* (see later).

Müller cells are the principal retinal neuroglia. These cells, which have important structural and metabolic functions in the retina, have their nuclei located in the inner nuclear layer. An individual Müller cell stretches vertically from the inner surface of the retina (the inner limiting membrane) to the distal margin of the optic nerve fibers (outer limiting membrane) (Figure 6.2).

Knowledge of the pattern of decussation of ganglion cell axons is essential to a thorough understanding of the organization of the central visual pathways. This topic, including how visual images project on the retina, is considered next. Later in this chapter we return to the pattern of retinal projections in greater detail when knowledge of the anatomical organization of the visual system is exploited to identify the location of central nervous system damage.

The Optical Properties of the Eye Transform Visual Stimuli

The combined field of view of both eyes when their position remains fixed is called the *visual field* (Figure 6.4; see also Figure 6.16). The field of view of each eye is not simply one half of the total visual field. Instead, the visual field of each eye overlaps extensively with that of the other eye (Figure 6.4A and B) to form the total visual field. The total visual field (or simply the visual field) is the sum of the right and left hemifields and consists of a central overlap (binocular) zone, which is seen by both eyes, and two monocular zones, which are seen by each eye separately. The visual field is divided into symmetrical right and left halves. The retina is also divided in half by a vertical line passing through the fovea into a *nasal hemiretina* and a *temporal hemiretina*. Each hemiretina includes one half of the fovea and the remaining peripheral retina.

Because of the lens, a visual image becomes inverted and reversed when it is projected on the retina (Figure 6.4B). The image reversal causes the right half of a visual image to fall on the left half of the retina of each eye—the *left temporal hemiretina* and the *right nasal hemiretina*. Conversely, the left half of an image falls on the right half of the retina of each eye— the right temporal hemiretina and the left nasal hemiretina. Ganglion cells of each *nasal hemiretina*, including both the foveal and peripheral portions, project to other components of the diencephalon and to the midbrain. Their axons decussate in the *optic chiasm*. Ganglion cells of each *temporal hemiretina* do not decussate, but pass to the *ipsilateral* diencephalon and midbrain. This pattern of incomplete decussation of ganglion cell axons does not violate the rule that sensory information decussates en route to processing by central nervous system structures because visual information from *one half of the visual field* is processed within the *contralateral central nervous system*.

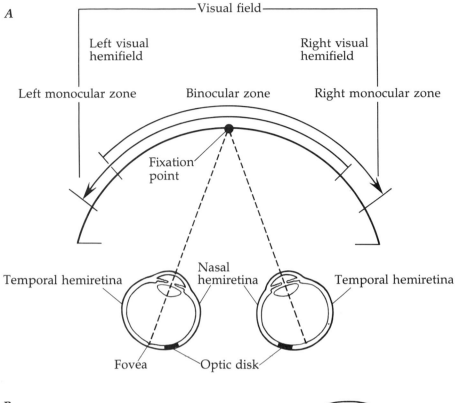

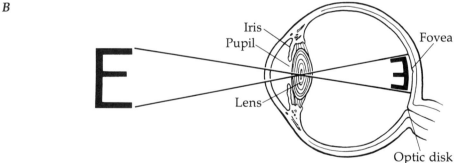

Figure 6.4 *A.* Horizontal view of the relationship between the location of the visual fields for each eye, an image in space, and how the image falls on the retina. *B.* Sagittal view shows the key features of the optical properties of the eye. (Adapted from Kandel, E. R., and Schwartz, J. H. 1985. Principles of Neural Science. New York: Elsevier.)

The Superior Colliculus Is Important in Oculomotor Control and Orientation

The optic tract axons that terminate in the superior colliculus course in a path on the diencephalic and brain stem surfaces called the *brachium of the superior colliculus* (Figure 6.5). The axons in this tract skirt the lateral geniculate nucleus and pass over the dorsal surface of the medial geniculate nucleus, which is the thalamic auditory nucleus (Chapter 7). The superior colliculus is synonymous with the tectum of the rostral midbrain. Throughout phylogeny the superior colliculus (termed the *optic tectum* in lower vertebrates) subserves visual function, and, in addition, its *laminated arrangement of neurons* remains remarkably similar from amphibians to humans. However, the relative size of the superior colliculus in relation to the brain decreases in proportion to the increase in size of the visual cortex. In lower vertebrates, the superior colliculus subserves both form vision and visual reflex function. In higher vertebrates, form vision is one

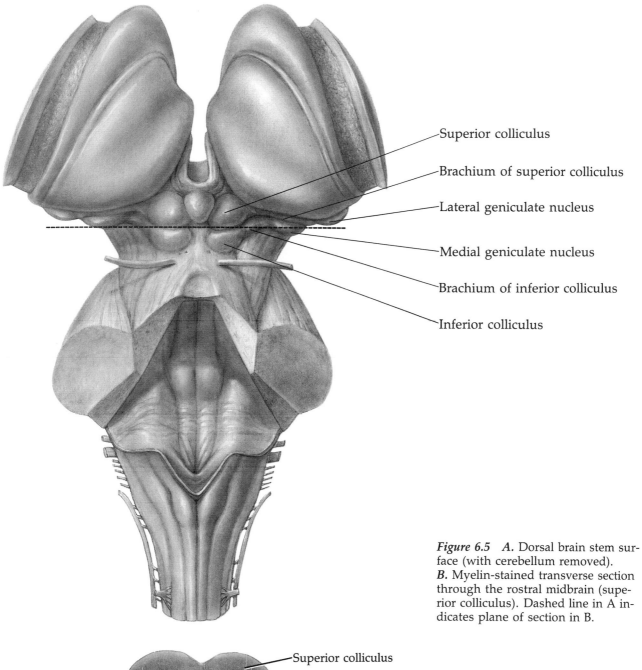

Superior colliculus

Brachium of superior colliculus

Lateral geniculate nucleus

Medial geniculate nucleus

Brachium of inferior colliculus

Inferior colliculus

Figure 6.5 *A.* Dorsal brain stem surface (with cerebellum removed). *B.* Myelin-stained transverse section through the rostral midbrain (superior colliculus). Dashed line in A indicates plane of section in B.

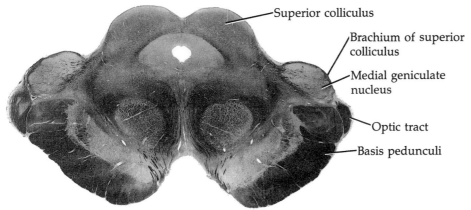

B

Superior colliculus

Brachium of superior colliculus

Medial geniculate nucleus

Optic tract

Basis pedunculi

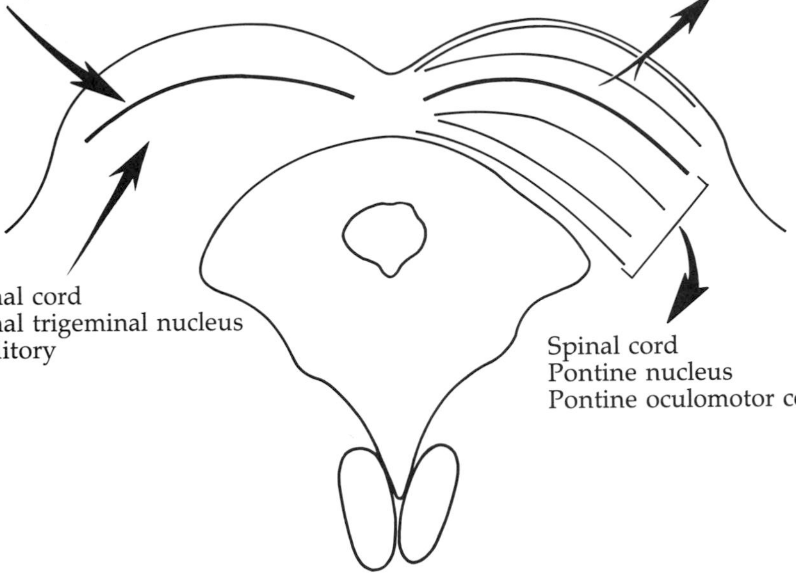

Afferent   Efferent

Retina
Primary visual cortex

Lateral posterior nucleus
Pulvinar

Spinal cord
Spinal trigeminal nucleus
Auditory

Spinal cord
Pontine nucleus
Pontine oculomotor centers

Figure 6.6 Schematic diagram illustrating the layers of the superior colliculus and their major input and output connections.

function of the visual cortex and the superior colliculus is more important in visuomotor function.

The superior colliculus of higher vertebrates consists of seven layers whose contents alternate between a predominance of neuronal cell bodies and a predominance of axons. Some of these layers are clearly visible in the myelin-stained section in Figure 6.5B. A schematic diagram of the lamination pattern in the superior colliculus and the connections of the various layers is shown in Figure 6.6. The dorsal three layers of the superior colliculus contain the neural apparatus for controlling rapid eye movements toward salient visual stimuli. The ventral four layers receive somatic sensory and auditory information in addition to input from other sources. The *spinotectal tract*, one component of the anterolateral system (Chapter 5), brings somatic sensory information to the superior colliculus. Certain neurons in these deeper layers project to the caudal brain stem and spinal cord and are involved in the *orientation of the head and body to important stimuli* (Chapter 9).

Ganglion Cell Axons from the Ipsilateral and Contralateral Retinae Terminate in Different Layers of the Lateral Geniculate Nucleus

The major retinal projection is to the *lateral geniculate nucleus* of the thalamus (Figure 6.7).[2] This large nucleus forms a surface landmark on the ventral diencephalon (Figure 6.5A). A coronal section through the

---

[2] This nucleus contains two separate divisions—dorsal and ventral. The dorsal division is the largest, projects to the primary visual cortex, and is the division that serves visual perception. The ventral division is a diffuse-projecting thalamic nucleus. Here, we focus on the dorsal division of the lateral geniculate nucleus, and refer to it simply as the lateral geniculate nucleus without the prefix indicating its location.

A

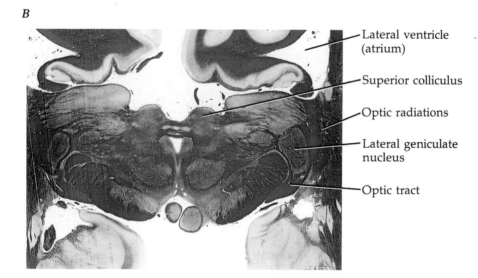

Medial geniculate nucleus

Lateral geniculate nucleus

Optic radiations

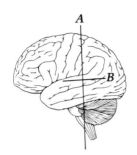

B

Lateral ventricle (atrium)

Superior colliculus

Optic radiations

Lateral geniculate nucleus

Optic tract

Figure 6.7 *A.* Myelin-stained coronal section through the lateral geniculate nucleus. *B.* Transverse section through the midbrain–diencephalic juncture. Inset shows planes of section.

lateral geniculate nucleus is shown in Figure 6.7A. In Figure 6.7B, which is a section sliced in a plane approximately orthogonal to the one in Figure 6.7A, the main portion of the optic tract appears to terminate in the lateral geniculate nucleus.

The lateral geniculate nucleus contains six major cell layers. All cell layers process input from the *contralateral visual field*, but each layer receives connections exclusively from either the *ipsilateral retina* or the *contralateral retina*. This pattern of connections is demonstrated in Figure 6.8A, an autoradiograph of the lateral geniculate nucleus of a rhesus monkey. To obtain this image, tritiated fucose was injected into the ipsilateral eye of the animal. The ganglion cells incorporated this radiolabeled material into glycoproteins, which were then carried to their terminals in

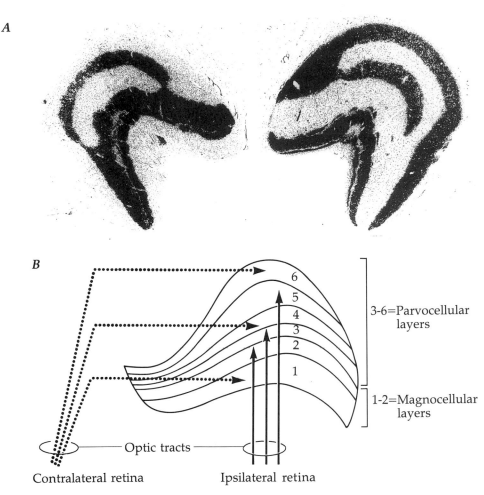

Figure 6.8 Each of the six cell layers of the lateral geniculate nucleus receives afferent input from either the ipsilateral or the contralateral eye. **A.** Autoradiograph of the monkey lateral geniculate nucleus. The left eye was injected with ^{3}H-fucose. Labelled regions are dark. The six principal layers of the lateral geniculate nucleus are labelled. For example, layers 1, 4, and 6 are labeled on the section of the lateral geniculate nucleus shown on right. In addition, there are thin subliminae that also receive retinal input. **B.** Schematic diagram of input connections of the human lateral geniculate nucleus. (**A,** Courtesy of Drs. David H. Hubel and Torsten N. Wiesel; from Hubel, D. H., and Wiesel, T. N. 1977. Ferrier Lecture: Functional architecture of macaque monkey visual cortex. Proc. R. Soc. Lond. B 198:1–59.)

the lateral geniculate nucleus by anterograde axonal transport. Exposing the tissue to photographic emulsion produced an autoradiograph that revealed the distribution of radiolabeled material.

Each layer of the lateral geniculate nucleus contains a complete and orderly representation of the contralateral visual field. An important aspect of the organization of this nucleus is that the representation of visual space in each of the various layers is in spatial register: *cells oriented along an axis orthogonal to the plane of the layers receive input from the same portion of the contralateral visual field*. In addition to receiving input from either the ipsilateral or the contralateral retina, neurons in these layers differ in at least two additional ways (Figure 6.8B). *First*, the dorsal four layers

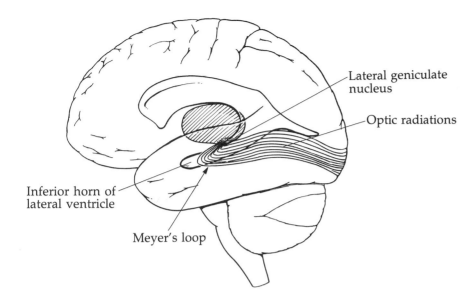

Figure 6.9 Course of the axons of the optic radiations from the lateral geniculate nucleus, over the lateral ventricle to reach the primary visual cortex. (Adapted from Brodal, A. 1981. Neurological Anatomy. New York: Oxford University Press.)

contain small neurons and therefore are termed the *parvocellular layers;* the ventral two layers contain large cells and are called the *magnocellular layers. Second,* the parvo- and magnocellular layers are believed to receive projections from different functional classes of retinal ganglion cells. Projection neurons in all six layers of the lateral geniculate nucleus send their axons to the primary visual cortex through the *optic radiations.*[3] Many of these axons take an indirect course around the lateral ventricle to reach their cortical target (Figure 6.9). As we will see in a later section of this chapter, some of these axons, subserving vision from a specific portion of the visual field, actually course rostrally within the temporal lobe (termed *Meyer's loop*), before coursing caudally to the primary visual cortex (Figure 6.9).

The Primary Visual Cortex Is Located in the Banks of the Calcarine Fissure

The primary visual cortex corresponds to Brodmann's cytoarchitectonic *area 17* (see Figure 3.16). Most of it is located on the medial surface of the cerebral hemispheres, in the banks of the *calcarine fissure* (Figure 6.10). The microscopic anatomy of the primary visual cortex is laminated (Figure 6.11) and, similar to that of the somatic sensory cortex, the various layers have different patterns of input and output connections. There are six principal layers, with layer IV subdivided into three sublaminae (Figure 6.11C). These layers can be seen in the schematic drawing of a Nissl-stained section through the primary visual cortex. Axons from the lateral geniculate nucleus principally terminate in layers IVa and IVc. Interneurons in these sublaminae, in turn, distribute information to other cortical layers (Figure 6.11C). Layer IVb is recognizable on myelin-stained sections by the presence of a dense plexus of myelinated axons, called the *stripe*

---

[3] The optic radiations are also termed the *geniculocalcarine tract* because they link the lateral geniculate nucleus with the visual cortex, which is located within and along the banks of the calcarine fissure.

Figure 6.10 The primary visual cortex is located predominantly on the medial surface of the cerebral hemisphere and within the calcarine fissure. *A.* Lateral view of the brain. *B.* Medial view of the brain.

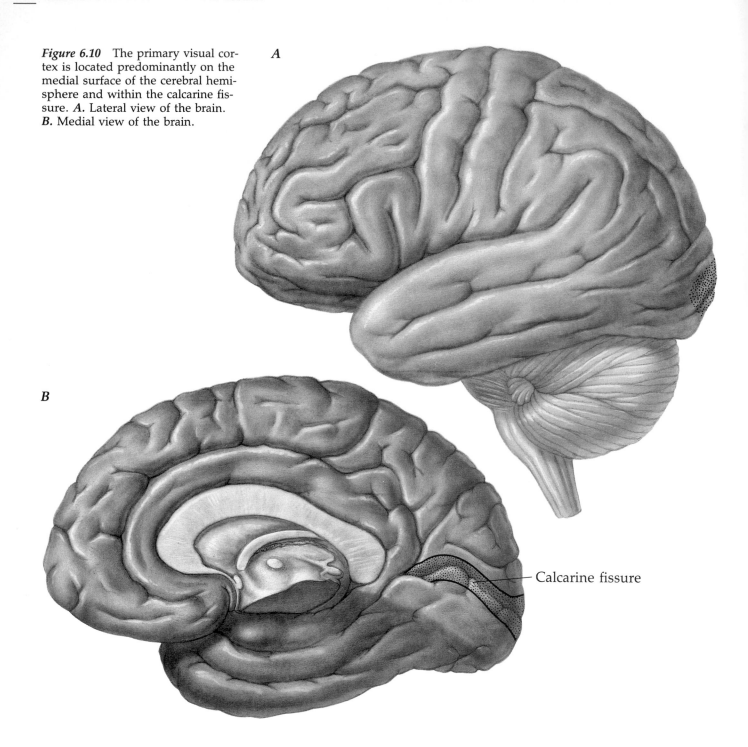

Calcarine fissure

of Gennari (Figure 6.11A), which are axon collaterals of primary visual cortical neurons. Another name for the primary visual cortex is the *striate cortex*. Layer IVb is so distinct that it actually can be observed in dissected, unstained, material. In addition, there is a small input from the lateral geniculate nucleus to layer III.

The cerebral cortex has a columnar organization. For example, in the primary somatic sensory cortex (Chapters 5), cortical neurons located above and below one another—yet in different layers—all process sen-

A

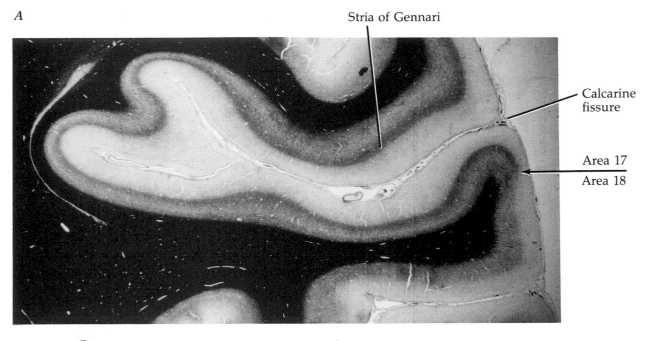

Stria of Gennari

Calcarine
fissure

Area 17

Area 18

B

C

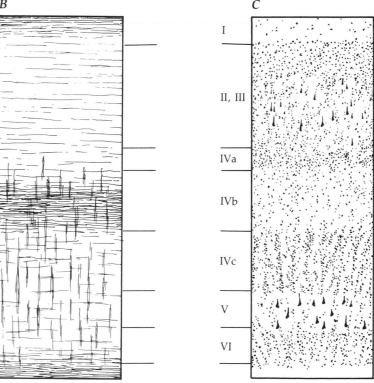

I

II, III

IVa

IVb

IVc

V

VI

Figure 6.11 The pattern of lamination in the primary visual cortex is
shown in myelin-stained section *A.*
Schematic drawing of a myelin-
stained section through the striate
cortex (*B*) and a Nissl-stained section
(*C*) illustrating the cytoarchitecture of
the primary visual cortex.

sory input from the same *peripheral location* and the same type of *sensory
receptor*. In the primary visual cortex there are at least two types of columns: (1) *ocular dominance columns*, where neurons receive visual input
from either the ipsilateral or the contralateral eye, and (2) *orientation columns*, where neurons are maximally sensitive to visual stimuli with similar
spatial orientations.

Input from the Lateral Geniculate Nucleus Is Segregated into Separate Ocular Dominance Columns in the Primary Visual Cortex

The projection from individual layers in the lateral geniculate nucleus, each of which receives either ipsilateral or contralateral retinal inputs, remains segregated as alternating bands in layer IV of the primary visual cortex. As a consequence, neurons in layer IV receive input either from one eye or the other eye. This segregated pattern of lateral geniculate axon terminations forms the anatomical basis of the *ocular dominance columns*. Other neurons in a column that are located in layers above and below layer IV receive input from both eyes, but preferentially from the same eye that projected information to layer IV. These binocular interactions point to a potentially important functional role of ocular dominance columns in binocular vision. Ocular dominance columns that serve a particular retinal location in one eye alternate with columns serving the corresponding location in the other eye. The system of ocular dominance columns in layer IV can be visualized using the autoradiographic technique shown in Figure 6.8. In sections perpendicular to the pial surface of the cortex, the columns appear as patches of radioactive label (Figure 6.12A). When a section is taken through layer IV, in a plane tangential to the cortical surface, the ocular dominance columns form stripes (Figure 12B; inset indicates the planes of sections shown in A and B).

Centered within the ocular dominance columns are aggregates of neurons sensitive to the wavelength of the visual stimulus. These color-sensitive neurons are assembled into clusters that spare layer I and a portion of layer IV. Neurons in these clusters are thought to receive a direct input from the lateral geniculate nucleus. The locations of these color sensitive cells correspond to regions of primary visual cortex that have high levels of activity of the mitochondrial enzyme *cytochrome oxidase* Figure 6.13. These cell clusters were termed *blobs* by their discoverers Margaret Livingstone and David Hubel at Harvard University. The color "blobs" can be identified using a method for histochemical localization of cytochrome oxidase activity. Figure 6.13 illustrates two tangential sections through layers II and III of the primary visual cortex of the squirrel monkey (left) and rhesus monkey (right). Cytochrome oxidase is a metabolic enzyme and it is reasoned that the color-sensitive cortical neurons, or the terminals of lateral geniculate neurons from which they receive a projection, are metabolically more active than surrounding regions. The functional significance of an increased level of metabolic activity in neurons mediating color vision is not known.

Orientation Columns Are Revealed by an Autoradiographic Mapping Technique That Images Functional Organization

Unlike ocular dominance, which is a columnar attribute based on *anatomical connections from one eye or the other*, orientation specificity is believed to be mediated by interconnections between cortical neurons themselves. Standard, and even sophisticated, anatomical staining techniques do not reveal these connections and thus do not distinguish between orientation columns. To reveal orientation columns, a technique must be used that images neuronal activity in response to a visual stimulus with a particular orientation. A method that accomplishes this purpose uses a radiolabeled glucose analog, 2-deoxyglucose, to produce an

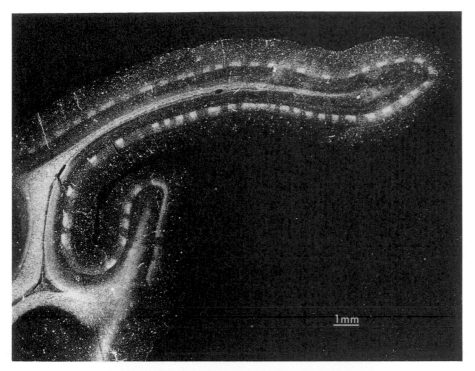

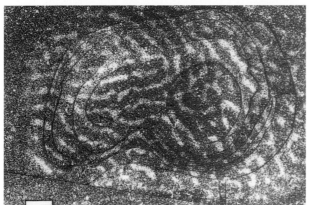

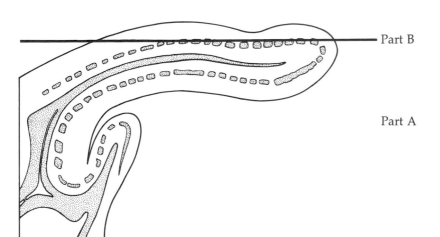

Part B

Part A

Figure 6.12 Ocular dominance columns can be demonstrated using autoradiography. *A.* The section was cut orthogonal to pial surface. *B.* A histological reconstruction in a plane parallel to the pial surface. Inset is a schematic drawing of the section shown in A indicating the plane of reconstruction in B. (*A,* From Hubel, D. H., and Wiesel, T. N. 1977. Ferrier Lecture: Functional architecture of macaque monkey visual cortex. Proc. R. Soc. Lond. B 198:1–59. *B,* From Hubel, D. H., Wiesel, T. N., and LeVay S. 1977. Plasticity of ocular dominance columns in monkey striate cortex. Philos. Trans. R. Soc. Lond. B 278:377–409)

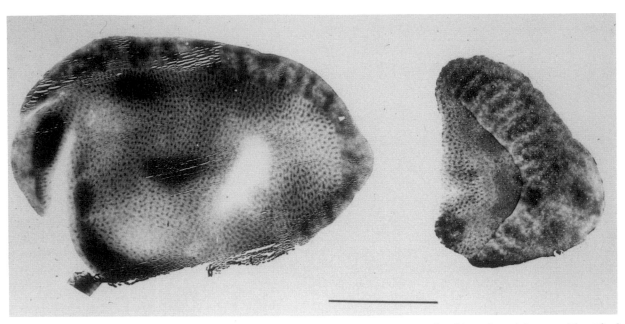

Figure 6.13 Clusters of neurons that are involved in color vision are identified by histochemical localization of cytochrome oxidase. The sections were cut parallel to the pial surface and predominantly through layers 2 and 3 of the occipital lobe of a rhesus monkey (left) and a squirrel monkey (right). Cytochrome oxidase activity is greater in the dark regions than in the lighter regions. In area 17 (primary visual cortex), regions that have high cytochrome oxidase activity have a spherical shape in cross section and are cylindrical in three dimensions. Cytochrome oxidase staining in area 18 (secondary visual cortex) reveals stripes rather than the polka-dot pattern shown in A. Bar indicates 5 mm. (Courtesy of Drs. Margaret Livingstone and David Hubel, Harvard University.)

image that reflects neuronal glucose utilization. Glucose utilization is proportional to neural activity because glucose is the energy source for the brain. Active neurons incorporate 2-deoxyglucose as if it were glucose. However, 2-deoxyglucose will become trapped within the cell because metabolic enzymes cannot further metabolize it. As the 2-deoxyglucose is radiolabeled, its location can be determined using autoradiographic methods. Orientation columns in the primary visual cortex of the rhesus monkey are illustrated in Figure 6.14, which is an autoradiograph obtained after visual stimulation at one stimulus orientation. As in Figure 6.13, the plane of section is parallel to the surface of the cortex. Orientation columns are located from layer II to layer VI, and spare a portion of layer IV, which contains neurons that are insensitive to orientation of a visual stimulus.

Higher Order Visual Cortical Areas and the Association Cortex Receive Input from the Primary Visual Cortex

The higher order visual areas and association areas are located in the occipital, temporal, and parietal lobes (Figure 6.15B) and each area contains a separate representation of visual space. Although their functions and interrelationships are extraordinarily complex, a simplifying scheme has recently been proposed in which most of the areas are *hierarchically* related to one or another area. According to this scheme, one structure projects on another in a *feedforward* manner (Figure 6.15A1). This

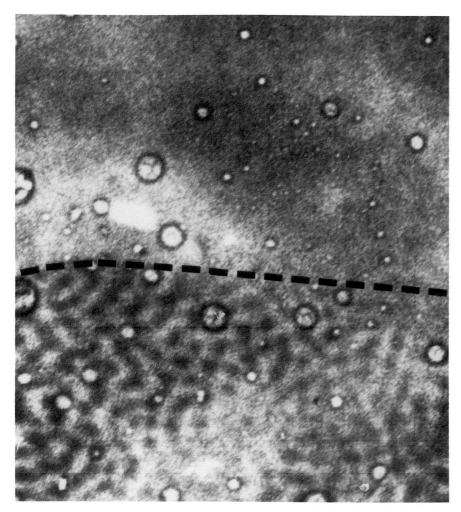

Figure 6.14 This 2-deoxyglucose autoradiograph illustrates the orientation columns in the primary visual cortex of the rhesus monkey. Vertical black and white stripes were presented to one portion of the visual field (upper field) and stripes of all orientations were presented to an adjacent portion of the visual field (lower field). This pattern of stimulation resulted in deoxyglucose-labeled orientation columns in the cortical representation of the upper visual field, which is in the region of autoradiograph below the dashed line, and no orientation columns in the lower visual field representation, which is the region above the dashed line. Plane of section is similar to that shown in Figure 6.13. (Autoradiograph courtesy of Dr. Roger Tootell, Harvard University.)

projection originates from neurons in the superficial cortical layers, and is directed to layer IV in the next higher level in the hierarchy (for example, from primary to secondary visual cortical areas). Each structure in the hierarchy also receives a *feedback* projection (Figure 6.15A2) from the next higher level. The feedback path originates from neurons mostly in the deeper layers and, to a lesser extent, in the superficial layers, and is directed to neurons in both superficial and deeper layers in the next lower level in the hierarchy (for example, from secondary to primary visual cortical areas). Out of the myriad of corticocortical projections from the primary and secondary visual areas, two functionally different parallel pathways emerge. One pathway analyzes the *form and color* of visual stim-

Figure 6.15 Projections from primary visual cortex. **A.** Feedforward and feedback paths, which are based on the patterns of anterograde and retrograde axon transport. **B.** Separate pathways are thought to mediate spatial vision (the analysis of motion and location of visual stimuli) and object vision (the analysis of form and color of visual stimuli). (**A,** Adapted from Maunsell, J. H. R., and Van Essen, D. C. 1983. The connections of the middle temporal visual area (MT) and their relationship to a cortical hierarchy in the macaque monkey. J. Neurosci. 3:2563–2568.)

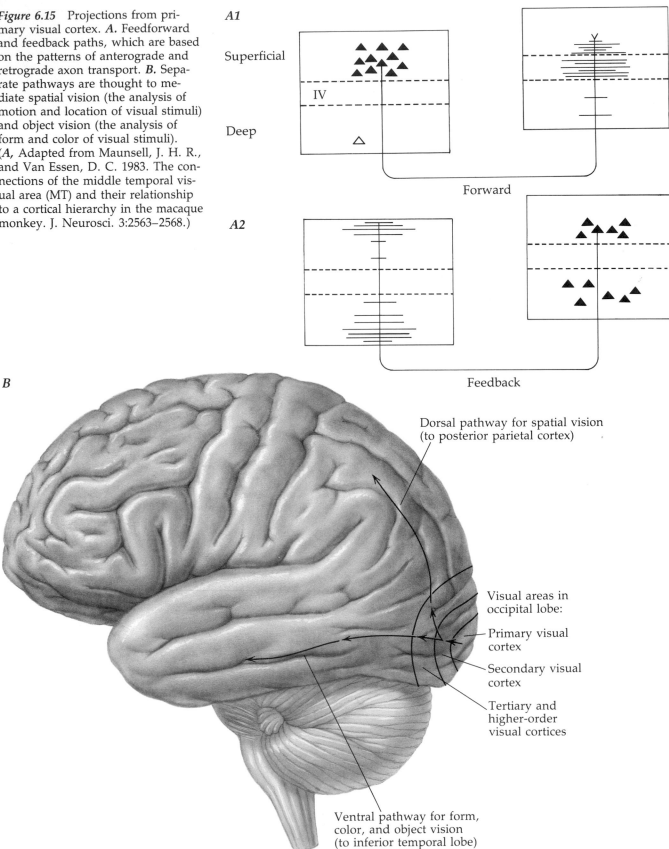

uli. This pathway courses ventrally and ultimately projects to visual areas in the *inferior temporal lobe* (Figure 6.15B). A second pathway, projecting to the posterior parietal cortex, analyzes the location and motion of visual stimuli. The pathway to the temporal lobe may mediate *object vision* and the path to the parietal lobe may participate in *spatial vision* (Figure 6.15B).

The Visual Field Changes in Characteristic Ways after Damage to the Visual System

The precise pattern of projection of retinal ganglion cells to the lateral geniculate nucleus and the projection of these thalamic neurons to the cerebral cortex are exploited by the clinician to help identify the location of central nervous system damage. Damage at specific locations in the visual path produces characteristic changes in visual perception. Here, the topography of retinal projections is examined in greater detail and from a clinical perspective. (In Chapter 13 the characteristic deficits in visual reflex and visuomotor functions that occur when specific midbrain structures become damaged will be examined.)

Recall that the total field of view of both eyes when their position remains fixed is called the *visual field* (Figure 6.16) and that the visual field of each eye overlaps extensively with that of the other eye (Figures 6.4 and 6.16A). The visual field of each eye can be mapped and recorded by having the patient fixate his or her gaze at a site on a tangent screen with one eye closed (Figure 6.16). (The patient, in doing so, positions the eyes such that the fixation point falls on the fovea.) By moving a visual target of a particular size horizontally and laterally from the fixation point, the *blind spot* can be identified (Figure 6.16B). The perimeter of the visual field of the eye can be defined by moving the visual target from outside the field to inside. The extreme temporal portions of the visual fields, called the *temporal crescents*, are viewed *monocularly* by the ipsilateral eye. The nose prevents images in this portion of the visual field from reaching the contralateral retina. The visual field has an irregular rather than a circular shape because other facial structures (supraorbital ridge and eyebrow), in addition to the nose, block portions of the light path.

A change in the size and shape of the visual field (visual field defect) is often a signature of specific pathological processes (Table 6.1). Visual field defects after damage to six key components of the visual system are considered: (1) the optic nerve, (2) the optic chiasm, (3) the optic tract or the lateral geniculate nucleus, (5) the optic radiations, (6) the primary visual cortex (Figure 6.17). In addition, we also consider briefly the changes in visual perception after lesion of the association cortex.

Optic Nerve. Complete destruction of the optic nerve produces blindness in one eye (Figure 6.17A, Table 6.1). However, when a tumor or other pathological process infringes on the optic nerve from one side, a specific diminution of the visual field will follow, because ganglion cells in the various portions of the retina have a specific pattern of projection into the optic nerve. Often a *scotoma*, an area devoid of vision, occurs after optic nerve damage. When a scotoma occurs in the central field of vision, the patient notices reduced visual acuity, but, remarkably, does not do so with a peripheral scotoma. Optic nerve damage also produces characteristic changes in the appearance of the optic disk (Figure 6.3A) because the ganglion cell axons degenerate.

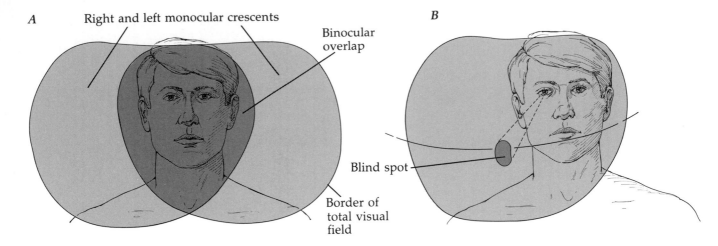

A Right and left monocular crescents

Binocular overlap

Blind spot

Border of total visual field

B

Figure 6.16 Schematic diagram of the visual field. *A.* Overlap of the visual fields of both eyes. *B.* Visual field for the right eye with the projection of the blind spot indicated. (Adapted from Patten, H. 1977. Neurological Differential Diagnosis. New York: Springer-Verlag.)

Optic Chiasm. Ganglion cell axons from the nasal retinae decussate in the optic chiasm (Figure 6.3B). These fibers transmit visual information from the temporal visual fields. The importance of knowing regional anatomy of the brain is clearly illustrated when injury to the optic chaism is considered. The pituitary gland is located ventral to the optic chiasm. It is common for pituitary tumors to damage the optic chiasm because, as the tumor grows, the bony floor of the sella (Figure 6.3B) forces the mass to expand dorsally, thereby encroaching on the optic chiasm from its ventral surface. This results in damage of the decussating fibers and produces a *bilateral temporal* visual field defect (Figure 6.17B, Table 6.1).

Table 6.1 Visual Field Defects[a]

Site of Lesion	Deficit
Optic nerve	Unilateral
Optic chiasm	Bitemporal heteronymous hemianopia
Contralateral Defects	
Optic tract	Homonymous hemianopia
Lateral geniculate nucleus	Homonymous hemianopia
Optic radiations	
Meyer's loop	Upper visual quadrant homonymous hemianopia
Main radiations	Homonymous hemianopia
Visual cortex	
Rostral	Homonymous hemianopia with macular sparing
Caudal	Homonymous hemianopia of the macular region

[a] Visual field defects are termed *homonymous* (or congruous) if they affect similar locations for the two eyes and are termed *heteronymous* (or incongruous) if they are different. Hemianopia is loss of half of the visual field in each eye.

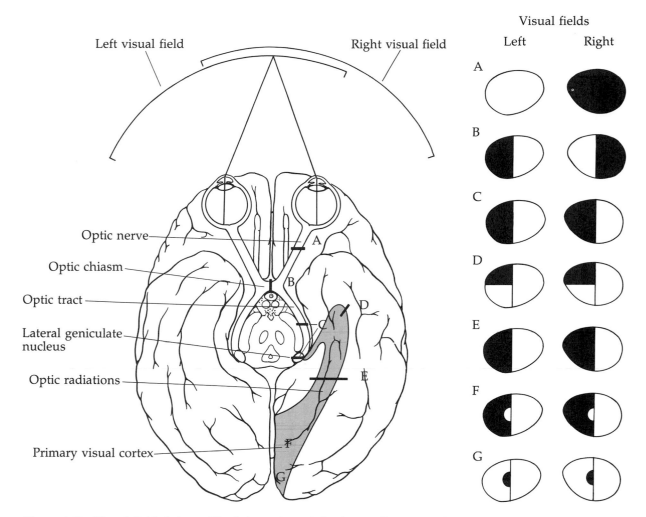

Figure 6.17 Visual field defects. The left portion of the figure illustrates schematically a horizontal view of the visual system. Visual field defects are shown
to the right. For each defect, the visual fields of the right and left eyes are separated. All defects as presented schematically. Rarely do such defects present
bilaterally symmetrical. **A.** Optic nerve; **B.** optic chiasm; **C.** optic tract (which is
similar to lateral geniculate nucleus; **D.** Meyer's loop component of optic radiations; **E.** main component of optic radiations; **F.** and **G.** primary visual cortex (F—
infarction producing macular sparing, G—direct trauma to the occipital pole).
(Adapted from Patten, H. 1977. Neurological Differential Diagnosis. New York:
Springer-Verlag.)

Optic Tract or the Lateral Geniculate Nucleus. Damage to the optic
tract or the lateral geniculate nucleus produces a defect in the *contralateral
visual field* (Figure 6.17C, Table 6.1).

Optic Radiations. Axons of lateral geniculate neurons course around
the rostral and lateral surfaces of the lateral ventricle (Figure 6.9) en route
to the primary visual cortex at the occipital pole. Neurons in the medial
portion of the lateral geniculate nucleus, which subserve vision from the
superior visual fields, have axons that course rostrally into the *temporal lobe*
before they course caudally to the primary visual cortex. This path is called
Meyer's loop. Temporal lobe lesions will result in a visual field defect lim-

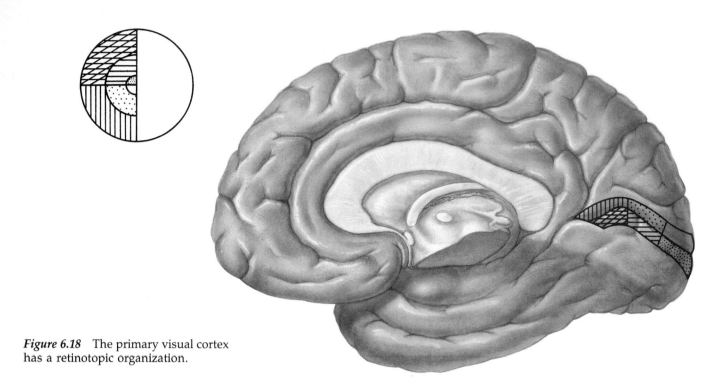

Figure 6.18   The primary visual cortex has a retinotopic organization.

ited to the *contralateral upper quadrant* of each visual field (Figure 6.17D, Table 6.1). This is sometimes referred to as a "pie in the sky" defect because it is often wedge-shaped. Neurons in the intermediate and lateral portions of the lateral geniculate nucleus, which subserve the macular region and the lower field, respectively, have a more direct course through the parietal lobe, where lesions on rare occasions produce visual field defects (Figure 6.17, Table 6.1).

Primary Visual Cortex.   Visual space is precisely represented in the primary visual cortex (Figure 6.18). The macular region is represented caudal to the perimacular and peripheral portions of the retina. The upper visual field is represented in the inferior bank of the calcarine fissure, and the lower visual field, in the superior bank. Whereas the macular region is a small portion of the retina, the area of primary visual cortex devoted to it is greatly expanded with respect to the remaining portions of the retina. This organization is similar to the overrepresentation of the fingertips in the primary somatic sensory cortex (Figure 5.17). The retinotopic organization of the primary visual cortex can be examined using PET. Figure 6.19 illustrates three PET scans obtained in sequence in the same individual. When presented with a stimulus to the macula portion of the retina (Figure 6.10A, top), there is increased emission of radioactive particles from the caudal portion of the visual cortex. The perimacula and peripheral stimuli result in emission of radioactive particles from progressively more rostral locations (Figure 6.19B and C). This illustrates a remarkable example in which the functional organization of the human cerebral cortex can be mapped with precision. Damage to the primary visual cortex, which commonly occurs after an infarction of the *posterior cerebral artery*, produces a contralateral visual field deficit that often spares the macular region of the visual field (Figure 6.17F, Table 6.1). Two factors

A   B   C

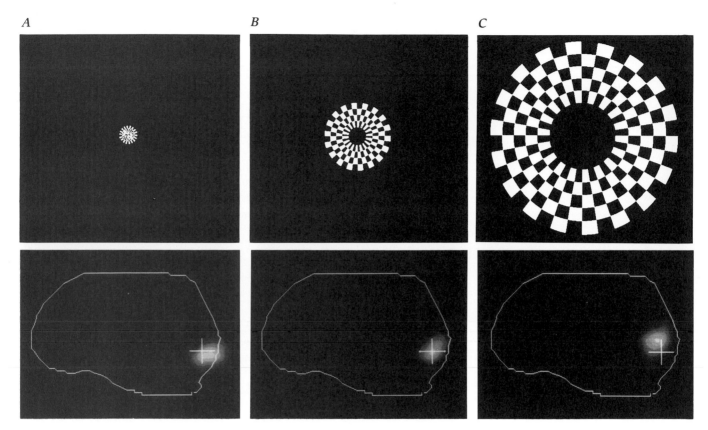

Figure 6.19   Positron emission tomography (PET) reveals the retinotopic organization of the human primary visual cortex. Top part of each panel illustrates
the particular stimulus the subject viewed while the scan (shown below) was
obtained. Bottom part of each panel is an ^{15}O-labeled water PET scan of a midsagittal slice. Each scan reflects the calculated difference between emission at rest
and during visual stimulation. *A.* Macular stimulation. *B.* Perimacular stimulation.
C. Peripheral stimulation. (Courtesy of Dr. Peter Fox, Washington University.)

contribute to macular sparing. First, the area of cortex that subserves
central vision is so large that a single infarction, or other pathological
process, rarely destroys it entirely. Second, in the case of infarctions, the
arterial supply to the cortical area that serves the macular region is provided primarily by the *posterior cerebral artery*, with a collateral supply
provided by the *middle cerebral artery*. Rarely will a traumatic injury to the
occipital pole produce a deficit involving the macular region only (Figure
6.17G, Table 6.1).

Higher Order Visual Areas and Association Cortex.   Alterations in visual
perception that are more complex than visual field defects are associated
with damage to the higher order visual areas and the association cortex.
Such deficits often involve more than one sensory modality and frequently differ in the two hemispheres. A particularly intriguing deficit is
called *sensory neglect*, which accompanies lesions of the posterior parietal
lobe in the nondominant hemisphere. In this condition a patient will
ignore visual information from the side contralateral to the lesion and

neglect that side of the body too. Other visual perceptual deficits involving the association areas of the parietal, temporal, and occipital lobes may result in spatial distortions or failure to recognize objects.

Summary

The retina is the peripheral portion of the visual system (Figures 6.1 and 6.2). Retinal neurons and their synaptic connections are organized into five layers. The cell bodies of photoreceptors are located in the *outer nuclear layer* (1): *cones* are the photoreceptors for *color vision and high-acuity vision, rods* are for *night vision*. Photoreceptors synapse on *bipolar cells* in the *outer synaptic (or plexiform) layer* (2), but their cell bodies are located in the *inner nuclear layer* (3). Bipolar cells, in turn, synapse on the *ganglion cells*—the output neurons of the retina—in the *inner synaptic (or plexiform) layer* (4). There are two additional retinal interneurons that mediate lateral interactions among photoreceptors, bipolar cells, and ganglion cells: amacrine cells and horizontal cells. A third interneuron, the *interplexiform cell*, transmits information from the inner synaptic layer to the outer synaptic layer. Ganglion cells are located in the *ganglion cell layer* (5) (Figure 6.2). Light must pass through the ganglion cells and interneurons before reaching the photoreceptors. Müller cells are the principal retinal neuroglia.

The retina receives a visual image that is transformed by the optical elements of the eye (Figure 6.4): the image becomes inverted and reversed. Images from one half of the *visual field* are projected on the *ipsilateral nasal hemiretina* and the *contralateral temporal hemiretina*. The axons from ganglion cells in the temporal hemiretina project into the *ipsilateral optic nerve* and *ipsilateral optic tract*. Ganglion cell axons from the nasal hemiretina project into the ipsilateral optic nerve, *decussate in the optic chiasm*, and course through the *contralateral optic tract*.

Ganglion cell axons destined for the midbrain leave the optic tract and course in the *brachium of the superior colliculus* (Figure 6.5A). A principal midbrain site for the ganglion cell axon terminals is the *superior colliculus*, a laminated structure. The *superficial layers* of the superior colliculus subserve *visuomotor and visual reflex function*, and the *deeper layers subserve orientation of the eyes, head, and body to salient stimuli*. The *pretectal nuclei*, where interneurons for the pupillary light reflex are located, also receive retinal input. The *lateral geniculate nucleus (dorsal division)* is the thalamic nucleus that receives the principal projection from the retina (Figure 6.7). Like other structures in the visual system, it too is laminated, and each of the *six layers* receives input from either the *ipsilateral or contralateral retina* (Figure 6.8), but visual information from the *contralateral visual hemifield*.

The lateral geniculate nucleus projects to the *primary visual cortex* (Figure 6.10) via the *optic radiations* (Figure 6.9), which course through the white matter of the temporal, parietal, and occipital lobes. Thalamic input terminates principally in *layer IV* (sublaminae a and c) of the primary visual cortex, and input from the ipsilateral and contralateral eyes remains segregated in this layer (Figure 6.11). This is the anatomical substrate of the *ocular dominance columns* (Figure 6.12). Clusters of neurons centered in the ocular dominance columns are color sensitive (Figure 6.13). The other type of column is the *orientation column* (Figure 6.14).

The primary visual cortex projects to the higher order visual areas of the occipital, parietal, and temporal lobes (Figure 6.15). At least two functional paths from the primary visual cortex are taken: one for *perception of stimulus form* and *color* (object recognition) and another for *perception of stimulus location and motion* (spatial vision).

Damage to the visual pathway produces characteristic changes in visual perception (Figures 6.17 and 6.18, Table 6.1): (1) complete transection of the optic nerve, *total blindness in the ipsilateral eye,* (2) optic chiasm, *bitemporal heteronymous hemianopia,* (3) optic tract and lateral geniculate nucleus, *contralateral homonymous hemianopia,* (4) optic radiation in temporal lobe (Meyer's loop), *contralateral upper quadrant homonymous hemianopia,* (5) optic radiations in parietal and occipital lobe, *contralateral homonymous hemianopia,* (6) primary visual cortex, *contralateral homonymous hemianopia with macular sparing.* ■

References

Berne, R. M., and Levy, M. N. 1983. Physiology. St. Louis: Mosby.

Bishop, P. O. 1984. Processing of Visual Information Within the Retinostriate System. In Darian-Smith, I. (ed.), Handbook of Physiology, Section 1: The Nervous System, Vol. III. Sensory Processes. Bethesda, Md.: American Physiological Society, pp. 341–424.

Brodal, A. 1981. Neurological Anatomy. New York: Oxford University Press.

Dowling, J. E., and Boycott, B. B. 1966. Organization of the primate retina: Electron microscopy. Proc. R. Soc. Lond. B 166:80–111.

Fox, P. T., Miezin, F. M., Allman, J. M., et al. 1987. Retinotopic organization of human visual cortex mapped with positron emission tomography. J. Neurosci. 7:913–922.

Hubel, D. H., and Wiesel, T. N. 1977. Ferrier Lecture: Functional architecture of macaque monkey visual cortex. Proc. R. Soc. Lond. B 198:1–59.

Kelly, J. P. 1985. Anatomy of the visual system. In Kandel, E. R., and Schwartz, J. H., Principles of Neural Science. New York: Elsevier, pp. 356–365.

Livingstone, M. S., and Hubel, D. H. 1984. Anatomy and physiology of a color system in the primate visual cortex. J. Neurosci. 4:309–356.

Schiller, P. H. 1984. The Superior Colliculus and Visual Function. In Darian-Smith, I. (ed.), Handbook of Physiology, Section 1: The Nervous System, Vol. III. Sensory Processes. Bethesda, Md.: American Physiological Society, pp. 457–506.

Selected Readings

Bailey, C. H., and Gouras, P. 1985. The retina and phototransduction. In Kandel, E. R., and Schwartz, J. H., Principles of Neural Science. New York: Elsevier, pp. 344–355.

DeYoe, E. A., and Van Essen, D. C. 1988. Concurrent processing streams in monkey visual cortex. Trends in Neurosci. 11:219–226.

Dowling, J. E. 1987. The Retina: An approachable part of the brain. Cambridge, Mass.: Harvard University Press.

Hendrickson, A. 1985. Dots, stripes and columns in monkey visual cortex. Trends in Neurosci. 8:406–410.

Huerta, M. F., and Harting, J. K. 1984. Connectional organization of the superior colliculus. Trends in Neurosci. 7:286–289.

Kandel, E. R. 1985. Processing of form and movement in the visual system. In Kandel, E. R., and Schwartz, J. H., Principles of Neural Science. New York: Elsevier, pp. 366–383.

Mishkin, M., Ungerleider, L. G., and Macko, K. A. 1983. Object vision: Two cortical pathways. Trends in Neurosci. 6:414–416.

Patten, H. 1977. Neurological Differential Diagnosis. New York: Springer-Verlag.

Stein, B. E. 1984. Development of the superior colliculus. Ann. Rev. Neurosci. 7:95–125.

Van Essen, D. C. 1979. Visual areas of the mammalian cerebral cortex. Ann. Rev. Neurosci. 2:227–263.

Van Essen, D. C., and Maunsell, J. H. R. 1983. Hierarchical organization and functional streams in the visual cortex. Trends in Neurosci. 6:370–375.

The Auditory and
Vestibular Systems

7

The Auditory and Vestibular Systems

The auditory system mediates the sense of hearing. Similar to the visual and somatic sensory systems, the central auditory connections are determined largely by the organizational plan of the peripheral receptive sheet. In addition, the auditory system, similar to these other sensory systems, consists of multiple parallel pathways, each path is hierarchically organized and is thought to subserve different aspects of auditory sensation. The vestibular system contributes to the sense of balance which, in contrast to hearing, is an aspect of sensation that is perceived only in special circumstances. However, the vestibular system plays a crucial role in the reflex control of limb, axial, and extraocular muscles, and the major central connection of the vestibular system reflects this function. The vestibulocochlear nerve (cranial nerve VIII) carries afferent information from the peripheral components of the auditory and vestibular systems, via separate cochlear and vestibular divisions, to the central nervous system.

In this chapter we first consider the general organizational plan of the auditory and vestibular systems. Then we examine key levels through the brain stem, levels in which structures that process auditory and vestibular information are located. Because motor pathways (the vestibulospinal tracts and the medial longitudinal fasciculus) originate from the vestibular nuclei, we will examine the central vestibular connections in greater detail in Chapter 9, when the motor systems are considered. Finally, the connections of the auditory system with the thalamus and cerebral cortex are examined.

Parallel Ascending Auditory Pathways May Be Involved in Different Aspects of Hearing

The auditory receptors, the *hair cells*, are located within the temporal bone in a structure called the *cochlea* (Figure 7.2). There is a systematic relationship between the location of a hair cell in the cochlea (see later) and the tonal frequency to which it is most sensitive. This differential frequency sensitivity of hair cells is the basis of the *tonotopic organization* of the receptive sheet, an organization that is present at virtually every level of the auditory system. Hair cells are innervated by the distal processes of bipolar neurons, and the central processes of the bipolar neurons form the *cochlear division* of the *vestibulocochlear (eighth cranial) nerve.* These axons project to the *cochlear nuclei,* which are located in the rostral medulla (Figure 7.1A). There are two divisions of the cochlear nuclei: *dorsal* and *ventral cochlear nuclei.* Both divisions ultimately project to the *inferior colliculus,* which is located in the midbrain. However, the routes by which the connections are made between the cochlear nuclei and the inferior colliculus differ. Both the dorsal and the ventral cochlear nuclei project to the contralateral inferior colliculus via an ascending pathway called the *lateral lemniscus.* In addition, the ventral cochlear nucleus projects to the *superior olivary complex,* a cluster of nuclei in the caudal pons. Neurons in this pontine nuclear complex, in turn, project to the inferior colliculus bilaterally. The projection from the ventral cochlear nucleus to the superior olivary complex is thought to be important in *localizing sound,* whereas the projection from the dorsal and ventral cochlear nuclei that ascend directly to the inferior colliculus may be important in other aspects of auditory perception, for example, *recognizing patterns of sound.* The ascending auditory paths on each side of the brain stem carry information from both ears. This is because there are several levels at which auditory information crosses the midline through decussations and commissures. The clinical significance of this organization is that brain stem damage on one side, unless it destroys the cochlear nuclei (or nerve), cannot cause deafness in one ear.

In sequence, the next segment of the ascending auditory pathway is from the inferior colliculus to the thalamic auditory nucleus, the *medial geniculate nucleus.* The projection from the medial geniculate nucleus to the primary auditory cortex, which is called the *auditory radiations,* terminates within the lateral sulcus (also called the Sylvian fissure) on the superior surface of the temporal lobe. The primary auditory cortex is located on two gyri (see Figure 7.9) that are oriented approximately orthogonal to the temporal lobe gyri visible on the surface of the cerebral hemisphere, the *Heschl's gyri.* The primary auditory cortex is surrounded by *higher order cortical auditory areas,* which are located on both the superior and the lateral surfaces of the temporal lobe in the superior temporal gyrus.

The Vestibular Nuclei Receive Monosynaptic Input from the Vestibular Division of the Eighth Cranial Nerve

The peripheral vestibular apparatus (Figure 7.2) includes the semicircular canals, the utricle, and the saccule. These structures are innervated by the *vestibular division* of the eighth cranial nerve. The pattern of afferent innervation of the receptor cells by the *vestibular bipolar neurons* is similar to that of the cochlea. The vestibular division of the eighth cranial nerve courses with the cochlear division and enters the brain stem at the lateral pontomedullary junction. The vestibular division terminates principally in four nuclei in the rostral medulla and caudal pons, the *vestibular nuclei* (Figure 7.1A, B). Thus, the terminations of the vestibular and cochlear divisions are separate and distinct. The efferent projections from the vestibular nuclei are complex. The major projections are to the spinal cord and to brain stem nuclei involved in the control of extraocular muscles. These projections are better described as *motor pathways* than ascending sensory pathways. The projections of the vestibular nuclei to the spinal cord, which form the vestibulospinal tracts, are described in Chapter 9. The connections of the vestibular nuclei with the extraocular nuclei are considered in Chapter 13. The vestibular system is unique in that it is the only sensory system whose primary sensory neurons project directly to the cerebellum (Chapter 10).

In addition to the "motor" projections of the vestibular nuclei, there is also a small ascending, or "sensory," projection to the cerebral cortex. The pathway is not well understood, but the thalamic relay nucleus is a portion of the *ventral posterior nucleus.* The vestibular cortex is located in the parietal lobe (Figure 7.9) in cytoarchitectonic area 5, which is directly behind the primary somatic sensory cortex (see Figure 5.18). In Chapter 5 we saw that the ventral posterior nucleus is the somatic sensory relay

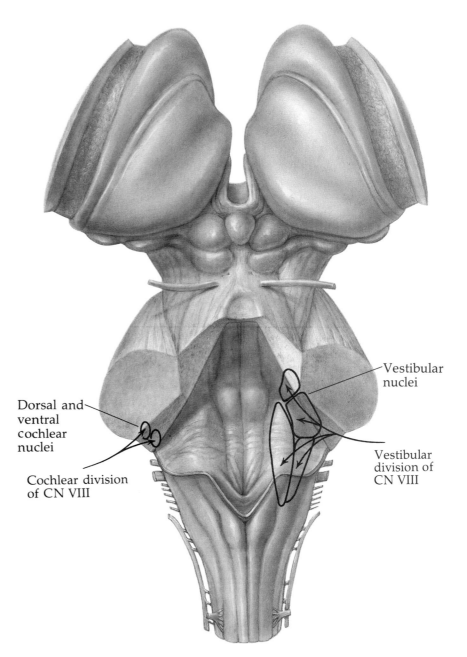

Vestibular nuclei

Dorsal and ventral cochlear nuclei

Cochlear division of CN VIII

Vestibular division of CN VIII

Figure 7.1 *A.* Brain stem projections of the cochlear division (left) and the vestibular division (left) of the vestibulocochlear nerve. *B.* General organization of the auditory system. *C.* General organization of the vestibular system.

nucleus. One function of the vestibular projection to the parietal lobe may be to integrate vestibular information with somatic sensory information. This convergence of sensory information may be important in the perception of the position of the body in space and for controlling body movements. This ascending vestibular pathway may also be important in the perception of body acceleration or vertigo.

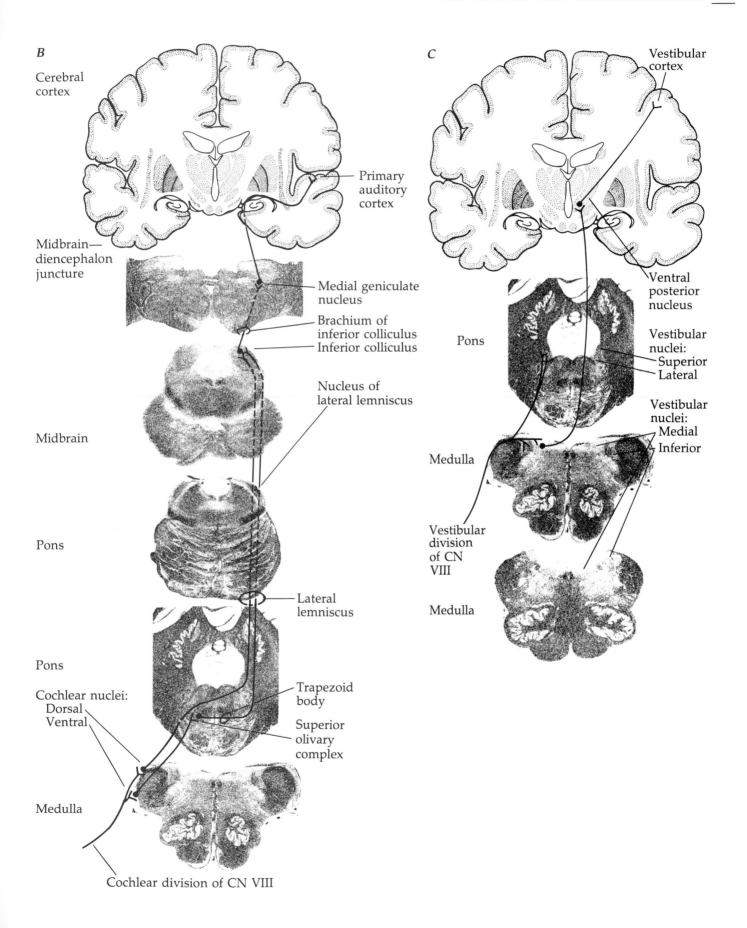

B

Cerebral cortex

Midbrain—diencephalon juncture

Midbrain

Pons

Pons

Cochlear nuclei:
Dorsal
Ventral

Medulla

Primary auditory cortex

Medial geniculate nucleus

Brachium of inferior colliculus

Inferior colliculus

Nucleus of lateral lemniscus

Lateral lemniscus

Trapezoid body

Superior olivary complex

Cochlear division of CN VIII

C

Vestibular cortex

Pons

Medulla

Vestibular division of CN VIII

Medulla

Ventral posterior nucleus

Vestibular nuclei:
Superior
Lateral

Vestibular nuclei:
Medial
Inferior

A

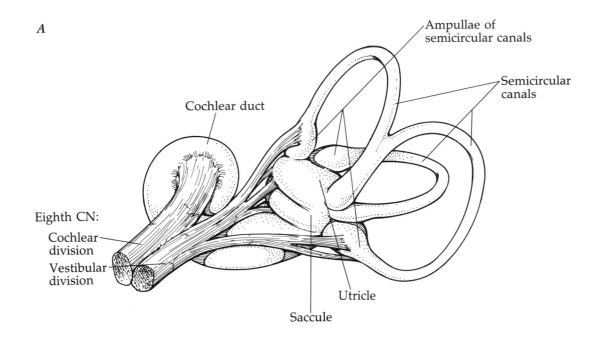

Cochlear duct

Ampullae of
semicircular canals

Semicircular
canals

Eighth CN:

Cochlear
division

Vestibular
division

Utricle

Saccule

B

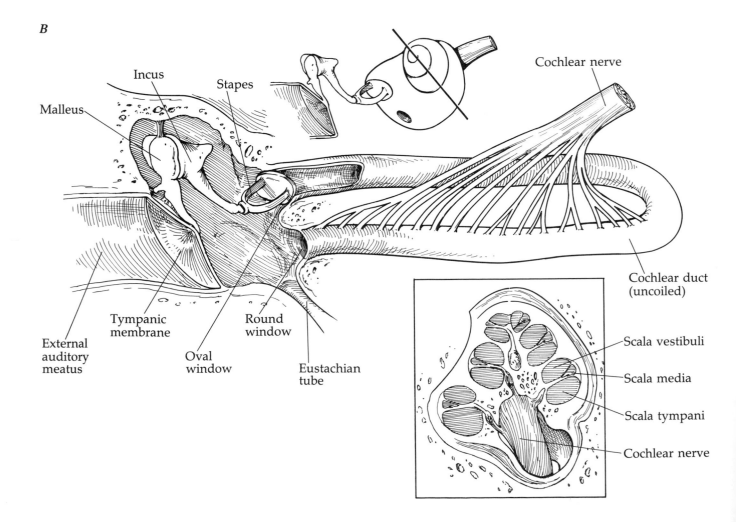

Incus

Stapes

Cochlear nerve

Malleus

Tympanic
membrane

Round
window

External
auditory
meatus

Oval
window

Eustachian
tube

Cochlear duct
(uncoiled)

Scala vestibuli

Scala media

Scala tympani

Cochlear nerve

C

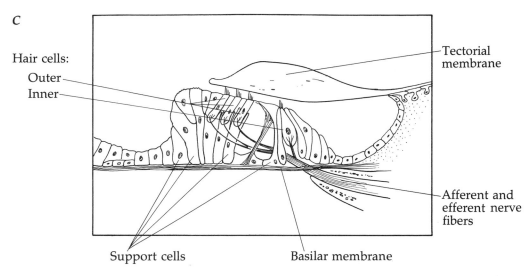

Hair cells:
Outer
Inner

Tectorial
membrane

Afferent and
efferent nerve
fibers

Support cells   Basilar membrane

Figure 7.2   *A.* The peripheral auditory and vestibular structures and innervation
by the cochlear and vestibular divisions of CN VIII. *B.* The middle ear and inner
ear. A straightened out and schematic view of the cochlea is depicted with innervation by the cochlear nerve. The upper inset in part B shows the coiled cochlear and the line indicates the plane of the section shown in the inset in the lower
portion of part B. *C.* Expanded view of a section through the cochlear duct illustrating the organ of Corti. (*C,* Adapted from Dallos, P. 1984. Peripheral mechanisms of hearing. In Darian-Smith, I. (ed.), Handbook of Physiology, Section 1:
The Nervous System, Vol. 3. Sensory Processes. Bethesda, Md.: American Physiological Society, pp. 595–637.)

The Membranous Labyrinth Contains the Peripheral
Auditory Apparatus and Vestibular Apparatus

The peripheral auditory apparatus and vestibular apparatus are located in the inner ear which consists of (1) *bony labyrinth,* cavities in
petrous portion of the temporal bone, and (2) *membranous labyrinth,* a
complex sac within the bony labyrinth (Figure 7.2A). Much of the membranous labyrinth is filled with *endolymph,* a fluid resembling intracellular
fluid in its ionic constituents. In contrast, *perilymph,* a fluid resembling
extracellular fluid and cerebrospinal fluid, is external to the membranous
labyrinth. The membranous labyrinth contains the cochlear duct, the
three semicircular canals, and the saccule and utricle (Figure 7.2A). Another name for the semicircular canals, utricle, and saccule is the *vestibular
labyrinth.*

The cochlear duct is a coiled structure within the temporal bone
(Figure 7.2A). It is drawn uncoiled in Figure 7.2B. Located within the
cochlear duct is the organ of Corti (Figure 7.2C), the component of the
auditory system that transduces sounds into neuronal potentials. The
organ of Corti consists of the auditory receptor cells, termed *hair cells,*
arranged in a spiral. It rests on the basilar membrane and is covered by
the tectorial membrane (see later). There are two kinds of hair cells in
the organ of Corti and their names reflect their position with respect to
the axis of the coiled cochlea: *inner* and *outer hair cells.* The inner hair cells
are arranged in a single row, whereas the outer hair cells are arranged
in three rows. Compared with the outer hair cells, the inner hair cells are
much fewer in number. An important research goal is to determine the
functions of the two classes of hair cells. The hair cells are innervated by

bipolar neurons, whose cell bodies are located in the *spiral ganglion.* The central axons of bipolar cells course in the *cochlear* division of the *eighth* cranial (*vestibulocochlear*) nerve. Most axons in the cochlear division innervate the inner hair cells, which may receive convergent input from 10 fibers. In contrast, the outer hair cells are innervated by a minority of nerve fibers.

The transductive process is largely related to the mechanical properties of the cochlea. Briefly, pressure changes, resulting from sound waves, are conducted by the *tympanic membrane* and the *middle ear ossicles* into the fluid-filled *scala vestibuli* of the inner ear (Figure 7.2B). The other two compartments of the inner ear, the *scala media* and the *scala tympani,* are also filled with fluid (Figure 7.2B). Pressure changes are conducted from the scala vestibuli through the scala media to the scala tympani. This conduction of pressure changes sets up a traveling wave in the compliant *basilar membrane* (Figure 7.2C), on which the hair cells and their support structures rest. The traveling wave results in the generation of shearing forces between the basilar membrane and the less compliant *tectorial membrane.* The receptor cells have stereocilia that are embedded in the tectorial membrane.[1] When the stereocilia are bent by the shearing forces, changes in membrane conductance of hair cells occur.

Sounds establish a complex traveling wave on the basilar membrane. *High-frequency sounds* generate a wave on the basilar membrane with a peak amplitude close to the base of the cochlea, and consequently these sounds activate the *basal* hair cells. As the frequency of the sound source decreases, the location of the peak amplitude of the wave on the basilar membrane shifts continuously toward the cochlear apex. This results in the activation of hair cells that are located closer to the *apex of the cochlea.* Thus, the mechanical properties of the basilar membrane determine the *tonotopic organization* of the receptive sheet. We will see that this organization underlies the topography of connections in the central auditory pathways.

Receptor cells are also located in specialized regions of the semicircular canals (termed *ampulae*) and the saccule and utricle (termed *maculae*). Like the auditory receptor cells, the vestibular receptors are also hair cells, and they are innervated by the distal processes of bipolar neurons, but these receptor cells are located in *Scarpa's ganglion.* The mechanism by which vestibular receptors are activated is different from that of the auditory receptors. The hair cells of the semicircular canals are covered by a gelatinous mass (termed the cupula). Head movement induces the endolymph within the canals to flow, displacing the gelatinous mass, which in turn deflects the hair cell stereocilia. The utricle and saccule also have a gelatinous covering over their maculae. Calcium carbonate crystals, embedded in the gelatin, rest on the stereocilia of the hair cells. Head movement causes the crystals to deform the gelatinous mass thereby deflecting the stereocilia.[2] The semicircular canals, utricle, and saccule each have a different orientation thereby conferring selective sensitivity to head movement in different directions. In the following sections we examine the central connections of the vestibular and cochlear divisions of the eighth cranial nerve.

---

[1] It is believed that only the stereocilia of the outer hair cells embed in the tectorial membrane.

[2] The saccule and utricle are sometimes called the otolith organs because otolith is the term for the calcium carbonate crystals.

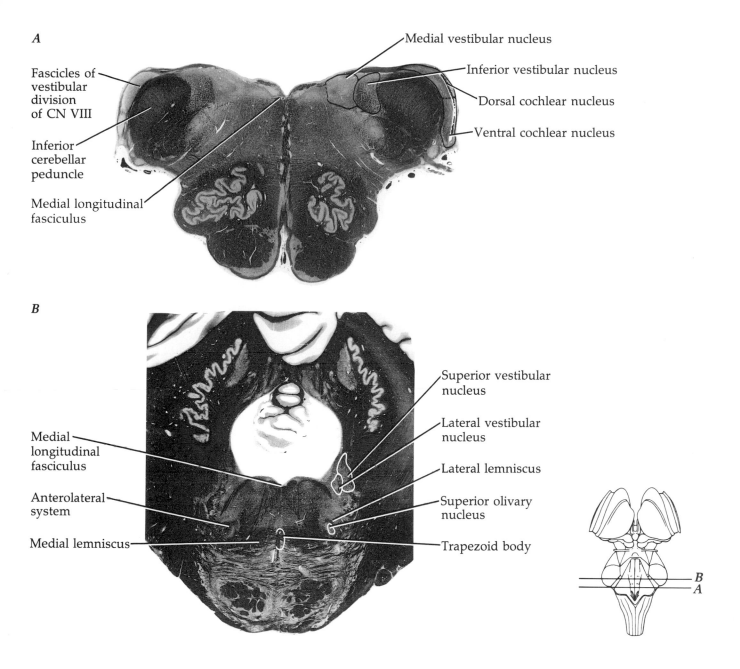

A

Fascicles of vestibular division of CN VIII

Inferior cerebellar peduncle

Medial longitudinal fasciculus

Medial vestibular nucleus

Inferior vestibular nucleus

Dorsal cochlear nucleus

Ventral cochlear nucleus

B

Medial longitudinal fasciculus

Anterolateral system

Medial lemniscus

Superior vestibular nucleus

Lateral vestibular nucleus

Lateral lemniscus

Superior olivary nucleus

Trapezoid body

The Vestibular Nuclei Contribute Axons to the Medial Longitudinal Fasciculus

The vestibular nuclei occupy the floor of the fourth ventricle in the dorsolateral medulla and pons (Figure 7.1A). There are four separate vestibular nuclei: (1) inferior, (2) medial, (3) lateral, (4) superior (Figure 7.3). The vestibular nuclei contribute axons to the vestibulospinal tracts, which are important in the maintenance of balance (Chapter 9). The vestibular nuclei also contribute axons to the *medial longitudinal fasciculus*, which is a brain stem path that interconnects nuclei that play essential roles in the control of eye movements. It is not yet understood which vestibular nucleus gives rise to the ascending "sensory" pathway to the ventral posterior nucleus of the thalamus. In both medulla and pons, the sulcus

Figure 7.3 Myelin-stained transverse sections through the medulla, at the level of the cochlear nuclei *(A)* and caudal pons *(B)*. Inset shows planes of sections.

limitans (Chapter 2) marks the medial boundary of the vestibular nuclei. Note in Figure 7.3B that the vestibular nuclei are adjacent to the cerebellum; this can also be appreciated in Figure 7.1A, where the cerebellum has been removed but portions of the cerebellar peduncles remain. This general region is termed the *cerebellopontine angle*. The cochlear nuclei also are located in this region (as are other cranial nuclei and nerves—Chapter 13). As a consequence of the localization of various cranial nerves, and associated nuclei, the growth of tumors in the cerebellopontine angle produces a somewhat characteristic set of neurological signs.

The Topography of Connections between Brain Stem Auditory Nuclei Provides Insight into the Functions of Parallel Ascending Auditory Pathways

An understanding of the functions of the lower order auditory relay nuclei can be gained by considering the connections between the various nuclei. The cochlear division of the vestibulocochlear nerve terminates in the cochlear nuclei. There are two other major groups of auditory relay nuclei in the brain stem: the superior olivary nuclei and the inferior colliculus. Each of these nuclei is located in a different division of the brain stem. The cochlear nuclei are located in the medulla; the superior olivary nuclei, in the pons; and the inferior colliculus, in the midbrain. Although the connections among the cochlear nuclei, superior olive, and inferior colliculus are complex, they provide important insights into the function of parallel auditory pathways originating from these nuclei, insights that are an essential first step toward understanding the anatomical substrates of auditory perception.

The Cochlear Nuclei Are the First Central Nervous System Relays for Auditory Information

There are two cochlear nuclei, the *dorsal and ventral cochlear nuclei*,[3] and they are located in the rostral medulla on the lateral surface of the inferior cerebellar peduncle (Figures 7.1A and 7.3A). The dorsal and ventral cochlear nuclei have different patterns of efferent connections. Neurons in the ventral cochlear nucleus project to the *superior olivary complex* (Figure 7.3B), the first site in the auditory pathway for *binaural convergence*, and to the *inferior colliculus*. Neurons in the dorsal cochlear nucleus bypass the superior olivary complex and synapse in the contralateral inferior colliculus. The direct projections to the inferior colliculus from the dorsal and ventral cochlear nuclei are largely *monaural*.

The Superior Olivary Complex Is the First Site for Binaural Convergence

The superior olivary complex is located in the caudal pons, lateral to the medial lemniscus and dorsal to the spinal anterolateral fibers (Fig-

---

[3] The ventral cochlear nucleus is separated into two subdivisions, the *anteroventral* and *posteroventral* cochlear nuclei, by the entering eighth nerve fibers.

ure 7.3B). The nuclear complex contains three components: the *medial superior olivary nucleus,* the *lateral superior olivary nucleus,* and the *nucleus of the trapezoid body.* (The superior olivary nuclei should be distinguished from the inferior olivary nucleus [Figure 7.3A] which contains neurons that project to the cerebellum.) The superior olivary complex is important in the localization of sounds. To understand how the anatomical connections between the ventral cochlear nucleus and the superior olivary complex contribute to this function we must first briefly consider how sound is localized. A sound source is localized, from one side or the other, by two means depending on its frequency: (1) *low-frequency* sounds activate the two ears at somewhat different times (*interaural time differences*): (2) *high-frequency* sounds activate the two ears with somewhat different intensities (*interaural intensity differences*). This is the "duplex theory" of sound localization.

Neurons in the *medial superior olivary nucleus* are tuned to low-frequency stimuli. They are sensitive to *interaural time differences,* and the projection from the ventral cochlear nucleus is thought to contribute to this sensitivity. Individual neurons in the medial superior olive receive monosynaptic connections from the ventral cochlear nuclei on both sides, and these inputs are *spatially segregated on their dendrites* (Figure 7.4A). In contrast, the neurons in the *lateral superior olivary nucleus* are tuned to high-frequency stimuli and are sensitive to *interaural intensity differences.* The anatomical connections that this nucleus makes with other auditory nuclei contribute to the sensitivity of its neurons to interaural intensity differences. The lateral superior olive receives a monosynaptic excitatory connection from the ipsilateral ventral cochlear nucleus and a disynaptic inhibitory connection from the contralateral ventral cochlear nucleus, relayed through the nucleus of the trapezoid body (Figure 7.4A). The components of the ventral cochlear nucleus that provide the auditory input to the superior olivary complex are thought to play an important role in sound localization. Conversely, because the projections of the dorsal cochlear nucleus spare the superior olivary complex, it is believed not to function in the localization of sounds. For other reasons, based in part on the complex physiological properties of its constituent neurons, the dorsal cochlear nucleus is thought to function in *pattern recognition.* The neurons of the ventral cochlear nucleus that project directly to the contralateral inferior colliculus may also function in auditory pattern recognition.

The paths by which the neurons of the dorsal and ventral cochlear nuclei reach the superior olivary complex or the inferior colliculus are dissimilar. The axons of cells in the dorsal cochlear nucleus course in the *dorsal acoustic stria,* one of three paths that auditory fibers take to decussate. The other two paths for decussating axons, the *intermediate acoustic stria* and the *trapezoid body,* are taken by neurons of the ventral cochlear nuclei. The locations of these paths are shown in Figure 7.4B, a simplified drawing of the caudal pontine section. The trapezoid body is the largest of the three paths and is the only one visible on sections through the caudal pons (Figure 7.3B). Axons of the trapezoid body intersect the medial lemniscus, making it difficult to see in some levels. The dorsal and intermediate acoustic striae and the trapezoid body converge to form the *lateral lemniscus,* a pathway that is present from the caudal pons (Figure 7.3B) to the midbrain.

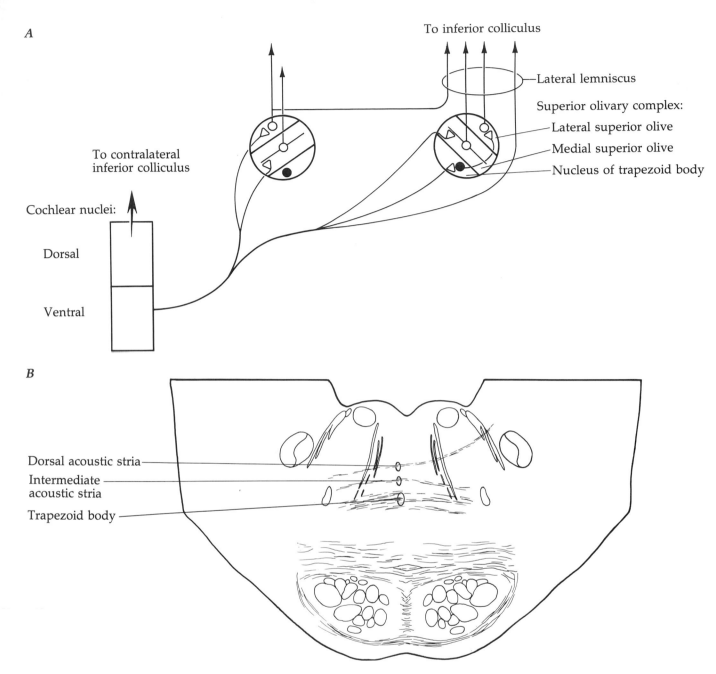

Figure 7.4 A. Key connections between the cochlear nuclei in the medulla and the superior olivary complex in the pons. The axons of the dorsal cochlear nucleus decussate in the dorsal acoustic stria en route to the inferior colliculus; the decussating axons of the ventral cochlear nucleus and superior olivary complex course in the intermediate acoustic stria and the trapezoid body. *B.* Paths taken by decussating auditory axons in the pons.

The Vestibulocochlear Nerve Also Contains Efferent Fibers

A small number of neurons in the superior olivary complex give rise to axons that project back to the cochlea, via the vestibulocochlear nerve. This efferent pathway is called the *olivocochlear bundle.* The neurons that contribute to this efferent path are located in the superior olivary complex on both the *ipsilateral* and *contralateral* sides with respect to the cochlea to which these axons project. The neurons contributing axons to the olivocochlear bundle receive auditory input directly from the cochlear nuclei, as well as auditory information relayed from higher levels of the auditory pathway. The axons of the olivocochlear bundle innervate both inner and outer hair cells. The precise function of the olivocochlear bundle remains a mystery. It is thought to regulate the flow of auditory information into the central nervous system because electrical stimulation of its fibers suppresses auditory responses in the cochlear nerve. The mechanism by which this suppression occurs may involve a change in the mechanical coupling of the auditory receptor with the basilar membrane. Outer hair cells actually contract when acetylcholine, which is thought to be the neurotransmitter of the olivocochlear bundle, is directly applied in in vitro examination. This mechanical change, if it also occurs *in vivo*, would be likely to cause the stereocilia to withdraw somewhat from the tectorial membrane.

Auditory Brain Stem Pathways Ascend in the Lateral Lemniscus

The *lateral lemniscus* is a discrete bundle of axons in the caudal pons (Figure 7.3B), but it is clearly visualized as a separate tract only in the rostral pons (Figure 7.5) and midbrain (Figure 7.6B). (The lateral lemniscus should be distinguished from the medial lemniscus [Figure 7.5], which relays somatic sensory information to the thalamus.) Virtually all of the fibers in the lateral lemniscus terminate in the inferior colliculus but many also send branches into the *nucleus of the lateral lemniscus,* which is centered within the structure for which it is named (Figure 7.5). (The nucleus of the lateral lemniscus also sends many of its axons to the inferior colliculus and even some directly to the medial geniculate nucleus.) At this rostral pontine level (Figure 7.5), the ascending somatic sensory pathways—the medial lemniscus and the anterolateral system—join with the lateral lemniscus to form a continuous band of myelinated axons that roughly divides the pontine tegmentum from the basal region. Recall that the tectum of the brain stem is the component located dorsal to the cerebral aqueduct. The pontine tectum is poorly developed compared with the midbrain tectum (see next section).

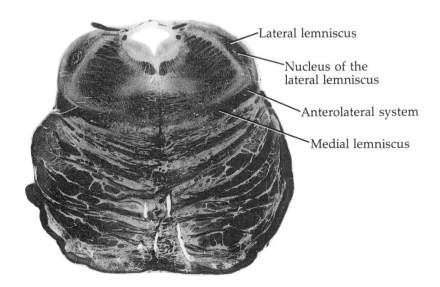

- Lateral lemniscus
- Nucleus of the lateral lemniscus
- Anterolateral system
- Medial lemniscus

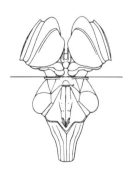

Figure 7.5 Myelin-stained transverse section through the rostral pons. Inset shows plane of section.

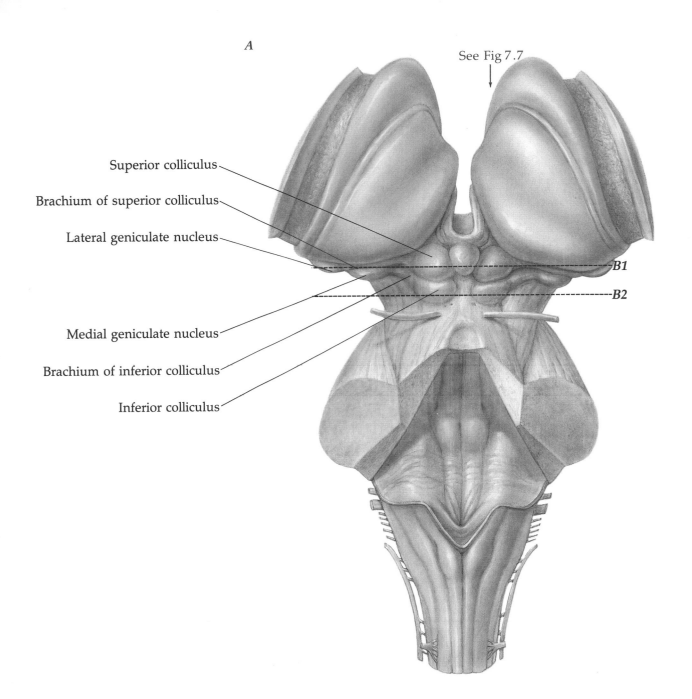

A

See Fig 7.7

Superior colliculus

Brachium of superior colliculus

Lateral geniculate nucleus

B1

B2

Medial geniculate nucleus

Brachium of inferior colliculus

Inferior colliculus

The Inferior Colliculus Is Located in the Midbrain Tectum

The inferior colliculus is located on the dorsal surface of the midbrain, caudal to the superior colliculus (Figure 7.6A). Even though both colliculi are located in the midbrain tectum, their roles in stimulus processing are fundamentally different. The superior colliculus is a component of the visual system (Chapter 6). It receives visual input in parallel with the lateral geniculate nucleus and functions in visuomotor control. In contrast, the inferior colliculus is an auditory relay nucleus. Here, the regional anatomy of the midbrain is briefly considered followed by a discussion of the organization of the inferior colliculus.

B1

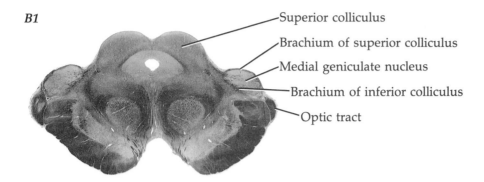

Superior colliculus

Brachium of superior colliculus

Medial geniculate nucleus

Brachium of inferior colliculus

Optic tract

B2

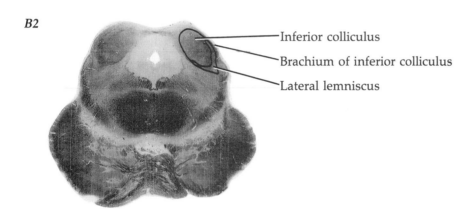

Inferior colliculus

Brachium of inferior colliculus

Lateral lemniscus

Figure 7.6 The inferior colliculi and medial geniculate nuclei are shown on the surface of the brain stem view *(A)* and in myelin-stained transverse sections through the rostral *(B1)* and caudal *(B2)* midbrain. The dashed lines indicate the planes of section in part B. The arrow in A indicates the plane of section in Figure 7.7.

The internal structure of the rostral and caudal portions of the midbrain is easier to distinguish than the various levels of the medulla or pons because of the presence of two landmarks in the tegmentum: the *decussation of the superior cerebellar peduncle,* and the *red nuclei* (Figure 7.6B). Both of these structures are key components of the motor system and will be discussed in Chapters 9 and 10. The decussation of the superior cerebellar peduncle is a white matter structure centered over the midline and clearly distinguishable from the two red nuclei, which are roughly spherical in cross section. (Because of the juxtaposition of these structures, the decussation of the superior cerebellar peduncle is sometimes called the "white nucleus" even though it does not contain neuronal cell bodies.)

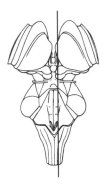

Figure 7.7 The superior and inferior colliculi can be identified on this sagittal section through the brain stem. The plane of section is indicated by the arrow in Figure 7.6.

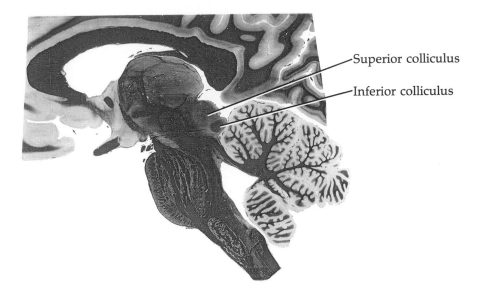

Superior colliculus

Inferior colliculus

We see that the presence of the decussation of the superior cerebellar peduncle marks the level at which the inferior colliculus is located, whereas the red nuclei mark the level of the superior colliculus. Ventrally, these two levels of the midbrain each contain the basis pedunculi and the substantia nigra. The superior and inferior colliculi are cut parasagittally in Figure 7.7; the plane of section is indicated in Figure 7.6A by the arrow.

The inferior colliculus contains three component nuclei: the central nucleus of the inferior colliculus, the external nucleus, and the pericentral nucleus. The central nucleus of the inferior colliculus is the principal nucleus. It receives convergent input from three sources: (1) the direct pathway from the *contralateral dorsal and ventral cochlear* nuclei, (2) pathways originating from the *ipsilateral and contralateral superior olivary nuclei*, and (3) axons from the *nucleus of the lateral lemniscus*. All of these projections, however, ascend from the medulla and pons in the lateral lemniscus. The function of the *central nucleus* is to process the physical characteristics of sounds for auditory perception. This nucleus is the only component of the inferior colliculus that is *laminated*. Lamination is a way of packaging neurons with similar functional attributes or connections. For example, in the dorsal horn of the spinal cord (Chapter 5), neurons in lamina I relay information from nociceptors and thermoreceptors to the ventral posterior lateral nucleus of the thalamus, whereas lamina II contains interneurons. In the lateral geniculate nucleus (Chapter 6), neurons in different laminae receive input from one eye or the other. In the central nucleus of the inferior colliculus, neurons in a single lamina are maximally sensitive to *similar tonal frequencies*. The function of the other nuclei of the inferior colliculus is much less clear. Studies in which lesions are placed in the various inferior colliculus nuclei of experimental animals suggest that the *external* and *pericentral nuclei* play a role in *acousticomotor function*, such as the orientation of the head and body axis to auditory stimuli.

The inferior colliculus projects to the thalamus via a tract that is located just below the dorsal surface of the midbrain, the *brachium of the inferior colliculus* (Figure 7.6A). As different as the superior and inferior colliculi are, so too are their brachia. The brachium of the superior colliculus brings afferent information to the superior colliculus, whereas the brachium of the inferior colliculus is an efferent pathway carrying axons to the medial geniculate nucleus (see next section).

The Medial Geniculate Nucleus Contains a Laminated Division That Is Tonotopically Organized

The *medial geniculate nucleus* is a landmark on the inferior surface of the thalamus, medial to the lateral geniculate nucleus and rostral to the superior colliculus (Figure 7.6A). The medial geniculate nucleus is composed of several divisions. The principal auditory relay nucleus is the *ventral medial geniculate nucleus* (Figures 7.6B and 7.8). It is often referred to as the medial geniculate nucleus without reference to its location. The spatial relationships between the medial and lateral geniculate nuclei and the superior colliculus can be appreciated by examining the dorsal view of the brain stem (Figure 7.6A) and the sections through the rostral midbrain (Figure 7.6B1), the midbrain–diencephalic junction, and the caudal diencephalon. A coronal section through the ventral division of the medial geniculate nucleus (Figure 7.8A) shows that it is interposed between the lateral geniculate nucleus and the main portion of the ventral thalamus. The section in Figure 7.8B is a transverse section through the midbrain–diencephalic junction (it is cut approximately orthogonal to the one shown in Figure 7.8A; see inset). Comparison of these two sections may help to create a "mind's eye" reconstruction of the spatial relations of these nuclei in three dimensions.

Although not observable on the myelin-stained sections shown in Figures 7.6B1 and 7.8, the ventral division of the medial geniculate nucleus is *laminated*. It receives the major ascending auditory projection from the central nucleus of the inferior colliculus which also is laminated. As the central nucleus of the inferior colliculus is tonotopically organized, so too is the ventral division of the medial geniculate nucleus. For both structures, lamination is a morphological correlate of precise tonotopic organization. In contrast, the dorsal division of the medial geniculate nucleus is not laminated. The dorsal division receives its major input from the pericentral nucleus of the inferior colliculus, which is not laminated. The ventral medial geniculate nucleus, in turn, projects to the *primary auditory cortex*, which is also tonotopically organized. By contrast, the dorsal medial geniculate nucleus projects to higher order auditory cortical areas, areas that do not have the precise tonotopic organization that the primary area does. The *auditory radiations*, the projections from the medial geniculate nuclei to the auditory cortical areas in the lateral sulcus, pass through the *sublenticular* portion of the internal capsule (see Figure 11.6). This portion is termed sublenticular because it lies beneath the lenticular nucleus, which is composed of the putamen and the globus pallidus (Chapter 11). Recall that the projection from the ventral posterior nucleus (Chapter 5) to the primary somatic sensory cortex is through the posterior limb of the internal capsule.

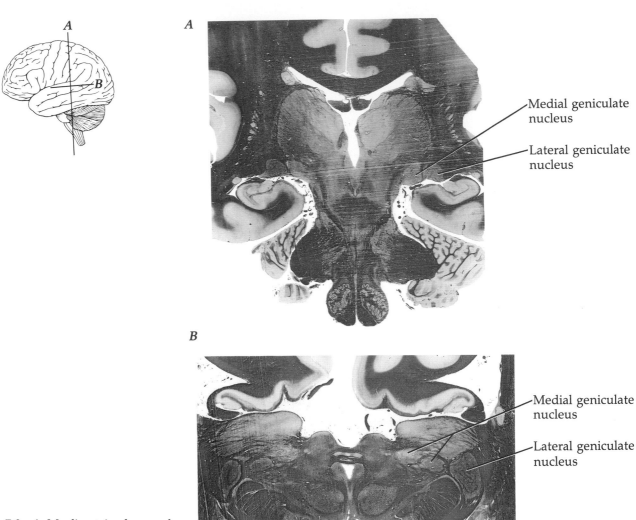

A

Medial geniculate
nucleus

Lateral geniculate
nucleus

B

Medial geniculate
nucleus

Lateral geniculate
nucleus

Figure 7.8 A. Myelin-stained coronal section through the medial geniculate nucleus. *B.* Transverse section through the midbrain–diencephalic juncture. Inset shows planes of section.

The Auditory Cortical Areas Are Located on the Superior Surface of the Temporal Lobe

The *primary auditory cortex* is located on *Heschl's gyri* in the temporal lobe and corresponds to cytoarchitectonic area 41. These gyri are located largely within the lateral sulcus (Figure 7.9). The primary auditory cortex, like other areas of the cerebral cortex, has a columnar organization. At least two types of columns have been identified. *Isofrequency columns* form long strips, and *binaural columns* are oriented at a right angle to them. The anatomical basis of the isofrequency strips is the tonotopically organized projection from the laminated portion of the medial geniculate nucleus. This is a dense projection and is directed predominantly to layers

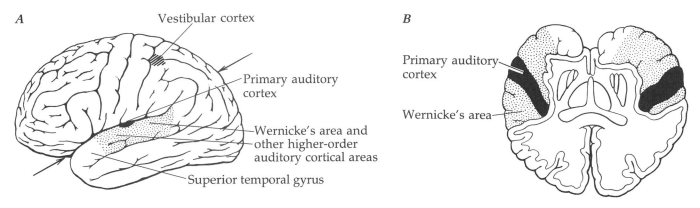

Figure 7.9 The locations of the primary and higher order auditory cortical areas are shown on the lateral cerebral hemisphere view *(A)* and in schematic horizontal cut through the cerebral hemisphere *(B)*. The primary auditory cortex corresponds approximately to the blackened region; the higher order auditory areas are stippled. Wernicke's area is located caudal to the primary auditory cortex on the left side in most individuals. The plane of section for the cut illustrated in B is indicated by the arrows in A. The vestibular cortex is indicated by cross hatching. It is located at the intersection of the postcentral and intraparietal sulci. *(B.* Adapted from Geschwind, N., and Levitsky, W. 1968. Human brain: Left-right assymmetries in temporal speech region. Science 161: 186–187.)

III and IV. The binaural columns, which bring together input from both ears, are formed largely by the projection from the medial geniculate nucleus that relays binaural input to the cortex. As a consequence of this binaural subcortical projection, damage to one primary auditory cortex cannot cause deafness in one ear. The higher order auditory cortical areas (*cytoarchitectonic areas 22 and 42*) partially encircle the primary auditory cortex on the superior and lateral surfaces of the temporal lobe (Figure 7.9). The higher order auditory areas are distinguished morphologically from the primary area because only the primary area has a prominent layer IV; this is a characteristic morphological feature of primary sensory areas.

Knowledge of the organization of the auditory cortical areas in human beings provides insight into general principles governing the anatomical substrates of higher brain function. Although the two cerebral hemispheres appear symmetrical in terms of their gross anatomy, they are not. The lateral sulcus is longer on the left side of the cerebral hemisphere than on the right side. This gross anatomical difference in the two cerebral hemispheres is paralleled by important functional differences. In the majority of human brains, the left cerebral hemisphere is specialized for *linguistic function*.[4] In the depths of the lateral sulcus on the left side and extending onto the lateral surface of the hemisphere on the *superior temporal gyrus* is a higher order auditory area, termed *Wernicke's area* (cytoarchitectonic area 22), which is important in *interpretive* (i.e., *sensory*) *speech mechanisms*. In the right temporal lobe, this area is

---

[4] It is interesting to note that the differences in the length of the lateral sulcus are present in the cerebral hemispheres of orangutans as well as Neanderthal man (determined by endocranial casts).

simply a higher order auditory area thought to be involved in nonlinguistic function. An important projection of Wernicke's area is to the motor speech area, *Broca's area*, in the frontal lobe via a corticocortical association pathway called the *arcuate fasciculus*. The arcuate fasciculus courses in the white matter of the temporal, parietal, and frontal lobes. This pathway provides the connection between the cortical locus for interpretation of spoken language (Wernicke's area) and the motor speech area (Broca's area). (Broca's area is located on the frontal operculum, corresponding approximately to the opercular and triangular parts of the inferior frontal gyrus [Appendix I.1].)

Summary

The auditory transductive apparatus, the *organ of Corti*, is located in the *cochlea*, a coiled canal in the temporal bone (Figure 7.2). The *hair cells* are the auditory receptors. They are organized into a sheet within the cochlea. This receptive sheet has a precise *tonotopic organization*: receptors sensitive to high frequencies are located near the cochlear base, and those sensitive to low frequencies, near the apex. The hair cells are innervated by the peripheral processes of *bipolar cells*, whose cell bodies are located in the *spiral ganglion*. The central processes of the bipolar cells collect into the *cochlear division* of the *vestibulocochlear nerve* (*cranial nerve* VIII) and terminate in the *cochlear nuclei*.

The cochlear nuclei (Figure 7.3A), which are located in the *rostral medulla*, have two main divisions: (1) the *dorsal cochlear nucleus* and (2) the *ventral cochlear nucleus*. Neurons in both the dorsal and ventral cochlear nuclei (Figure 7.4) give rise to axons that decussate and then ascend in the *lateral lemniscus* (Figure 7.5) to terminate in the *inferior colliculus* (Figure 7.6). Many neurons in the ventral cochlear nucleus project to the *superior olivary complex* in the pons (Figure 7.3B), on either the ipsilateral or the contralateral side (Figure 7.4). Neurons in the superior olivary complex project to either the ipsilateral or the contralateral inferior colliculus, via the lateral lemniscus. Certain of these decussating axons form a discrete commissure, the *trapezoid body* (Figures 7.3 and 7.4B).

The inferior colliculus (Figures 7.6B2 and 7.7) contains three main nuclei. The *central nucleus* (1), the principal auditory relay nucleus in the inferior colliculus, is *laminated* and has a *precise tonotopic organization*. It projects to the *laminated portion* of the medial geniculate nucleus (Figure 7.8), which in turn projects to the *primary auditory cortex* (cytoarchitectonic area 41) (Figure 7.9). The *pericentral* (2) and the *external* (3) nuclei of the inferior colliculus project to the *nonlaminated* portions of the medial geniculate nucleus, which in turn projects to *higher order auditory areas* (Figure 7.9). In human beings, primary auditory cortex is located largely on the superior surface of the temporal lobe, in *Heschl's gyri* (Figure 7.9). The higher order auditory areas encircle the primary area (Figure 7.9). The temporal lobes on the right and left cerebral hemispheres are not symmetrical. The higher order auditory cortex located caudal to the primary auditory cortex of the left hemisphere is *Wernicke's area* (Figure 7.9), which is specialized for the interpretation of language.

The vestibular apparatus includes the *semicircular canals*, *utricle*, and *saccule*. Receptor cells, located in specialized regions of the vestibular apparatus, are innervated by the distal processes of bipolar neurons located in *Scarpa's ganglion*. The central processes of these bipolar neurons form the *vestibular division* of the eighth cranial nerve. These fibers terminate in the vestibular nuclei, located beneath the floor of the fourth ventricle in the rostral medulla and caudal pons (Figure 7.1A). There are four separate nuclei: (1) *inferior vestibular nucleus*, (2) *medial vestibular nucleus*, (3) *lateral vestibular nucleus*, and (4) *superior vestibular nucleus* (Figure 7.3). Most of the efferent projections of the vestibular nuclei form major motor pathways for controlling axial, limb, and extraocular muscles. The ascending "sensory" pathway from the vestibular nuclei terminates in a portion of the *ventral posterior nucleus*, which, in turn, projects to the parietal lobe. The *vestibular cortex* is located caudal to the primary somatic sensory cortex, in cytoarchitectonic area (Figure 7.9A; see Figure 5.18). This pathway may be important in the perception of vestibular information. ■

References

Economo, C. von, and Horn, J. 1930. Über Windungsrelief, Masse und Rinderarchitektonik der Supratemporalfläche, ihre individuellen und ihre Seitenunterschiede. Z. ges Neurol. Psychiat. 130:678–757.

Geschwind, N., and Levitsky, W. 1968. Human brain: Left-right assymmetries in temporal speech region. Science 161:186–187.

Imig, T. J., Ruggero, M. A., Kitzes, L. M., et al. 1977. Organization of auditory cortex in the owl monkey (*Aotus Trivirgatus*). J. Comp. Neurol. 171:111–128.

Kelly, J. P. 1985. Auditory system. In Kandel, E. R., and Schwartz, J. H., Principles of Neural Science. New York: Elsevier, pp. 396–408.

Merzenich, M. M., and Brugge, J. F. 1973. Representation of the cochlear partition on the superior temporal plane of the macaque monkey. Brain Res. 50:275–296.

Moore, J. K., and Osen, K. K. 1979. The Human Cochlear Nuclei. In Creutzfeldt, O., Scheich, H., and Schreiner, C. (eds.), Hearing Mechanisms and Speech. Berlin: Springer-Verlag, pp. 36–44.

Roth, G. L., Aitkin, L. M., Andersen, R. A., et al. 1978. Some features of the spatial organization of the central nucleus of the inferior colliculus of the cat. J. Comp. Neurol. 182:661–680.

Strominger, N. L., Nelson, L. R., and Dougherty, W. J. 1977. Second order auditory pathways in the chimpanzee. J. Comp. Neurol. 172:349–366.

Selected Readings

Aitkin, L. M., Irvine, D. R. F., and Webster, W. R. 1984. Central neural mechanisms of hearing. In Darian-Smith, I. (ed.), Handbook of Physiology, Section 1: The Nervous System, Vol. III. Sensory Processes. Bethesda, Md.: American Physiological Society, pp. 675–737.

Dallos, P. 1984. Peripheral Mechanisms of Hearing. In Darian-Smith, I. (ed.), Handbook of Physiology, Section 1: The Nervous System, Vol. III. Sensory Processes. Bethesda, Md.: American Physiological Society, pp. 595–637.

Fredrickson, J. M., and Rubin, A. M. 1984. Vestibular cortex. In Jones, E. G., and Peters, A. (eds.), Cerebral Cortex. Vol. 5. Sensory-motor Areas and Aspects of Cortical Connectivity. New York: Plenum Press, pp. 99–111.

Imig, T. H., and Morel, A. 1983. Organization of the thalamocortical auditory system in the cat. Ann. Rev. Neurosci. 6:95–120.

The Gustatory and Olfactory Systems

8

The Gustatory and Olfactory Systems

The chemical senses, taste and smell, are mediated by four cranial nerves (CNs). Taste, or gustation, is mediated by the facial (CN VII), glossopharyngeal (CN IX), and vagus (CN X) nerves. Smell, or olfaction, is mediated by the olfactory nerve (CN I). Although anatomically separate, gustatory and olfactory systems work jointly in perception of certain chemical stimuli. For example, even though the gustatory system is concerned with the four primary taste sensations—sweet, sour, salty, and bitter—the perception of richer and more complex flavors such as chocolate and vanilla is dependent on a properly functioning olfactory system. Damage to the olfactory system, as a result of head trauma or even the common cold, can result in a change in the "taste" of foods while the sensations of sweet, sour, salty, and bitter are preserved. The anatomy of the central gustatory and olfactory pathways has a unique property: their connections with the central nervous system are largely ipsilateral, in contrast to other sensory modalities, which are predominantly crossed. In addition, the sense of smell is further distinguished because many areas of the cerebral cortex that subserve olfaction receive a projection that does not relay in the thalamus.

In this chapter, the gustatory system is examined first. The central connections of the afferent fibers that innervate the gut, the cardiovascular system, and the lungs are also considered because they are similar to those of the gustatory system. The olfactory system is considered next. The study of the olfactory system provides us with the opportunity to examine a region of the ventral surface of the cerebral hemisphere that was considered only briefly in Chapter 1. As in the previous chapters on the sensory systems, the general organization of each system is considered before examining the brain regions that process gustatory and olfactory stimuli.

Gustatory System

The facial (CN VII), glossopharyngeal (CN IX), and vagus (CN X) nerves mediate the sense of taste. Taste is a *special visceral afferent* modality. These nerves also have a *general somatic sensory* component that innervates the skin of the ear and the posterior oral cavity (Chapter 12). The afferent innervation of the *gut, cardiovascular system, and lungs* is mediated in large measure by the glossopharyngeal and vagus nerves. This innervation provides the central nervous system with information about the internal state of the body, for example, blood pressure. Innervation of the viscera is a *general visceral afferent* modality. The viscera are also innervated by spinal nerves that synapse on neurons in the dorsal horn. This component of the innervation of the viscera will not be considered.

There Are Separate Gustatory and Viscerosensory Ascending Pathways

Gustatory receptors are clustered in the *taste buds,* which are complex gustatory sensory organs located on the tongue, soft palate, pharynx, epiglottis, and larynx. Unlike innervation of the skin and mucous membranes, where generally the *terminal portion* of the pseudounipolar afferent fiber is sensitive to stimulus energy, gustatory receptors are *separate cells* from the primary afferent fibers which relay the sensory information to the central nervous system (Figure 8.1A, inset). Gustatory receptors are innervated by the distal branches of the primary afferent fibers in the facial, glossopharyngeal, and vagus nerves (Figure 8.1A). The central branches of the afferent fibers, after entering the brain stem, collect into a tract in the dorsal medulla, the *solitary tract*. The solitary tract is surrounded by a nucleus, called the *solitary nucleus*, in which the afferent fibers terminate. Gustatory afferent fibers synapse principally in the *rostral solitary nucleus*. The axons of second-order neurons in this nucleus ascend *ipsilaterally* in the brain stem and terminate in the most *medial portion of the ventral posterior medial nucleus*, in the *parvocellular* component. From the thalamus, third-order neurons project to the frontal operculum and the anterior portion of the insular cortex where the gustatory cortical areas are located. This pathway is thought to mediate the *discriminative aspects of taste*.

Other visceral afferent input, for example, information from the gut, contributes to a second ascending pathway. This pathway is thought to be involved in coordinating autonomic and endocrine function and in mediating the affective consequences of viscerosensory information. Neurons in the *caudal portion* of the solitary nucleus give rise to the viscerosensory path, which projects to the *parabrachial nucleus* of the pons. The parabrachial nucleus, in turn, transmits this information to the *amygdala* and *hypothalamus*, two structures that are recognized to play a key role in visceral function and food intake. In addition, in the rat the parabrachial nucleus also transmits viscerosensory information to the thalamus (to a region adjacent to the thalamic gustatory nucleus). This thalamic viscerosensory relay nucleus, in turn, projects to a more *posterior* portion of the insular cortex that contains a viscerotopic sensory representation. This pathway may participate in the perception of viscerosensory information. The caudal solitary nucleus also participates in the reflex control of respiration, swallowing, and cardiovascular function. The control of these essential body functions is mediated by projections of the caudal solitary nucleus with autonomic preganglionic neurons and the medullary reticular formation. Neural connections for processing viscerosensory information are illustrated in Figure 8.1C.

In the next three sections, the peripheral components of the gustatory and viscerosensory systems are considered first, followed by the central relay nuclei and, then, the cortical areas.

The Facial, Glossopharyngeal, and Vagus Nerves Innervate Different Parts of the Oral Cavity

The chorda tympani branch of the facial nerve innervates gustatory receptors that are located in taste buds in fungiform papillae of the *anterior two thirds of the tongue*. The glossopharyngeal nerve supplies taste buds in foliate and circumvallate papillae on the *posterior one third of the tongue* (Figure 8.2), and the vagus nerve, innervates taste buds on the epiglottis, pharynx, and larynx. The greater superficial petrosal nerve (a branch of the facial nerve) innervates taste buds on the palate. The glossopharyngeal and vagus nerves have other visceral afferent fibers that innervate arterial blood pressure receptors (baroreceptors) in the carotid sinus and

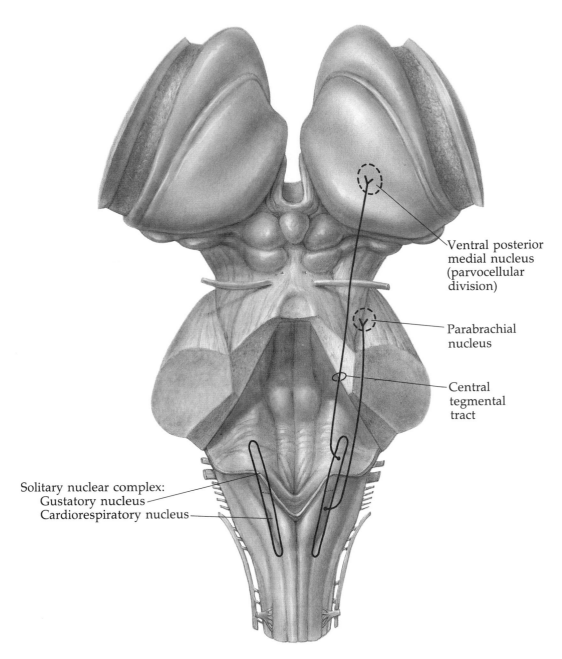

Ventral posterior medial nucleus (parvocellular division)

Parabrachial nucleus

Central tegmental tract

Solitary nuclear complex:
Gustatory nucleus
Cardiorespiratory nucleus

Figure 8.1 General organization of the gustatory and viscerosensory systems. *A.* Dorsal view of brain stem illustrating the location of the solitary nucleus and the differential projections form the rostral and caudal divisions. *B.* Ascending gustatory pathway. Inset illustrates a taste bud. *C.* Ascending viscerosensory pathway. (*A.* Adapted from Beckstead, R. M., Morse, J. R., and Norgren, R. 1980. The nucleus of the solitary tract in the monkey: Projections to the thalamus and brain stem nuclei. J. Comp. Neurol. 190:259–282.)

aortic arch. The vagus nerve also provides a general visceral afferent innervation, serving respiratory structures and most of the gut. Visceral afferent fibers are pseudounipolar neurons, like other primary afferent fibers (see Figure 12.2). The cell bodies of the afferent fibers in the facial,

B

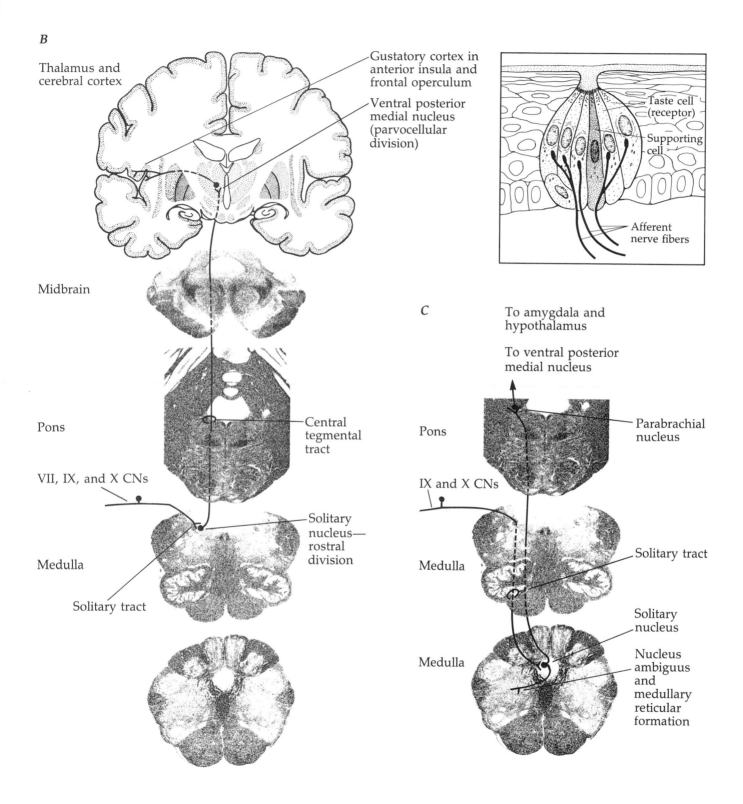

Thalamus and
cerebral cortex

Gustatory cortex in
anterior insula and
frontal operculum

Ventral posterior
medial nucleus
(parvocellular
division)

Taste cell
(receptor)

Supporting
cell

Afferent
nerve fibers

Midbrain

C

To amygdala and
hypothalamus

To ventral posterior
medial nucleus

Pons

Central
tegmental
tract

Pons

Parabrachial
nucleus

VII, IX, and X CNs

IX and X CNs

Solitary
nucleus—
rostral
division

Solitary tract

Medulla

Medulla

Solitary tract

Solitary
nucleus

Nucleus
ambiguus
and
medullary
reticular
formation

Medulla

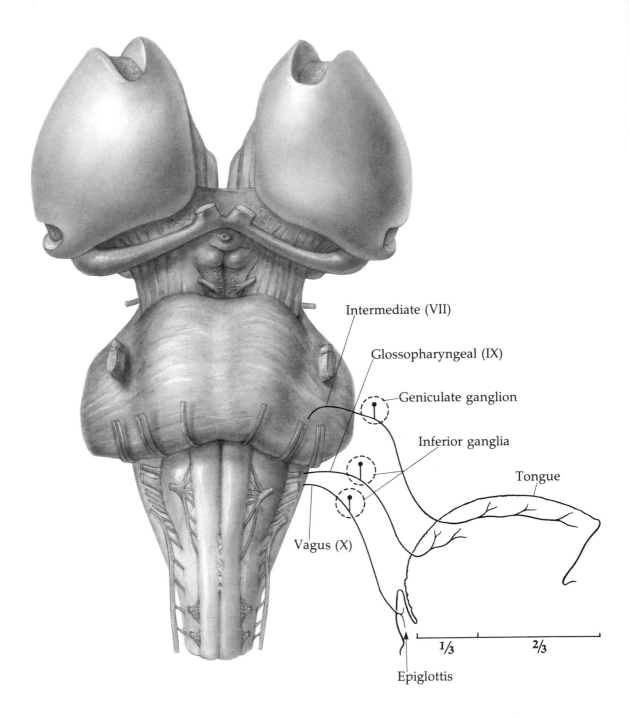

Intermediate (VII)

Glossopharyngeal (IX)

Geniculate ganglion

Inferior ganglia

Tongue

Vagus (X)

1/3 2/3

Epiglottis

Figure 8.2 Gustatory innervation of the oral cavity by the facial, glossopharyngeal, and vagus nerves.

glossopharyngeal, and vagus nerves are located in different peripheral sensory ganglia. The cell bodies of facial nerve afferent fibers are located in the *geniculate ganglion*, whereas those of the vagus and glossopharyngeal nerves are located in their respective *inferior ganglia*. (The superior ganglia of the glossopharyngeal and vagus nerves contain cell bodies of general somatic afferents.[1])

[1] There is an alternate nomenclature for the sensory ganglia of the glossopharyngeal and vagus nerves. The superior ganglia are also termed the jugular ganglia, the inferior ganglion of CN IX is also termed the petrosal ganglion, and the inferior ganglion of CN X, the nodose ganglion.

The afferent fibers of the facial nerve collect in a separate root from the somatic motor axons (Figure 8.2) called the *intermediate nerve*. It enters the brain stem immediately lateral to the somatic motor root at the *pontomedullary junction*. The intermediate nerve is smaller than the motor root of the facial nerve. Unlike the sensory fibers of the facial nerve, those of the glossopharyngeal and vagus nerves do not form a separate root. The glossopharyngeal and vagus nerves enter the brain stem in the rostral medulla (Figure 8.2).

The Solitary Nucleus Is the First Central Nervous System Relay for Taste and Viscerosensory Information

The solitary tract contains the central branches of pseudounipolar neurons whose cell bodies are located in the geniculate and inferior ganglia. The solitary nucleus (Figure 8.3) is divided into functionally distinct rostral and caudal subdivisions (Figure 8.1A). The boundary between these divisions is approximately at the level at which most of the vagus nerve fibers enter the medulla. The rostral subdivision of the solitary nucleus receives input primarily from the facial and glossopharyngeal nerves. This subdivision is called the *gustatory nucleus* (Figure 8.3) because it is the relay nucleus for taste perception. Axons from the gustatory nucleus ascend in the ipsilateral *central tegmental tract* (Figure 8.4) and terminate in the most medial portion of the ventral posterior medial nucleus of the thalamus (see later). The medial lemniscus, which carries the ascending somatic sensory projection from the dorsal column nuclei, is located ventral to the central tegmental tract at the levels shown in Figure 8.4.

The caudal subdivision of the solitary nucleus, termed the *cardiorespiratory nucleus*, receives input from visceral receptors. There is reason to believe that this portion of the solitary nucleus plays a dual function: (1) it transmits viscerosensory information to the *parabrachial nucleus*,

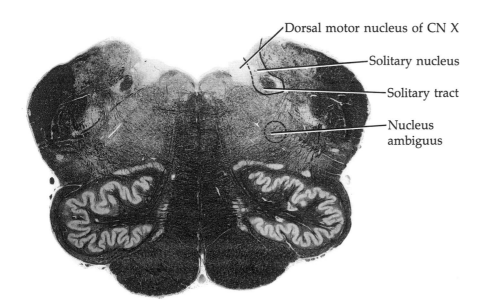

Dorsal motor nucleus of CN X

Solitary nucleus

Solitary tract

Nucleus ambiguus

Figure 8.3 The gustatory component of the solitary nucleus is illustrated in this myelin-stained transverse section through the medulla. Inset shows plane of section.

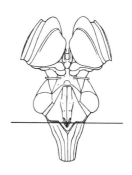

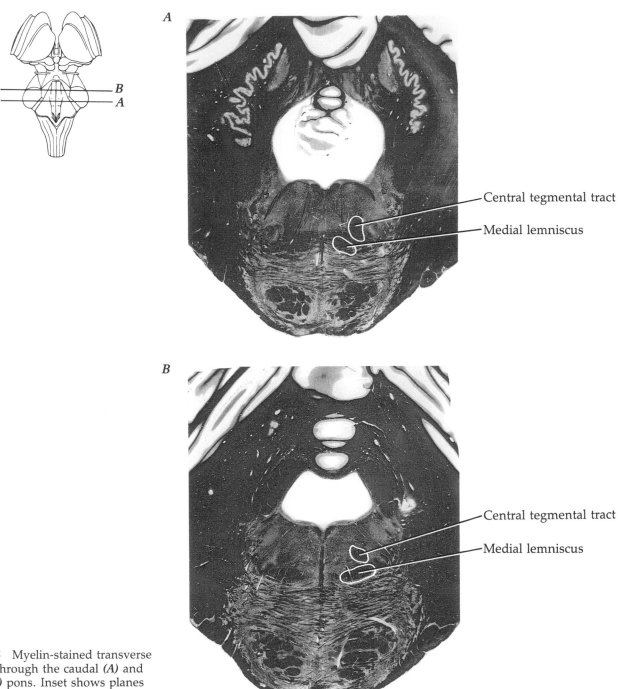

Figure 8.4 Myelin-stained transverse sections through the caudal *(A)* and rostral *(B)* pons. Inset shows planes of section.

which coordinates autonomic, endocrine, and other visceral functions, and (2) it participates in cardiovascular, respiratory, and other visceral reflexes via projections to the spinal cord and to other medullary neurons. The parabrachial nucleus is located in the pons adjacent to the principal output path of the cerebellum, the superior cerebellar peduncle (Chapter 10). (Another name for the superior cerebellar peduncle is the brachium conjunctivum; hence the term parabrachial.) The approximate location of the parabrachial nucleus is shown in Figure 8.1C. One important projection of the parabrachial nucleus is to transmit viscerosensory information farther rostrally to the hypothalamus. The parabrachial nucleus also projects to the amygdala, which is located in the temporal lobe (Figure 8.11). It will be shown in Chapter 15 that the amygdala is a component of the limbic system and that it is thought to participate in a variety of autonomic and endocrine functions, for example, feeding and reproductive behaviors. The other function of the caudal solitary nucleus is in regulation of the function of the autonomic nervous system, especially in cardiovascular regulation. Neurons in the caudal solitary nucleus project their axons to the nucleus ambiguus, the motor nuclei of the glossopharyngeal and vagus nerves (Figure 8.3, Chapter 13), as well as to medullary preganglionic parasympathetic neurons involved in cardiovascular function. The solitary nucleus projects directly, and indirectly via neurons in the ventral medulla, to the intermediolateral nucleus of the spinal cord, which is the location of sympathetic preganglionic neurons. Therefore, the local connections of the solitary nucleus as well as its ascending and descending projections are critically involved in integrating viscerosensory information and autonomic function.

The Parvocellular Portion of the Ventral Posterior Medial Nucleus Relays Gustatory Information to the Frontal Operculum and Anterior Insular Cortex

As with somatic sensation, vision, and audition there is an area of the cerebral cortex that processes gustatory information, and this information arrives via a particular thalamic relay nucleus. Gustatory information is processed by the *parvocellular division* of the *ventral posterior*

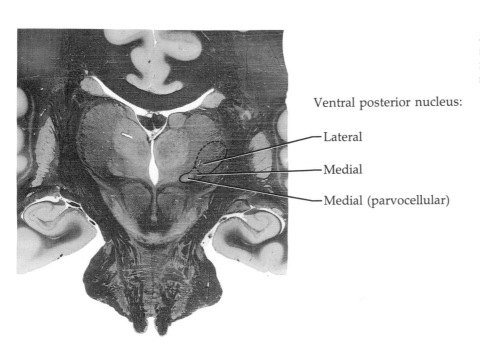

Ventral posterior nucleus:

Lateral

Medial

Medial (parvocellular)

Figure 8.5 A myelin-stained coronal section through the thalamic taste nucleus. Inset shows plane of section.

medial nucleus. This nucleus has a characteristic light appearance on myelin-stained sections (Figure 8.5). The axons of thalamocortical projection neurons in the parvocellular division of the ventral posterior medial nucleus project via the *posterior limb of the internal capsule* to the *frontal operculum and anterior insular cortex* (Figures 8.1A and 8.6A). Figure 8.6B is a schematic coronal section through the cerebral hemisphere revealing the operculum of the frontal and parietal lobes overlying the insular cortex.

The cortical gustatory area is separate from the face area of the primary and secondary somatic sensory cortical areas, where impulses from mechanoreceptors are relayed (Figure 8.6A). The presence of separate cortical areas for processing perioral tactile and gustatory stimuli is a reflection of an important principle of cortical organization: there is a separate cortical representation for each sensory modality. Tactile and proprioceptive information from the limbs and trunk are processed by the different cytoarchitectonic areas of the primary somatic sensory cortex (Chapter 5). Taste too is represented in a cortical location separate from tactile sense of the tongue, even though the sensory receptors mediating the two modalities are intermingled in the periphery.

Olfactory System

The Olfactory Projection to the Cerebral Cortex Does Not Relay in the Thalamus

Olfaction, similar to gustation, is a special visceral afferent modality. The primary olfactory neurons are located in the olfactory epithelium, which is located on the *superior nasal concha* as well as the septum and roof of the nasal cavity (Figure 8.7A). The primary olfactory neurons have a bipolar morphology (Figure 8.7A, inset) (see Figure 12.2). The peripheral portion of the primary olfactory neuron is *chemosensitive*, and the central process is an *unmyelinated axon* that projects to the central nervous system. Recall that the gustatory receptors and the primary afferent fibers are separate cells. The unmyelinated axons of the olfactory receptors collect into numerous small fascicles, which collectively form the *olfactory nerve*, the first cranial nerve. The olfactory nerve fascicles pass through foramina in a portion of the *ethmoid bone* termed the *cribriform plate* (Figure 8.7A) and synapse on neurons in the *olfactory bulb* (Figures 8.7 and 8.8). Head trauma frequently shears off these delicate fascicles as they traverse the bone, resulting in *anosmia*, the inability to perceive odors.

The next link in the olfactory pathway is the projection of second-order neurons in the olfactory bulb through the *olfactory tract* to five separate areas of the cerebral hemisphere (Figure 8.7B). The *anterior olfactory nucleus* (1) is made up of cells scattered along the olfactory tract which project to the contralateral olfactory bulb via the anterior commissure. The projection to the *amygdala* (2) and the *olfactory tubercle* (3) are thought to be important in the emotional, endocrine, and visceral consequences of odors. The projection to the *piriform cortex* (4), a part of the cerebral cortex of the medial temporal lobe, may be important for olfactory perception. The *entorhinal cortex* (5), which is also located in the medial temporal lobe, receives a projection from the olfactory bulb. This cortical

A

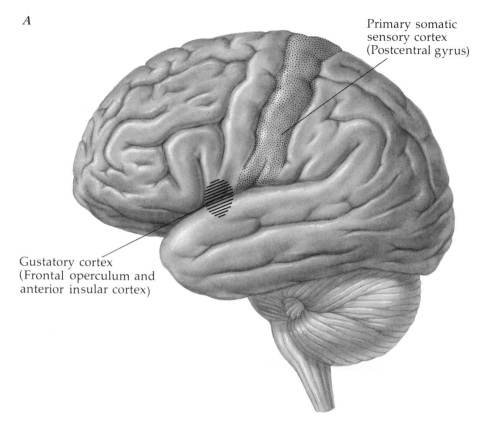

Primary somatic
sensory cortex
(Postcentral gyrus)

Gustatory cortex
(Frontal operculum and
anterior insular cortex)

Figure 8.6 Cortical gustatory area.
A. Lateral view of human cerebral
hemisphere, hatched field
corresponds approximately to
gustatory areas. These areas,
identified in the Rhesus monkey, are
located entirely beneath the cortical
surface on frontal operculum and
anterior insular cortex. The dotted
area corresponds to primary somatic
sensory cortex. *B.* Schematic coronal
section through the anterior insular
cortex and fronto-parietal operculum.

B

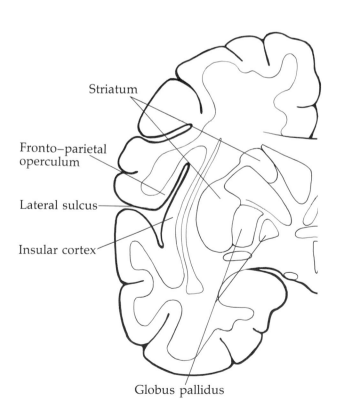

Striatum

Fronto–parietal
operculum

Lateral sulcus

Insular cortex

Globus pallidus

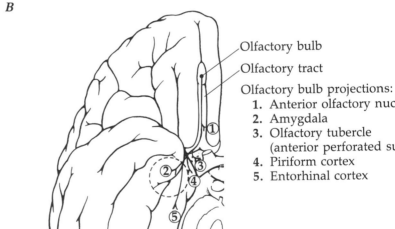

A

Fascicle of
olfactory nerve

Olfactory bulb
and tract

Cribriform plate
of ethmoid bone

Olfactory epithelium

B

Olfactory bulb

Olfactory tract

Olfactory bulb projections:
1. Anterior olfactory nucleus
2. Amygdala
3. Olfactory tubercle
   (anterior perforated substance)
4. Piriform cortex
5. Entorhinal cortex

Figure 8.7 Olfactory pathway.
A. Olfactory epithelium on the
superior nasal, with an expanded
region of the nasal epithelium. The
nasal septum is not shown.
B. Schematic of inferior surface of
cerebral hemisphere illustrating the 5
main termination sites of olfactory
tract fibers.

region, in turn, projects to the hippocampal formation, a structure important in memory (Chapter 15). The central projections of the olfactory bulb are not topographically organized. This is in contrast to the organization of the central projections of the other sensory systems, where projections between the receptive sheet and central structures have a precise topographic organization, for example, the retinotopic organization of the visual system.

In the following sections, we discuss first the peripheral components of the olfactory system and then the cortical olfactory areas.

The Olfactory Bulb Is the First Central Nervous System Relay for Olfactory Input

The olfactory bulb (Figures 8.7–8.9) develops from the telencephalon and is, therefore, a part of the cerebral hemisphere (Chapter 2). The central processes of olfactory receptors synapse on three types of neurons in the olfactory bulb (Figure 8.8): (1) *mitral cells,* (2) *tufted cells,* and (3) *periglomerular cells.* The olfactory receptor terminals and the dendrites of mitral and tufted cells form a morphological unit termed the *glomerulus.* The glomerulus is a common neuroanatomical solution to the problem of ensuring specificity of connections: certain presynaptic and postsynaptic elements are brought into close proximity and ensheathed by *glial cells.* The periglomerular cell is an inhibitory interneuron. This neuron inhibits mitral cells in the same and adjacent glomeruli. Another inhibitory interneuron in the olfactory bulb is the *granule cell.* The granule cell receives excitatory synaptic input from mitral cells to which it feeds back inhibition (Figure 8.8). Mitral and tufted cells are the projection neurons of the olfactory bulb. Their axons project from the olfactory bulb through the *olfactory tract* (Figures 8.7B, 8.9, and 8.10).

Figure 8.8   The axons of bipolar cells synapse on the projection neurons of the olfactory bulb, the mitral cells, and the tufted cells, as well as the periglomerular cells, a type of inhibitory interneuron. Also illustrated are the granule cells, another inhibitory interneuron. (Adapted from Shepard, G. M. 1972. Synaptic organization of the mammalian olfactory bulb. Physiol. Rev. 52:864–917.)

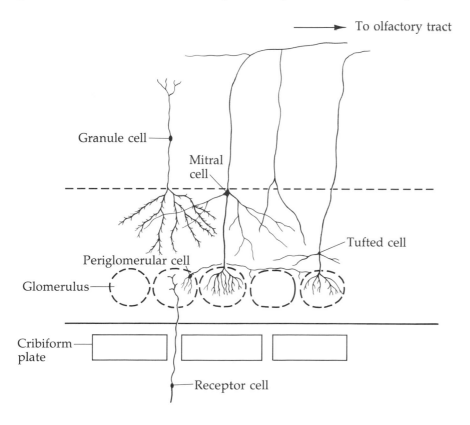

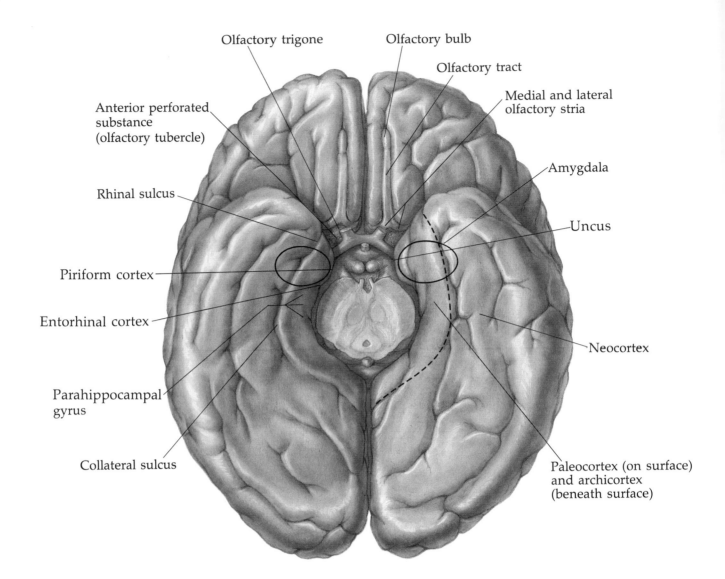

Olfactory trigone   Olfactory bulb

Olfactory tract

Medial and lateral olfactory stria

Anterior perforated substance (olfactory tubercle)

Amygdala

Rhinal sulcus

Uncus

Piriform cortex

Entorhinal cortex

Neocortex

Parahippocampal gyrus

Collateral sulcus

Paleocortex (on surface) and archicortex (beneath surface)

Figure 8.9 Ventral surface of the cerebral hemisphere. The parahippocampal gyrus contains numerous anatomical and functional divisions, two of which are the entorhinal cortex and piriform cortex. Paleocortex is located medial to the collateral sulcus and rhinal fissure. Approximate location of amygdala is indicated.

The Olfactory Bulb Projects to Structures on the Ventral Brain Surface

The anterior olfactory nucleus is located caudal to the olfactory bulb and is formed by cells scattered along the olfactory tract (Figure 8.9). This olfactory nucleus projects its axons primarily to the contralateral olfactory bulb. The olfactory tract runs along the ventral surface of the cerebral cortex (Figure 8.9). As the olfactory tract approaches its termination sites it bifurcates into a prominent *lateral olfactory stria* (Figures 8.9 and 8.10) and a small *medial olfactory stria*. A triangular-shaped region on the ventral brain surface, called the *olfactory trigone*, is formed by the olfactory striae. Caudal to the olfactory trigone is the *anterior perforated substance*. This region, named for its appearance, is the site where tiny branches of the anterior cerebral artery perforate the ventral brain surface to provide the arterial supply for parts of the basal ganglia and internal capsule. The

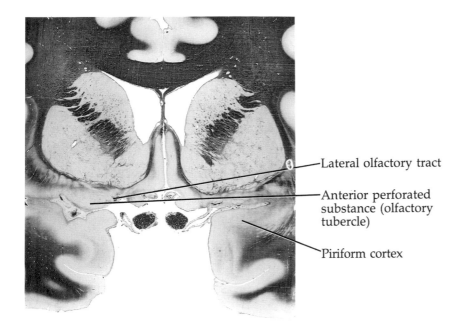

—Lateral olfactory tract

—Anterior perforated
substance (olfactory
tubercle)

—Piriform cortex

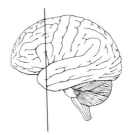

Figure 8.10 Myelin-stained coronal section through the region of the anterior perforated substances. Inset shows plane of section.

anterior perforated substance is gray matter,[2] whereas the olfactory stria are pathways on the brain surface. The *olfactory tubercle*, one region to which the olfactory bulb projects, is located in the anterior perforated substance (Figure 8.10). These structures are part of the *basal forebrain*, which is the area of the ventral cerebral hemisphere that is rostral to the hypothalamus. The basal forebrain is continuous with the cerebral cortex of the ventral frontal and temporal lobes (Figure 8.9).

Projections of the Olfactory Bulb to the Amygdala Are Important in Integrating Visceral Functions and in the Emotional Consequences of Olfactory Stimuli

A major subcortical projection of the olfactory tract is to the *amygdala* (Figures 8.9 and 8.11). The amygdala is also termed the *amygdaloid complex* because it is a heterogeneous structure with numerous component nuclei. This nuclear complex is sometimes considered as one component of the basal ganglia because it derives from the corpus striatum of the embryonic brain (Chapter 2). Its functions and anatomical connections are unlike those of the other corpus striatum derivatives, the caudate nucleus and putamen (Chapter 11), and it therefore makes little sense to group these structures together. The amygdala has three major nuclear divisions: corticomedial nuclear group, basolateral nuclear group, and central nucleus. The olfactory bulb projects to the *corticomedial* nuclear group. When it is considered that the corticomedial nuclei, in turn, project to the portion of the hypothalamus that is important in the control of feeding, insight is gained into the function of this olfactory projection. In addition, it is

---

[2] The anterior perforated substance is allocortex.

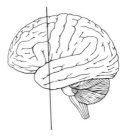

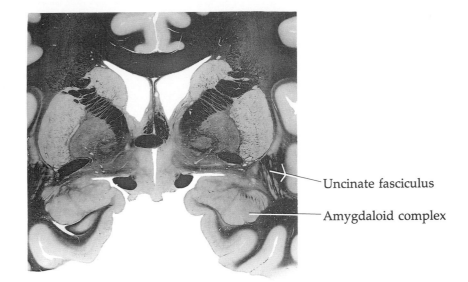

Uncinate fasciculus

Amygdaloid complex

Figure 8.11 Myelin-stained coronal section through the amygdala. Inset shows plane of section.

well known that odors influence behavior in animals, especially reproductive behavior. The amygdala has been shown to be essential for olfactory mediated reproductive behavior in certain rodents. The organization of the amygdala will be considered in detail in Chapter 15. Compared with the amygdala, primates have relatively few olfactory tract projections to the olfactory tubercle. This structure, which receives a major projection from the basolateral division of the amygdala, may be more involved in emotions than olfactory perception.

The Piriform and Entorhinal Areas of the Cerebral Cortex Receive Direct Projections from the Olfactory Bulb

Two cortical olfactory areas, the *piriform cortex* and the *entorhinal cortex,* are located on the medial portion of the temporal lobe (Figure 8.12). The piriform cortex is located on the rostral *parahippocampal gyrus* (Figure 8.9). A portion of the parahippocampal gyrus, termed the *uncus,* is a prominent landmark on the medial surface of the temporal lobe (Figure 8.9). The uncus protrudes toward the midline because the amygdala and the rostral portion of the hippocampal formation is located beneath it. This area of the cerebral cortex is termed *piriform* because it is shaped like a *pear* (Latin: *pirum,* pear) in the brains of certain mammals (for example, the cat). The piriform cortex has been termed the *primary olfactory cortex* because it is a cortical region that receives a major project from the olfactory bulb. However, unlike other primary cortical sensory areas, the input to the piriform cortex is *not relayed through the thalamus.* The *entorhinal cortex* is located more caudally in the parahippocampal gyrus (Figure 8.12). The lateral portion of the entorhinal cortex receives direct olfactory tract projections, albeit small in primates; the medial portion receives olfactory input from the piriform cortex. Most of the entorhinal cortex projects to the hippocampus, a structure involved in memory and not specifically in olfactory perception. The lateral entorhinal cortex projects

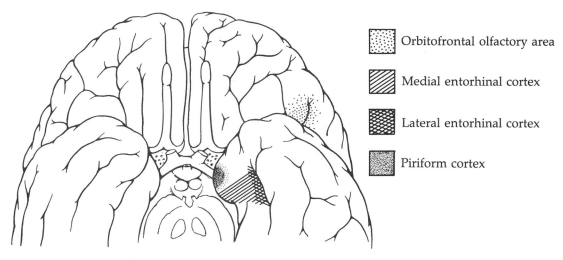

Orbitofrontal olfactory area

Medial entorhinal cortex

Lateral entorhinal cortex

Piriform cortex

Figure 8.12 Olfactory regions of the temporal and frontal lobes. The olfactory tract projects directly to the piriform cortex and lateral entorhinal cortex. The orbitofrontal olfactory area receives a projection from the lateral entorhinal cortex. The medial entorhinal cortex receives an olfactory projection from the piriform cortex.

to another cortical region, the *orbitofrontal cortex*, which may be important in olfactory perception. Lesions of the orbitofrontal olfactory area of cortex in monkeys produce an impairment in olfactory discrimination. The orbitofrontal cortex receives olfactory input from the entorhinal cortex (see Figure 8.12) via the *uncinate fasciculus* (Figure 8.11), a major pathway linking the orbitofrontal cortex with the rostral temporal lobe. In addition, the orbitofrontal cortex receives a projection from the *dorsal medial nucleus* of the thalamus. It is interesting that the portion of the dorsomedial nucleus that projects to the orbitofrontal olfactory area receives an olfactory projection directly from the piriform cortex. Because of its role in olfactory discrimination, this thalamocortical olfactory projection may be functionally similar to the thalamocortical projections of the visual, somatic sensory, gustatory, and auditory systems.

The Piriform Cortex Is an Example of Paleocortex

The olfactory cortical areas on the parahippocampal gyrus (Figures 8.9 and 8.12) have a cytoarchitecture that is characteristically different from the nonolfactory cortical regions located lateral to it. Most of the cerebral cortex has *six cell layers*. This morphological type of cortex is termed *neocortex*, because it is the type of cortex that dominates the brains of phylogenetically more recent animals. Somatic sensory, visual, and auditory cortical areas are part of the neocortex. In contrast, the olfactory cortex has less than six layers. Cortex with fewer than six layers is termed *allocortex*. There are two kinds of allocortex: (1) *paleocortex*, which is phylogenically older than neocortex, and (2) *archicortex*, which is the most primitive. The olfactory cortex is paleocortex. So too is the anterior perforated substance. Additional paleocortical regions are located caudally along the parahippocampal gyrus and retrosplenial cortex (the area of cortex located caudal to the splenium of the corpus callosum).[3] On the ventral brain surface, paleocortex remains medial to the *rhinal sulcus* and its caudal extension, the *collateral sulcus* (Figure 8.9). Archicortex is located in the hippocampal formation (see Chapter 15). (See Figure 3.15 for comparison of morphology of neocortex and allocortex.)

Summary

GUSTATORY SYSTEM.   Gustatory receptors are clustered in *taste buds*, which are located on the tongue, palate, pharynx, larynx, and epiglottis. The *facial nerve* (CN VII) subserves *taste* on the *anterior two thirds of the tongue* (chorda tympani branch) and the *palate* (greater superior petrosal branch); the *glossopharyngeal nerve* (CN IX), the *posterior one third of the tongue*; and the *vagus nerve* (CN X), the epiglottis, pharynx, and larynx (Figures 8.1 and 8.2). Afferent fibers of these nerves enter the solitary tract and terminate principally in the *rostral* portion of the *solitary nucleus*, also termed the *gustatory nucleus* (Figure 8.3). Projection neurons from the solitary nucleus ascend ipsilaterally, in the *central tegmental tract* (Figure 8.4), to the *parvocellular portion of the ventral posterior medial nucleus* (Figure 8.5). The cortical areas to which the thalamic neurons project are located on the *frontal operculum* and *anterior insular cortex*. These areas are separate from the representation of tactile sensation on the tongue (Figure 8.6).

The *caudal solitary nucleus* (Figure 8.1) does not receive gustatory input but rather receives visceral afferent input from cardiovascular, respiratory, and gastrointestinal structures. This portion is also termed the *cardiorespiratory nucleus* and it has a pattern of anatomical connections different from those of the gustatory nucleus. The axons of many projection neurons ascend ipsilaterally to the *parabrachial nucleus* (Figures 8.1A, C), which, in turn, projects to the hypothalamus and the amygdala. Other neurons in the caudal solitary nucleus project to *cranial nerve motor nuclei* and the reticular formation to mediate reflex functions (for example, blood pressure regulation).

OLFACTORY SYSTEM.   *Primary olfactory neurons*, located in the *olfactory epithelium*, are *bipolar neurons* (Figure 8.7A). The distal process is sensitive to chemical stimuli and the central process projects to the *olfactory bulb* (Figure 8.8) as the *olfactory nerve* (CN I). The olfactory nerve is formed by multiple small fascicles of axons of primary olfactory neurons that pass through foramina in a portion of the *ethmoid bone* termed the *cribriform plate* (Figure 8.7).

Olfactory nerve fibers synapse on *mitral* and *tufted cells*, the projection neurons of the *olfactory bulb* (Figure 8.8). The axons of mitral and tufted cells project via the *olfactory tract* to five regions of the cerebral hemisphere: (1) *anterior olfactory nucleus*, (2) *olfactory tubercle* (a portion of the *anterior perforated substance*) (Figures 8.9 and 8.12), (3) *amygdala* (Figure 8.11), (4) *piriform cortex* (Figures 8.10 and 8.12), and (5) *entorhinal cortex* (Figure 8.12). The piriform cortex is *paleocortex* and has fewer than six layers, similar to archicortex of the hippocampus, which has three layers. In contrast, *neocortex* has six layers. ■

---

[3] The cingulate gyrus, especially its rostral portion, is considered by many to be a form of cortex that is transitional between neocortex and paleocortex.

References

Beckstead, R. M., Morse, J. R., and Norgren, R. 1980. The nucleus of the solitary tract in the monkey: Projections to the thalamus and brain stem nuclei. J. Comp. Neurol. 190:259–282.

Cechetto, D. F., and Saper, C. B. 1987. Evidence for a viscerotopic sensory representation in the cortex and thalamus in the rat. J. Comp. Neurol. 262:27–45.

Nauta, W. J. H., and Haymaker, W. 1969. Hypothalamic Nuclei and Fiber Connections. In Haymaker, W., Anderson, E., Nauta, W. J. H. (eds.), The Hypothalamus. Springfield, Ill.: Charles C. Thomas, pp. 136–209.

Potter, H., and Nauta, W. J. H. 1979. A note on the problem of olfactory associations of the orbitofrontal cortex in the monkey. Neurosci. 4:361–367.

Pritchard, T. C., Hamilton, R. B., Morse, J. R., et al. 1986. Projections of thalamic gustatory and lingual areas in the monkey, Macaca fascicularis. J. Comp. Neurol. 244:213–228.

Reis, D. J., Ruggiero, D. A., and Granata, A. 1986. Central nervous system control of the heart: Brainstem mechanisms governing the tonic and reflex control of the circulation. In Stober, T., Schimrigk, K., Ganten, D., and Sherman, D.G. (eds.), Central Nervous System Control of the Heart. Boston: Martinus Nijhoff Publishing, pp. 19–36.

Selected Readings

Castellucci, V. F. 1985. The chemical senses: Taste and smell. In Kandel, E. R., and Schwartz, J. H., Principles of Neural Science. New York: Elsevier, pp. 409–425.

Finger, T. E. 1987. Gustatory Nuclei and Pathways in the Central Nervous System. In Finger, T. E., and Silver, W. L. (eds.), Neurobiology of Taste and Smell. New York: John Wiley and Sons, pp. 331–353.

Norgren, R. 1984. Central neural mechanisms of taste. In Darian-Smith, I. (ed.), Handbook of Physiology, Section 1: The Nervous System, Vol. III. Sensory Processes. Bethesda, Md.: American Physiological Society, pp. 1087–1128.

Price, J. L. 1987. The central olfactory and accessory olfactory systems. In Finger, T. E., and Silver, W. L. (eds.), Neurobiology of Taste and Smell. New York: John Wiley and Sons, pp. 179–203.

Shepard, G. M. 1972. Synaptic organization of the mammalian olfactory bulb. Physiol. Rev. 52:864–917.

Descending Projection Systems and the Motor Function of the Spinal Cord

9

Descending Projection Systems

The motor system consists of those parts of the brain and spinal cord that control skeletal muscle. Traditionally, four anatomically separate components of the motor system are recognized. The first component is part of the gray matter of the spinal cord, specifically the intermediate zone and the ventral horn, as well as the equivalent cell groups in the brain stem. Motor neurons are located in the ventral horn and cranial nerve motor nuclei and interneurons that synapse on spinal motor neurons are located in the intermediate zone. The second component of the motor system is, collectively, the regions of the cerebral cortex and brain stem that contribute to the descending projection pathways. This component is organized similarly to the sensory pathways, but rather than beginning in the periphery and ascending to the brain, the descending pathways have the reverse organization. *Descending projection neurons* in the cerebral cortex and brain stem either synapse directly on motor neurons or on interneurons that, in turn, synapse on motor neurons. The third and fourth components of the motor system are the cerebellum and the basal ganglia (Chapters 10 and 11). The roles of the cerebellum and basal ganglia in motor behavior are exerted through their actions on the descending pathways.

In this chapter, the descending motor pathways that project to the spinal cord are examined. The organization of the spinal cord motor nuclei is also considered because knowledge of their organization will help in understanding the anatomy and function of the descending pathways. First, we survey the key features of the descending pathways. Then, we explore the anatomy of the different levels of the motor system, levels containing neurons that contribute to the descending systems as well as levels through which the descending systems course en route to the spinal cord. The pathways that control skeletal muscles of the head, as well as the cranial nerve motor nuclei, will be considered in Chapter 13.

There Are Three Functional Classes of Descending Pathways

The descending pathways can be classified as (1) motor control pathways, (2) pathways that regulate sensory processing, and (3) pathways that regulate the functions of the autonomic nervous system. *Motor control pathways* originate in the cerebral cortex and brain stem and ultimately terminate on motor neurons that innervate skeletal muscle. These pathways mediate voluntary control of movement and regulate reflexes. The pathways that are involved in control of limb and axial muscles synapse in the motor nuclei of the spinal cord, where the motor neurons are located. Motor control pathways also terminate in regions of the ventral horn and intermediate zone where interneurons that synapse on motor neurons are located. The pathways for controlling cranial muscles terminate in cranial nerve motor nuclei in the brain stem. The descending pathways that regulate *somatic sensory processing* originate in the cerebral cortex and brain stem, similar to the motor control pathways, but terminate on dorsal horn neurons and in brain stem sensory nuclei. These pathways are important in controlling the flow of somatic sensory information into the central nervous system. For example, the raphe spinal path mediates pain suppression (Chapter 5). The descending pathways

Table 9.1

Tract	Site of Origin	Decussation	Spinal Cord Column	Site of Termination	Function
Cerebral Cortex					
Corticospinal					
Lateral	Areas 6, 4, 1, 2, 3, 5, 7	Crossed—Pyramidal decussation	Lateral	Dorsal horn, lateral intermediate zone, ventral horn	Sensory control, voluntary movement (limb muscles)
Ventral	Areas 6, 4	Uncrossed[a]	Ventral	Medial intermediate zone, ventral horn	Voluntary movement (axial muscles)
Corticobulbar	Areas 6, 4, 1, 2, 3, 5, 7	Crossed and uncrossed[b]	Brain stem only	Cranial nerve sensory and motor nuclei, reticular formation	Sensory control, voluntary movement (cranial muscles)
Brain Stem					
Rubrospinal	Red nucleus (magnocellular)	Ventral tegmentum	Lateral	Lateral intermediate zone and ventral horn	Voluntary movement, limb muscles
Vestibulospinal					
Lateral	Deiters' nucleus (lateral vestibular nucleus)	Ipsilateral[a]	Ventral	Medial intermediate zone and ventral horn	Balance
Medial	Medial vestibular nucleus	Bilateral	Ventral	Medial intermediate zone and ventral horn	Head position/neck muscles
Reticulospinal					
Pontine	Pontine reticular formation	Ipsilateral[a]	Ventral	Medial intermediate zone and ventral horn	Involuntary movement, axial and limb muscles
Medullary	Medullary reticular formation	Ipsilateral[a]	Ventrolateral	Medial intermediate zone and ventral horn	Involuntary movement, axial and limb muscle
Tectospinal	Deep superior colliculus	Dorsal tegmentum	Ventral	Medial intermediate zone and ventral horn	Coordinates neck with eye movements

[a] Whereas these tracts descend ipsilaterally, they terminate on interneurons that decussate in the ventral commissure and thus influence axial musculature bilaterally.

[b] The projections to the hypoglossal nucleus are crossed; those to the part of the facial nucleus that innervates upper facial muscles are bilateral and those to the lower facial muscles are contralateral. Projections to the trigeminal motor nucleus are bilateral.

that regulate the *functions of the autonomic nervous system* originate primarily in the hypothalamus and terminate in brain stem and spinal cord parasympathetic and sympathetic nuclei (Chapter 14). In this chapter we consider only the anatomical organization of the projections to the intermediate zone and ventral horn, projections that are important in the control of limb and trunk musculature (see later).

There are seven major descending motor control pathways, and they originate in cerebral cortex and in various nuclei in the brain stem (Table 9.1). Three of these pathways originate primarily in the frontal lobe: (1) *lateral corticospinal tract*, (2) *ventral (or anterior) corticospinal tract*, and (3) *corticobulbar tract*. The corticobulbar tract terminates in the caudal brain stem (pons and medulla) motor nuclei. It has an organization similar to that of the lateral and ventral corticospinal tracts and will be considered in Chapter 13. The remaining four pathways originate from brain stem nuclei: (4) *rubospinal tract*, (5) *reticulospinal tracts*, (6) *vestibulospinal tracts*, and (7) *tectospinal tract*. Before the anatomy of the descending motor pathways is considered, we briefly examine one important aspect of their general organization, the manner in which connections are made between descending projection neurons and motor neurons.

Descending Motor Control Pathways Synapse on Spinal Cord Interneurons and Motor Neurons

Each of the descending motor control pathways influence skeletal muscle via *monosynaptic connections* between descending projection neurons and *motor neurons* and through *di- and polysynaptic* paths. Typically, the axon of a descending projection neuron makes both monosynaptic connections with motor neurons, which are located in the motor nuclei in the ventral horn, and polysynaptic connections. The polysynaptic connections are mediated by two kinds of spinal cord neurons. One type is the *segmental interneuron* (sometimes termed *intrasegmental neuron*) which has a short axon that distributes branches within a single spinal cord segment. The second type of interneuron, the *propriospinal neuron*, has an axon that projects for many segments. The cell body of a propriospinal neuron is located two or more segments away from the motor neurons with which it synapses. Another name for the propriospinal neuron is *intersegmental neuron*. These segmental interneurons and propriospinal neurons are located primarily in the intermediate zone and the ventral horn.

In addition to receiving input from the descending pathways, motor neurons, propriospinal neurons, and segmental interneurons receive sensory input from the various functional categories of primary afferent fibers, input that is important for mediating reflexes. This sensory input is relayed either monosynaptically or polysynaptically via interneurons. Motor neurons receive monosynaptic input from only one functional afferent fiber category, Group Ia (or A-alpha) fibers, which carry action potentials from the *primary muscle spindle receptors* to the spinal cord. This monosynaptic input is the basis of the knee jerk reflex (Chapter 3). Segmental interneurons and propriospinal neurons receive monosynaptic input from virtually all afferent fiber classes: mechanoreceptors, thermoreceptors, and nociceptors. This difference in the patterns of afferent input onto motor neurons and interneurons is significant. The primary muscle spindle receptors have privileged access to the motor neurons. In contrast, other kinds of sensory input to motor neurons are subject to further control, through regulation of the excitability of the interneurons that transmit this sensory information to the motor neurons.

The Location of Descending Pathways in the Spinal Cord Provides Insights into Their Function

Motor control pathways that descend in the *lateral* portion of the spinal cord white matter primarily control *distal limb muscles*. In contrast, those that descend in the *medial* portion of the white matter primarily control *axial* and *girdle muscles*. In fact, there is a correspondence between key features of the anatomy of the motor pathways, spinal cord neurons, and muscles: 1) the locations of the various descending motor pathways in the spinal cord white matter, 2) the locations of the motor neurons and interneurons they innervate, and 3) the particular muscles controlled. The motor neurons innervating *distal muscles*, and the interneurons from which they receive input, are located in the *lateral ventral horn and intermediate zone*. These neurons receive input from the lateral descending pathways, pathways that course in the lateral column. In contrast, motor

A

B

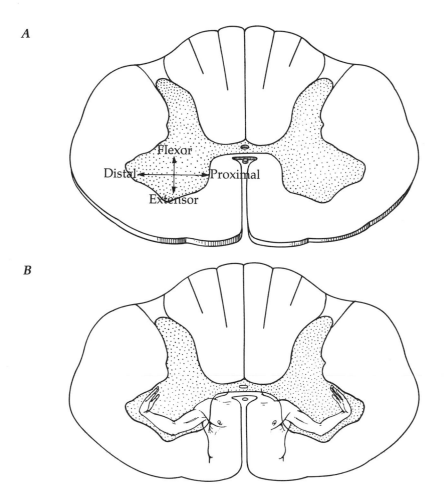

Figure 9.1 The somatotopic organization of the ventral horn. *A.* Schematic diagram of the spinal cord, indicating the general locations of motor neurons innervating limb and axial muscles and flexor and extensor muscles. *B.* A partial "homunculus" is superimposed on the ventral horns. (*B.* Adapted from Crosby, E. C., Humphrey, T., and Lauer, E. W. 1962. Correlative Anatomy of the Nervous System. New York: Macmillan.)

neurons innervating *axial and girdle muscles,* and their associated interneurons, are located in the medial part of the gray matter and receive their major input from the medial descending pathways. These pathways course in the ventral column and the ventromedial part of the lateral column. Motor neurons that innervate flexor or extensor muscles have different spinal cord locations. Flexor muscles are innervated by motor neurons that are located dorsal to extensor motor neurons. The mediolateral somatotopic organization and dorsoventral flexor and extensor organization are easy to remember when it is understood that the functional organization of the intermediate zone and ventral horn mimics the form of the body (Figure 9.1). It is interesting to note that the snake, which just has axial muscles, has only medial motor nuclei.

The Laterally Descending Pathways Control Limb Muscles

There are two laterally descending pathways: lateral corticospinal tract and rubrospinal tract. These pathways play a key role in voluntary limb movements. The *lateral corticospinal tract* originates in the *cerebral cortex*. This is the principal motor control pathway in humans. The other lateral pathway, the *rubrospinal tract*, originates in a midbrain nucleus, the *red nucleus* (see later). The neurons that give rise to these pathways are *somatotopically* organized. Moreover, the lateral corticospinal and rubrospinal tracts control muscles on the *contralateral* side of the body. Deficits in the ability to control *limb muscles* (opposed to axial and girdle muscles) accompany lesions of the lateral corticospinal tract and rubrospinal tract. One such motor deficit is the loss of *fractionation*, which is the ability to control an individual muscle independently from other muscles. Normal manual dexterity is dependent on fractionation.

Two areas of the frontal lobe contribute most of the axons to the lateral corticospinal tract: the *primary motor cortex* (Brodmann's area 4), which is part of the *precentral gyrus* (Figure 9.2A), and the *supplementary motor area* (a portion of area 6). The parietal lobe also contributes axons to the lateral corticospinal tract, and by some estimates, similar numbers are contributed by the primary motor cortex, the supplementary motor area, and the parietal lobe. In contrast to motor cortex and the supplementary motor area, whose descending projections terminate in the intermediate zone and the ventral horn, the projection from the parietal lobe terminates primarily in the dorsal horn. The projection from the parietal lobe to the dorsal horn may regulate somatic sensory input to the central nervous system (Chapter 5).

The lateral corticospinal tract descends within the cerebral hemisphere in the *internal capsule* and, in the midbrain, on its ventral surface, in the *basis pedunculi* (Figure 9.2A). Next on its caudal course, the tract disappears beneath the ventral surface of the pons only to reappear on the ventral surface of the medulla, as the *pyramid*. At the junction of the spinal cord and medulla, the axons *decussate* and descend in the dorsolateral portion of the *lateral* column of the spinal cord white matter. Hence the name lateral corticospinal tract (see Figure 9.4). This pathway terminates in the lateral portions of the intermediate zone and ventral horn. These are the locations of the spinal cord neural circuitry for controlling distal limb muscles.

The *rubrospinal tract* is the second laterally descending pathway (Figure 9.2B) and has fewer axons than the corticospinal tract. The rubrospinal tract originates from neurons in the caudal portion of the *red nucleus*. This portion is termed *magnocellular* because rubrospinal tract neurons are characteristically large. The rubrospinal tract decussates in the midbrain and descends in the dorsolateral portion of the brain stem. Like the lateral corticospinal tract, the rubrospinal tract is located in the dorsal portion of the lateral column (Figure 9.4) and it terminates in the *lateral portions of the intermediate zone and ventral horn*. Despite its small size, the rubro-

Figure 9.2 Laterally descending pathways. *A.* Lateral corticospinal tract. *B.* Rubrospinal tract. Note that the lateral corticospinal tract also originates from neurons located in the supplementary motor area and the parietal lobe. ▷

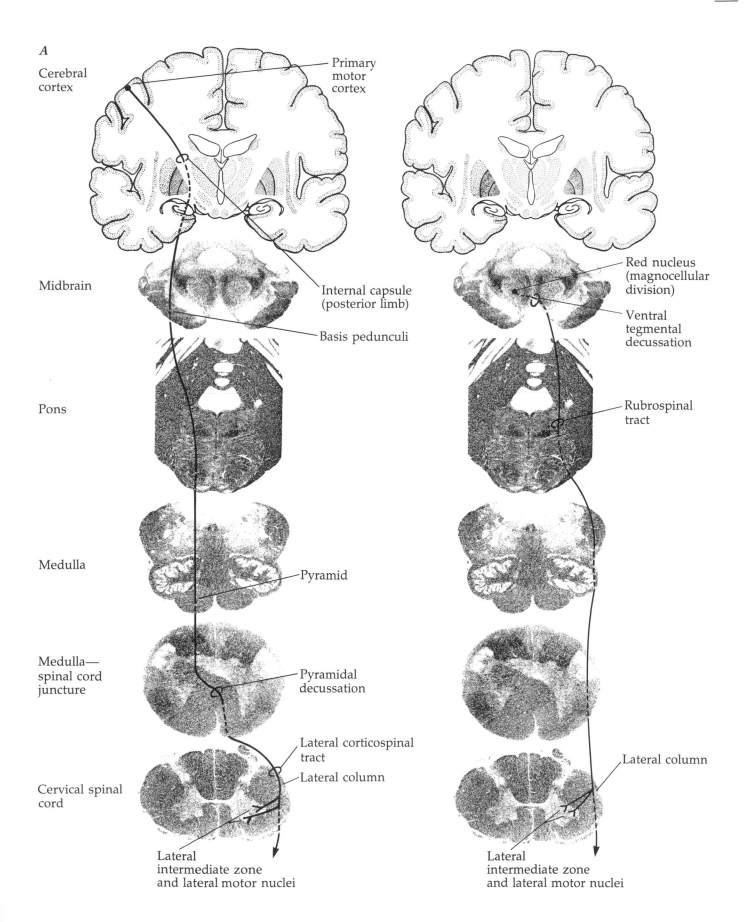

A

Cerebral cortex

Primary motor cortex

Midbrain

Internal capsule (posterior limb)

Basis pedunculi

Red nucleus (magnocellular division)

Ventral tegmental decussation

Pons

Rubrospinal tract

Medulla

Pyramid

Medulla— spinal cord juncture

Pyramidal decussation

Cervical spinal cord

Lateral corticospinal tract

Lateral column

Lateral column

Lateral intermediate zone and lateral motor nuclei

Lateral intermediate zone and lateral motor nuclei

Figure 9.3 Medially descending pathways. *A.* Ventral corticospinal tract. *B.* Tectospinal tract, pontine, and medullary reticulospinal tracts. *C.* Lateral and medial vestibulospinal tracts. Another name for the medial vestibulospinal tract is the descending medial longitudinal fasciculus.

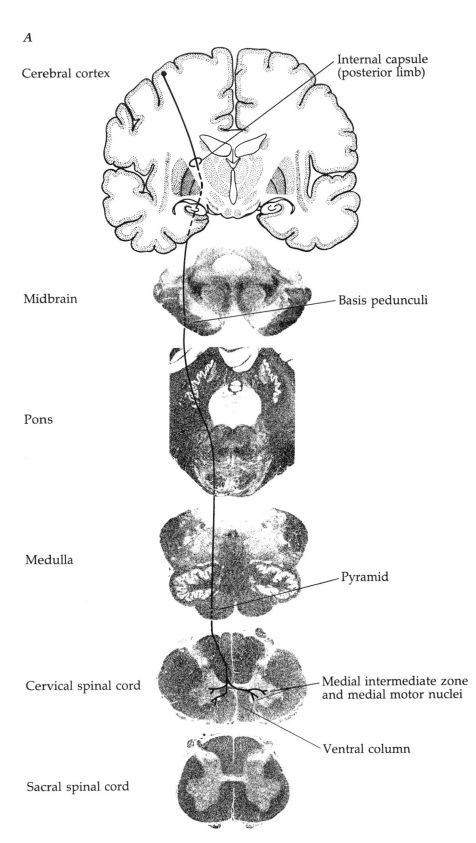

A

Cerebral cortex

Internal capsule (posterior limb)

Midbrain

Basis pedunculi

Pons

Medulla

Pyramid

Cervical spinal cord

Medial intermediate zone and medial motor nuclei

Ventral column

Sacral spinal cord

B

C

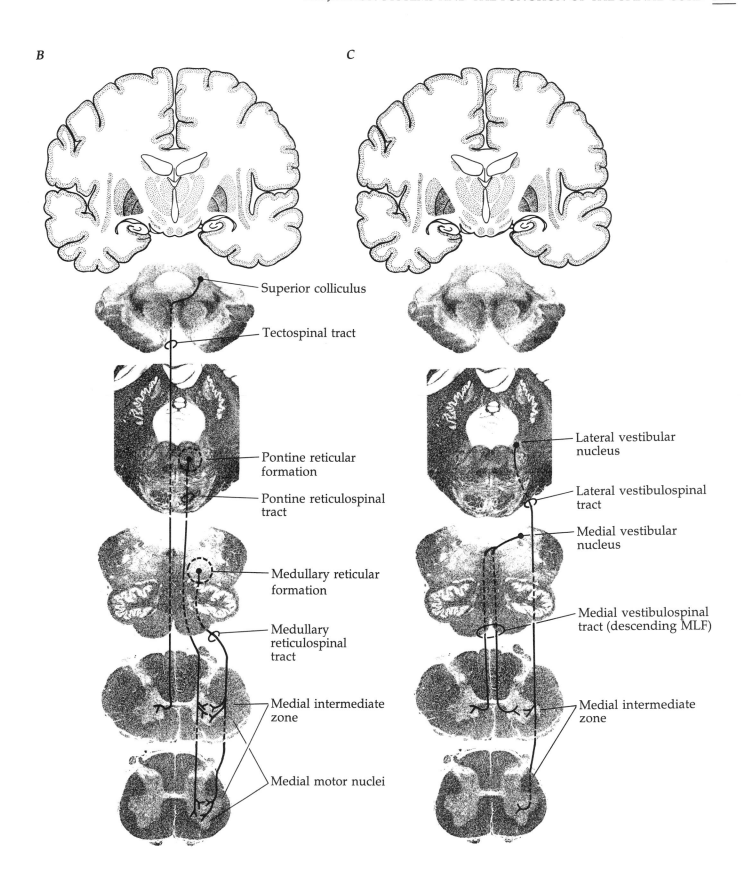

Superior colliculus

Tectospinal tract

Pontine reticular formation

Pontine reticulospinal tract

Medullary reticular formation

Medullary reticulospinal tract

Medial intermediate zone

Medial motor nuclei

Lateral vestibular nucleus

Lateral vestibulospinal tract

Medial vestibular nucleus

Medial vestibulospinal tract (descending MLF)

Medial intermediate zone

Medial motor nuclei

spinal tract is clinically important because it is thought to subserve some residual motor function after damage of the lateral corticospinal tract. The red nucleus is one of the largest midbrain nuclei (see Figure 9.9), yet in humans the magnocellular division is much smaller than the other component of the red nucleus, the *parvocellular* (or small-celled) division. Neurons of the parvocellular division are part of a multisynaptic pathway from the cerebral cortex to the cerebellum (see Chapter 10).

The Medially Descending Pathways Control Axial and Girdle Muscles

Axial and girdle muscles are controlled primarily by the four medially descending pathways: *ventral corticospinal tract*, the *reticulospinal tracts, vestibulospinal tracts,* and *tectospinal tract* (Table 9.1). A characteristic feature of the medially descending pathways is *bilateral control* of axial and girdle muscles. This is in contrast to the lateral corticospinal tract and the rubrospinal tract, which have a predominantly contralateral spinal cord projection. An important clinical consequence of this organization is that *unilateral* brain stem or cerebral cortical lesions that interrupt descending motor pathways do not produce profound axial motor control deficits because of the sustaining contralateral projection of the medially descending systems. Limb motor control, however, is profoundly affected. An interesting feature of the medially descending pathways is that many have projections to restricted rostrocaudal levels of the spinal cord and function in the control of neck, upper trunk, and shoulder musculature.

The *ventral corticospinal tract* (Figure 9.3A) originates predominantly from the *primary motor cortex* and the *supplementary motor area*. This pathway follows a descending course through the internal capsule, the basis pedunculi, the ventral pons, and the medullary pyramid. At the junction of the spinal cord and the medulla, where the lateral corticospinal tract decussates, the ventral corticospinal tract descends without decussating in the *ipsilateral ventral column* of the spinal cord (Figure 9.4). Similar to its medial descent in the spinal cord white matter, the terminations of the ventral corticospinal tract are located in the medial gray matter. This pathway synapses on motor neurons in the *medial* ventral horn and segmental interneurons and propriospinal neurons in the *medial* intermediate zone. Many ventral corticospinal tract axons have branches that decussate in the spinal cord. As a consequence, the ventral corticospinal tract on one side influences axial and girdle muscles bilaterally. The major projections of the ventral corticospinal tract do not extend beyond the thoracic spinal cord. On the basis of this limited rostrocaudal projection, it is preferentially involved in the control of the neck, shoulder, and upper trunk muscles rather than lower trunk and hip muscles.

There are two separate reticulospinal tracts (Figure 9.3B) and they originate from different regions of the *reticular formation*: the *pontine reticulospinal tract* and the *medullary reticulospinal tract* (Figure 9.4). Fewer neurons from the midbrain reticular formation project to the spinal cord. The pontine reticulospinal tract descends in the ventral column of the spinal cord, whereas the medullary reticulospinal tract descends in the ventrolateral quadrant of the lateral column. The reticulospinal tracts descend predominantly in the ipsilateral spinal cord, and are thought to participate in more automatic, sometimes considered involuntary movements such as posture and locomotion.

The *tectospinal tract* (Figure 9.3B) originates primarily from neurons of the deeper layers of the superior colliculus, or *tectum*, of the rostral midbrain. Like the ventral corticospinal tract, the tectospinal tract has a limited rostrocaudal distribution, projecting only to the cervical spinal segments. It therefore is believed to participate in the control of muscles of primarily the neck, shoulder, and upper trunk. Because the superior colliculus is also important in controlling eye movements (Chapter 6), it is believed that the tectospinal tract is important for *coordinating head movements with eye movements*.

There are two *vestibulospinal tracts* (Figure 9.3C) and they originate primarily from two of the four vestibular nuclei (see later). The *lateral vestibular nucleus* (also termed *Deiters' nucleus*) gives rise to the *lateral vestibulospinal tract*, which descends ipsilaterally. This pathway is important in maintaining balance. The *medial vestibular nucleus* gives rise to the *medial vestibulospinal tract*. Unlike the lateral vestibulospinal tract, which projects to all levels of the spinal cord on the ipsilateral side, the medial vestibulospinal tract descends bilaterally only to the cervical and upper thoracic spinal cord. As a consequence of its limited rostrocaudal distribution, the medial vestibulospinal tract influences neck and upper back muscles and may play a role in controlling the position of the head. Despite its name, the lateral vestibulospinal tract is classified as part of the group of medially descending pathways.

The locations of the different descending pathways in the spinal cord are illustrated on the right side of Figure 9.4. For comparison and review, the locations of the ascending somatic sensory pathways (Chapter 5) are illustrated on the left side of the figure. The two spinocerebellar pathways, which will be discussed in Chapter 10 also are illustrated.

Figure 9.4 Schematic diagram of the spinal cord indicating the locations of the ascending and descending pathways. Ascending pathways are stippled on left and descending pathways are stippled on right.

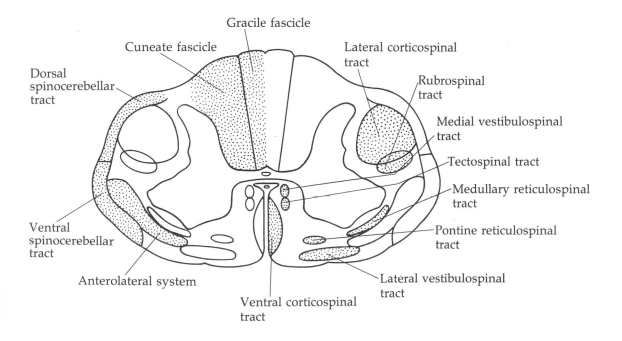

The Descending Pathways Have a Parallel and Hierarchical Organization

Up to now we have considered the organization of the descending projection systems as separate parallel motor control pathways. However, connections exist between the pathways that originate in the cerebral cortex and those that originate in the brain stem. The cerebral cortex controls motor neurons directly—through its connections with the spinal cord—and also indirectly—through its projections to brain stem nuclei that, in turn, give rise to descending motor pathways. The indirect path has a *hierarchical organization*: neurons of the cerebral cortex constitute the higher level in the sequence (or hierarchy), and brain stem nuclei, the lower level. One important hierarchically organized path is the projection from the motor cortex to the reticular formation and from there to the spinal cord. It is currently believed that this is an important route by which parts of the primary motor cortex that control distal limb muscles also influence axial and girdle muscles by synapsing on a component of the medial descending systems. Neurons of the primary motor cortex also project to the magnocellular component of the red nucleus, thereby constituting a second hierarchically organized pathway for controlling motor neurons, the *corticorubrospinal projection*.

In the remaining portions of this chapter we examine the different anatomical levels of the brain and spinal cord that are important in understanding the anatomy of the descending projection pathways. In the chapters on the sensory systems (Chapters 5–8), key sections through the brain and spinal cord were examined from caudal to rostral. Since the highest level of control of movement is exerted from the cerebral cortex, we begin examining sections with the most rostral and proceed caudally.

Motor Regions of the Cerebral Cortex Are Located in the Frontal Lobe

Three separate regions of the frontal lobe serve motor function (Figure 9.5A): *primary motor cortex*, *premotor cortex*, and *supplementary motor area*. The caudal part of the *precentral gyrus*, extending from the lateral sulcus to the medial surface of the cerebral hemisphere, is the *primary motor cortex* (*area 4*). The primary motor cortex plays a key role in the execution of skilled movement. Descending projection neurons in the primary motor cortex send their axons to the spinal cord via the lateral and ventral corticospinal tracts. These axons synapse on motor neurons and interneurons. The *premotor cortex* is located rostral to the primary motor cortex, in the *lateral part of area 6* (Figure 9.5A). The *supplementary motor area* is also located rostral to the motor cortex, but in *area 6* primarily on the *medial surface of the cerebral hemisphere* (Figure 9.5A). The premotor cortex and the supplementary motor area are the *higher order motor cortical regions*.[1] Through the study of the frontal lobe of the Rhesus monkey, it is now understood that the medial and lateral portions of area 6 each contain numerous anatomical divisions.

---

[1] Sometimes the entire area 6 is termed *premotor cortex* because both the medially located supplementary motor area and the laterally located "premotor cortex" contain neurons that send their axons to the primary motor cortex.

The primary motor cortex, premotor cortex, and the supplementary motor area each receive input from subcortical structures indirectly via *separate components of the ventral lateral nucleus of the thalamus* (Figure 9.8). Each of these motor areas of the frontal lobe also receives direct projections from other regions of the cerebral cortex. The primary motor cortex receives its principal subcortical input from the *cerebellum* (Chapter 10). The somatic sensory cortical areas (primary, secondary, and tertiary-cytoarchitectonic area 5) give rise to the major cortical projections to the primary motor cortex. The premotor cortex also receives its major subcortical input from the *cerebellum*. However, cerebellar projections to the premotor cortex originate from different portions of the cerebellum than those influencing the primary motor cortex. The projection to the premotor cortex is transmitted by a component of the ventral lateral nucleus separate from that which transmits information to the primary motor cortex. In contrast to the primary motor and premotor cortical areas, which receive input from the cerebellum, the supplementary motor area receives its subcortical input from the *basal ganglia* (Chapter 11). This projection remains segregated in the ventral lateral nucleus from the two cerebellar projections. The premotor cortex and supplementary motor area also receive sensory information from higher order sensory and association areas via a cascade of *corticocortical (association)* connections. Complex stimulus features, such as three-dimensional shapes of objects or the rate and direction of a moving visual stimulus, are transmitted by this path. The premotor cortex and supplementary motor area are in a unique position to integrate sensory information from higher order sensory areas and association cortex with information from subcortical motor structures. This information is then transmitted to the primary motor cortex. It is thought that this corticocortical path from the higher-order motor areas to the primary motor cortex is important in motor planning. These two higher-order motor cortical regions also have descending projections that allow them to influence other components of the motor system. As previously described, the supplementary motor area projects directly to the spinal cord and therefore may influence spinal motor neurons in parallel with the descending projection from the primary motor cortex. The major descending projection of the premotor cortex is not to the spinal cord but, rather, to the *reticular formation*. This path may be important for controlling the actions of girdle muscles by a projection to neurons that give rise to the *reticulospinal tracts*.

The Cytoarchitecture of the Motor Areas Differs from That of the Sensory Areas

The cytoarchitecture of the three motor areas of the frontal lobe is different from that of sensory areas in the parietal, temporal, and occipital lobes (see Figure 3.16). Whereas the sensory areas have a thick layer IV and a thin layer V, the motor areas have a *thin layer IV* and *thick layer V*. Recall that layer IV is the principal input layer of the cerebral cortex, where most of the axons from the thalamic relay nuclei terminate, and that layer V is the layer from which descending projections originate. In the motor areas, thalamic terminations have a wider laminar distribution than sensory areas.

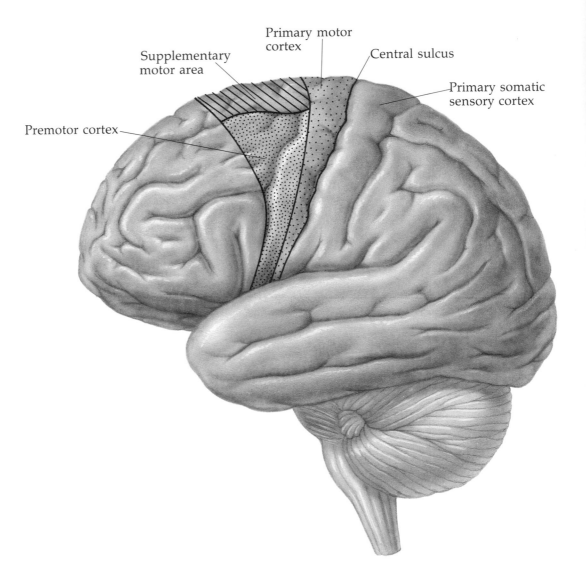

Figure 9.5 Lateral (***A***) and medial (***B***) views of the human brain, indicating the locations of the primary motor cortex, premotor cortex, and supplementary motor area.

The cytoarchitecture of the primary motor cortex is further distinguished from that of the other motor areas by the presence of *Betz cells*, which are large pyramidal cells in layer V. Betz cells are the largest neurons in the mammalian central nervous system. They were once thought to be the only cortical neuron to project to the spinal cord. However, on one side of the precentral gyrus there are only about 30,000 to 40,000 Betz

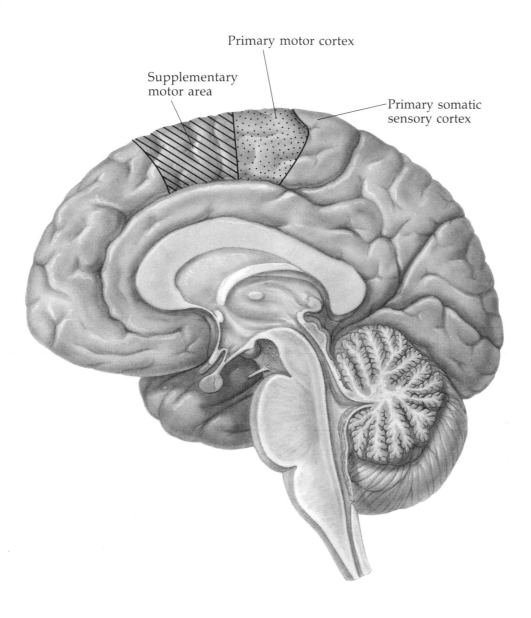

Supplementary
motor area

Primary motor cortex

Primary somatic
sensory cortex

cells, whereas there are about one millon axons in one medullary pyramid, suggesting that other cortical neurons contribute axons to the corticospinal tracts. The question of which motor cortex neurons project to the spinal cord is answered directly by using a modern neuroanatomical tracing technique. A retrograde tracer, for example horseradish peroxidase (see Chapter 1), is injected into the spinal cord gray matter. Cortical neurons that project to the spinal cord take the horseradish peroxidase into their terminals and retrogradely transport this material to the cell body. This experimental approach has confirmed that in addition to the larger Betz cells, smaller pyramidal cells also project to the spinal cord. This approach has confirmed that neurons from area 6 and the parietal lobe also project to the spinal cord.

The Primary Motor Cortex Is Somatotopically Organized

The primary motor cortex is somatotopically organized (Figure 9.6). In Chapter 5 we considered the somatotopic organization of the somatic sensory system. At all levels of the ascending somatic sensory pathways there is a representation of the receptive sheet in which neighborhood spatial relations are preserved. Sensory information from adjacent regions of the body surface is processed by adjacent regions of the somatic sensory system. In the primary somatic sensory cortex, there is a distorted map of the body surface, the *sensory homunculus*. In the primary motor cortex, muscle groups are represented somatotopically. Regions controlling facial muscles (through projections to the cranial nerve motor nuclei) are located in the lateral portion of the precentral gyrus, close to the lateral sulcus. Regions controlling other body parts are from lateral to medial, neck, arm, and trunk areas. The leg and foot areas are located on the medial surface of the brain. The motor representation in the precentral gyrus forms a *motor homunculus*, similar to the sensory homunculus of the postcentral gyrus (see Figure 5.17).

Figure 9.6 **A.** Somatotopic organization of the primary motor cortex. The descending pathways by which these areas of motor cortex influence motor neurons are indicated in **B.** (**A.** Adapted from Penfield, W., and Rasmussen, T. 1950. The Cerebral Cortex of Man: A Clinical Study of Localization of Function. New York: Macmillan.) Inset shows plane of schematic section in A and B.

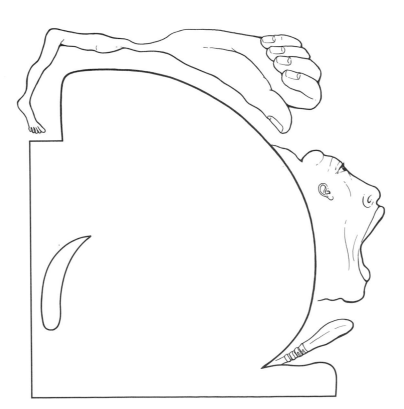

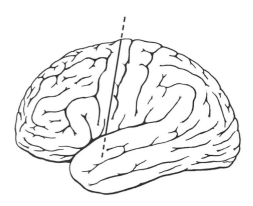

As a consequence of this somatotopic organization, different mediolateral regions of the primary motor cortex contribute differently to the three descending cortical paths: the lateral and ventral corticospinal tracts and the corticobulbar tract. As described before, limb muscles are preferentially controlled by the lateral corticospinal tract, and girdle and axial muscles, by the ventral corticospinal tract. Thus, the arm and leg areas contribute preferentially to the lateral corticospinal tract, whereas the neck, shoulder, and trunk regions contribute preferentially to the ventral corticospinal tract. The face area of motor cortex projects to the cranial nerve motor nuclei and thus gives rise to the corticobulbar projection (Chapter 13). Anatomical and physiological experiments in sub-human primates have shown that the higher order motor cortices, the supplementary motor area and the premotor cortex, are also somatotopically organized.

The Projection from Cortical Motor Regions Passes through the Internal Capsule en Route to the Brain Stem and Spinal Cord

Descending axons from the various motor areas course in the *internal capsule*. The internal capsule is shaped like a curved fan (Figure 9.7). It has three main components. The rostral component of the internal capsule is termed the *anterior limb*, and the caudal component is termed the *posterior limb*. Joining the two limbs is the *genu*. The three components of

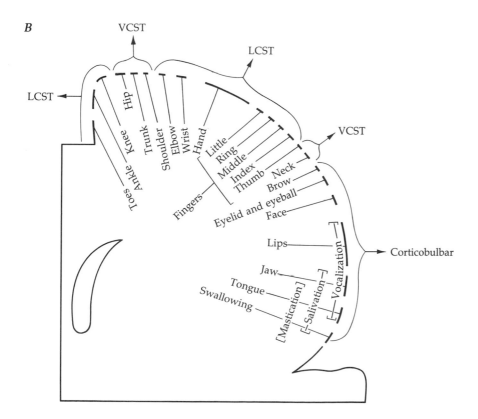

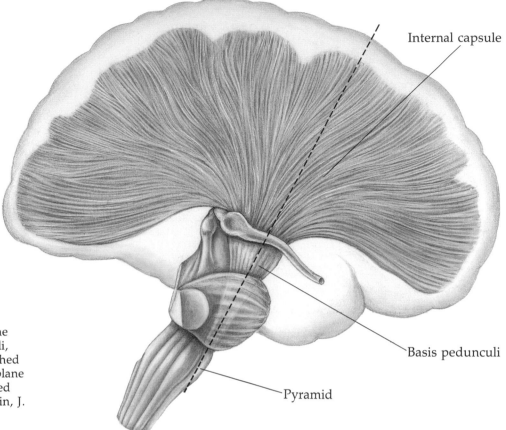

Internal capsule

Basis pedunculi

Pyramid

Figure 9.7 Three-dimensional view of fibers in the white matter of the cerebral cortex. The regions corresponding to the internal capsule, basis pedunculi, and pyramid are indicated. Dashed line indicates the approximate plane of section in Figure 9.9. (Adapted from Carpenter, M. B., and Sutin, J. 1983. Human Neuroanatomy. Baltimore: Williams & Wilkins.)

the internal capsule can be seen in Figure 9.8, which is a horizontal section through the cerebral hemisphere. The anterior limb separates the caudate nucleus and the putamen, the two principal components of the striatum. The posterior limb separates the caudate nucleus and thalamus from the putamen. Ascending thalamocortical projections, termed *thalamic radiations*, are located in the internal capsule. The projections from the ventral anterior and ventral lateral nuclei of the thalamus (Figure 9.8) course here. The ascending thalamocortical together with descending corticopontine projections form the bulk of the axons in the various component parts of the internal capsule. The descending motor projection to the spinal cord courses in the posterior limb (labeled A, T, L for arm, trunk, and leg in Figure 9.8), whereas the projection to the caudal brain stem—via the corticobulbar tract—descends in the genu (labeled F for face in Figure 9.8). The entire internal capsule appears to condense to form the *basis pedunculi* of the midbrain (Figure 9.7). The internal capsule is larger than the basis pedunculi because it contains both ascending thalamocortical fibers and descending cortical fibers, whereas the basis pedunculi contains only descending cortical fibers. Figure 9.9 is a coronal section through the *posterior limb* of the internal capsule. (The approximate level of this section is indicated by the arrow in Figure 9.8.) The descending cortical pathway can be followed from rostral to caudal (Figure 9.9): internal capsule, basis pedunculi, and medullary pyramids. The *red nucleus* can also be seen on the coronal section in Figure 9.9. The rubrospinal

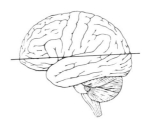

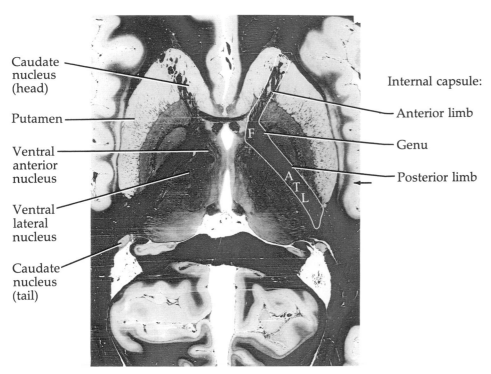

Caudate nucleus (head)

Putamen

Ventral anterior nucleus

Ventral lateral nucleus

Caudate nucleus (tail)

Internal capsule:

Anterior limb

Genu

Posterior limb

Figure 9.8 Myelin-stained horizontal section through the internal capsule. The somatotopic organization of the internal capsule is shown on the right. (Abbreviations: F, face; A, arm; T, trunk; L, leg.) Inset shows plane of section. Arrow indicates plane of section shown in Figure 9.9.

Figure 9.9 Myelin-stained coronal section through the posterior limb of the internal capsule. Note that the component of the internal capsule is identified as the posterior limb in this section because the thalamus is located medial to the internal capsule. In the horizontal section shown in Figure 9.8, note how the thalamus extends rostrally as far as the genu. The head of the caudate nucleus and the putamen are separated by the anterior limb of the internal capsule.

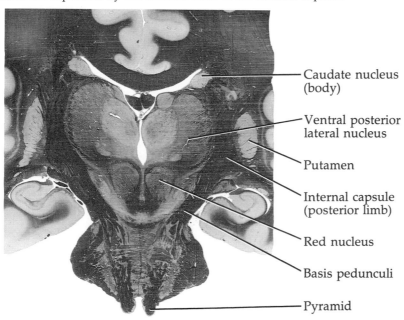

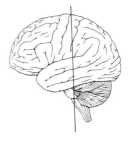

Caudate nucleus (body)

Ventral posterior lateral nucleus

Putamen

Internal capsule (posterior limb)

Red nucleus

Basis pedunculi

Pyramid

tract originates from neurons in the caudal portion of the red nucleus (magnocellular division).

Lesions of the Posterior Limb of the Internal Capsule Produce Spasticity

The arterial supply of the internal capsule is provided mainly by deep branches of the *middle cerebral artery* and, in its most inferior portions, by the *anterior choroidal artery* (a large branch of the internal carotid artery) (see Figure 4.7). Infarction of the posterior limb that destroys a large fraction of the corticospinal fibers is accompanied initially by flaccid paralysis (loss of muscle tone) of the contralateral arm and leg. However, it is rare for only the arm or leg to be affected by the infarction. This is because the axons that descend from the arm and leg areas of the primary motor cortex, even though their cells of origin are widely separated in the cortex, converge within a small space in the posterior limb of the internal capsule. In the period after the infarction, a consistent sequence of abnormal motor signs occurs with great regularity. First, the *Babinski sign* emerges (dorsiflexion of the big toe and fanning of the other toes in response to scratching of the lateral margin of the foot), then *increased myotactic reflexes* (for example, the knee jerk reflex) and *spasticity* (increased muscle tone and increased resistance to muscle stretch consequent to an increase in reflex activity) ensue. The spasticity is thought to result from damage of pathways other than the corticospinal tract because selective damage of a medullary pyramid in experimental animals produces decreased, not increased, muscle tone.

The Corticospinal Tract Courses in the Base of the Midbrain

Each division of the brain stem contains three regions from its dorsal to ventral surfaces: *tectum, tegmentum,* and *base* (Chapter 3). In the rostral midbrain (Figure 9.10), the tectum consists of the superior colliculus. This is a key level in the motor system because two prominent nuclei that subserve motor function are located in the midbrain tegmentum: the *red nucleus* (see later) and the *substantia nigra*. The substantia nigra is a component of the basal ganglia (Chapter 11). The midbrain base is termed the *basis pedunculi.*[2] Corticospinal tract axons are somatotopically organized. They course in the middle of the basis pedunculi, flanked medially and laterally by corticopontine axons (Chapter 10). Together, the tegmentum and basis pedunculi constitute the *cerebral peduncle.*

As we saw earlier, two descending brain stem pathways, the *rubrospinal tract* and the *tectospinal tract,* originate from neurons at this midbrain level (Figure 9.10). The rubrospinal tract originates from the *magnocellular portion of the red nucleus,* and the tectospinal tract originates from neurons in the deeper layers of the *superior colliculus* (Figure 9.10; see Figure 6.6). The tectospinal and rubrospinal tracts decussate in the midbrain, in the *dorsal tegmental* and *ventral tegmental decussations,* respectively.

---

[2] Another name for the basis pedunculi is the crus cerebri.

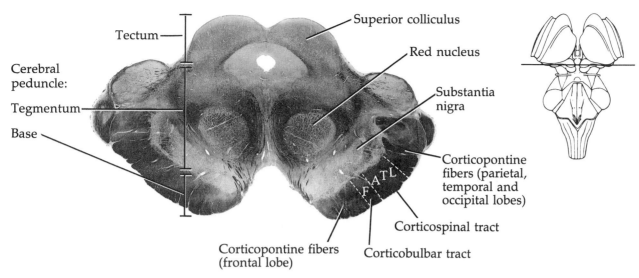

Figure 9.10 Myelin-stained transverse section through the rostral midbrain. The composition of axons in the basis pedunculi and the somatotopic organization of the corticospinal fibers are shown on right. (Abbreviations: F, face; A, arm; T, trunk; L, leg.) Inset shows plane of section.

Descending Cortical Fibers Separate into Small Fascicles in the Ventral Pons

Sections through the pons reveal that the descending cortical fibers no longer occupy the ventral brain stem surface, but rather are located deep within the base of the pons. The characteristic appearance of these fibers in the midbrain, as a discrete tract that is clearly separated from the other components of the midbrain, is no longer present in the rostral pons (Figure 9.11). The compact group of descending cortical fibers divides into many small fascicles, and each one is separated from the other by the pontine nuclei and the efferent axons of these nuclei, the ponto-

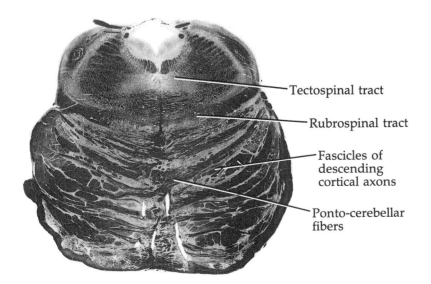

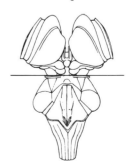

Figure 9.11 Myelin-stained transverse section through the rostral pons. Inset shows plane of section.

Tectospinal tract

Rubrospinal tract

Fascicles of descending cortical axons

Ponto-cerebellar fibers

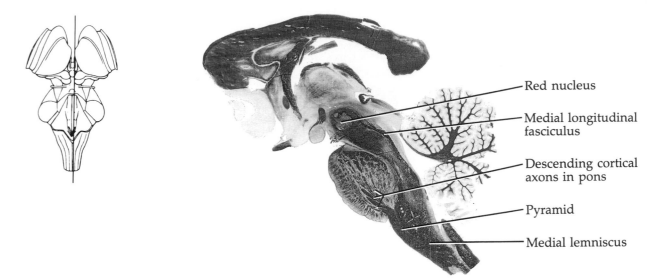

Figure 9.12 Myelin-stained sagittal section (close to the midline) through the brain stem. Inset shows plane of section.

cerebellar fibers (Figures 9.11 and 9.13B). Pontine nuclei receive their principal input from the cerebral cortex via fibers that course in the basis pedunculi (see Figure 9.10). The corticopontine projection is an important path by which information from diverse regions of the cerebral cortex influences the cerebellum (Chapter 10). In the caudal pons, fewer separate fascicles are apparent (Figures 9.12 and 9.13B1 and B2). This is largely a consequence of corticopontine axon terminations in the pontine nuclei. Note that the rubrospinal tract remains dorsal to the corticospinal tract throughout the brain stem, and the tectospinal tract is located dorsal and close to the midline (Figures 9.11 and 9.13). The path of the descending cortical fibers in the caudal brain stem can be followed in the sagittal section shown in Figure 9.12. Note that the numerous fascicles in the caudal pons collect to form the pyramid in the medulla.

The Vestibular Nuclei Are Located in the Dorsal Pons and Medulla

The vestibular nuclei are the first central nervous system relays for the vestibular labyrinth, the group of cranial sensory structures that contain receptors sensitive to position and movement of the head (Chapter 7). There are four vestibular nuclei (Figure 9.13A), and together they play a key role in maintaining balance by coordinating the contraction of axial and girdle muscles via the vestibulospinal tracts. The *lateral vestibular nucleus* (also termed *Deiters' nucleus*) gives rise to the *lateral vestibulospinal tract*, an ipsilateral descending pathway that projects to all levels of the spinal cord. The remaining three vestibular nuclei, the *medial, superior,* and *inferior vestibular nuclei*, give rise to the *medial vestibulospinal tract*, which descends bilaterally only as far as the cervical segments. However, the medial vestibular nucleus contributes most of the axons to the medial vestibulospinal tract. The medial vestibulospinal tract is the caudal extension of the *medial longitudinal fasciculus* (MLF), and as a consequence is also termed the *descending medial longitudinal fasciculus*. The medial longitudinal fasciculus, which is located close to the midline (Figure 9.12) is a brain stem pathway that contains axons from numerous sources that are crucial for controlling eye movements (Chapter 13). Lesions of the medial longitudinal fasciculus (or the nuclear regions contributing axons to it) produce characteristic deficits in eye movements. All four vestibular nuclei contribute ascending axons to the medial longitudinal fasciculus. Note that the tectospinal tract, which coordinates head movements with eye movements, is located ventral to the medial longitudinal fasciculus (Figure 9.13B1). (The MLF is present, but unlabeled, on the other sections in Figure 9.13B.)

Neurons in the pontine and medullary reticular formation (Figure 9.13) give rise to the *pontine* and *medullary reticulospinal tracts*, respectively. Whereas some fibers of the reticulospinal tracts originate from discrete nuclei, most fibers originate from neurons scattered in the medial tegmentum of the pons and medulla. The reticular formation and the intermediate zone of the spinal cord share two features. First, their locations are similar, forming the central region of the brain stem and spinal cord. Second, both the reticular formation and the intermediate zone contain neurons that have a widespread projection pattern that often includes an axon with both an ascending and a descending branch. The significance of this morphology is that such neurons simultaneously transmit information to spinal cord motor nuclei and to brain stem nuclei that are important for integrating sensory and motor information. As a consequence of their similarities, the reticular formation is considered to be the rostral extension of the intermediate zone.

The Lateral Corticospinal Tract Decussates in the Caudal Medulla

The *pyramids* are located on the ventral surface of the medulla (Figure 9.14). Each pyramid contains the axons of the lateral and ventral corticospinal tracts that originated from the *ipsilateral frontal lobe*. This is why the terms *corticospinal tract* and *pyramidal tract* are often used interchangeably. However, these terms are not synonymous because the pyramids also contain *corticobulbar fibers*, which terminate in the medulla. In transverse sections, the pyramids are triangle-shaped (Figure 9.14). The pyramidal decussation (of the lateral corticospinal tract) is seen in Figure 9.14B. Note that the decussation of internal arcuate fibers (Chapter 5), or "somatic sensory decussation" (Figure 9.14A), occurs rostral to the pyramidal or "motor" decussation. Positions of the other descending pathways are indicated. The rubrospinal tract, which is located *dorsolaterally* in the brain stem, joins with the lateral corticospinal tract at the medulla–spinal cord juncture and descends in the lateral column (Figure 9.4). In contrast, the vestibulospinal tracts, the reticulospinal tracts, and the tectospinal tract remain medial and assume a more ventral position as they descend in the spinal cord.

A

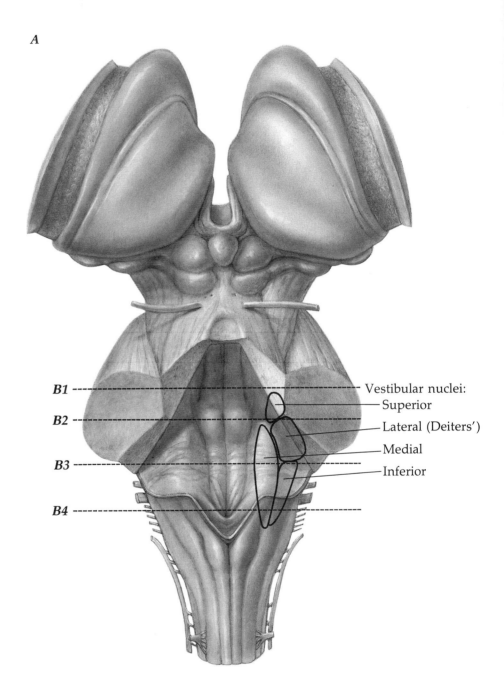

Vestibular nuclei:
Superior
Lateral (Deiters')
Medial
Inferior

Figure 9.13 *A.* Locations of the vestibular nuclei are shown in this dorsal view of the brain stem. *B.* Four myelin-stained transverse sections through the pons and medulla (B1–B4).

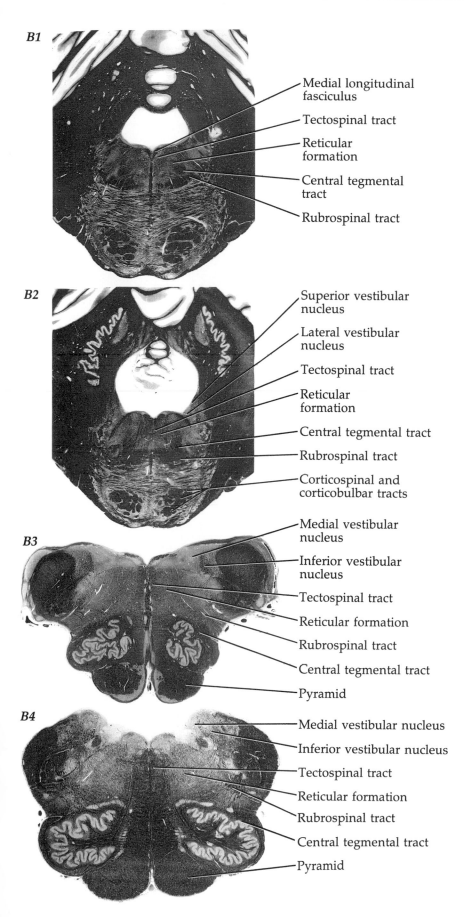

B1

Medial longitudinal fasciculus

Tectospinal tract

Reticular formation

Central tegmental tract

Rubrospinal tract

B2

Superior vestibular nucleus

Lateral vestibular nucleus

Tectospinal tract

Reticular formation

Central tegmental tract

Rubrospinal tract

Corticospinal and corticobulbar tracts

B3

Medial vestibular nucleus

Inferior vestibular nucleus

Tectospinal tract

Reticular formation

Rubrospinal tract

Central tegmental tract

Pyramid

B4

Medial vestibular nucleus

Inferior vestibular nucleus

Tectospinal tract

Reticular formation

Rubrospinal tract

Central tegmental tract

Pyramid

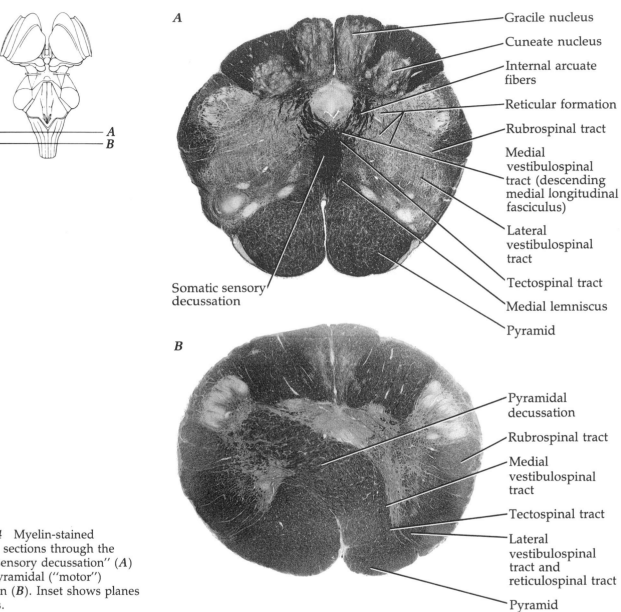

A

- Gracile nucleus
- Cuneate nucleus
- Internal arcuate fibers
- Reticular formation
- Rubrospinal tract
- Medial vestibulospinal tract (descending medial longitudinal fasciculus)
- Lateral vestibulospinal tract
- Tectospinal tract
- Medial lemniscus
- Pyramid

Somatic sensory decussation

B

- Pyramidal decussation
- Rubrospinal tract
- Medial vestibulospinal tract
- Tectospinal tract
- Lateral vestibulospinal tract and reticulospinal tract
- Pyramid

Figure 9.14 Myelin-stained transverse sections through the "somatic sensory decussation" (*A*) and the pyramidal ("motor") decussation (*B*). Inset shows planes of sections.

The Intermediate Zone and Ventral Horn of the Spinal Cord Receive Input from the Descending Pathways

The motor pathways descend in the ventral and lateral columns of the spinal cord (Figure 9.4) and synapse on motor neurons in the ventral horn and on segmental interneurons and propriospinal neurons in the intermediate zone (Figure 9.15). The gray matter of the spinal cord is organized into laminae that course rostrocaudally—the ten laminae of Rexed (see Table 5.1). The dorsal horn corresponds to Rexed's laminae I through VI, the intermediate zone to lamina VII, and the ventral horn to laminae VIII and IX. Lamina X surrounds the spinal cord central canal. Earlier we saw that the pathways that descend in the medial portion of the spinal cord white matter terminate in the medial portions of the in-

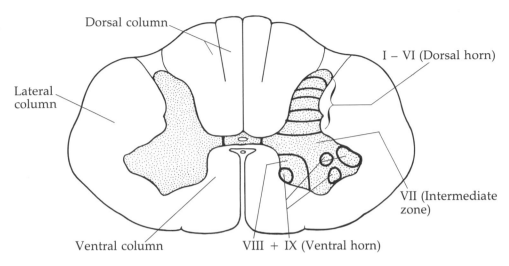

Figure 9.15 Schematic drawing of the general organization of the spinal cord gray matter and white matter.

termediate zone and ventral horn. These regions of the spinal cord gray matter contain the neuronal machinery for controlling girdle and axial muscles. Propriospinal neurons in the medial intermediate zone have long axons that project to many spinal cord segments, up to the entire length of the spinal cord. Many of these propriospinal neurons (as well as some segmental interneurons) have an axon branch that decussates in the ventral commissure of the spinal cord. This pattern of connectivity is thought to provide the anatomical linkages for the *coordinated contraction of axial and girdle muscles during postural adjustments*. In contrast, the lateral descending pathways terminate in the lateral parts of the intermediate zone and ventral horn, where neurons controlling distal limb muscles are located. Propriospinal neurons located laterally have short axons that course less than five segments.

The Lateral and Medial Motor Nuclei Have Different Rostrocaudal Distributions

Motor neurons in the cervical enlargement (which corresponds to C5–T1 in the human spinal cord) and in the lumbosacral enlargement (L1–S2) innervate distal limb muscles (lateral motor nuclei) as well as girdle and axial muscles (medial motor nuclei) (Figure 9.16). Between approximately T3 and T12 (Figure 9.16B), and at the extreme rostral and caudal poles of the spinal cord, only medial motor nuclei are present. There is a simple way of understanding the rostrocaudal organization of the motor nuclei. The medial motor nuclei form a column consisting of adjacent motor nuclei extending continuously from the cervical to the sacral segments. The lateral column of limb motor nuclei is interrupted in the thoracic regions and is present only in the cervical and lumbosacral enlargements. Autonomic preganglionic motor neurons are also arranged in columns oriented rostrocaudally (Chapter 14) and, together with the motor nuclei, have a three-dimensional organization that is reminiscent

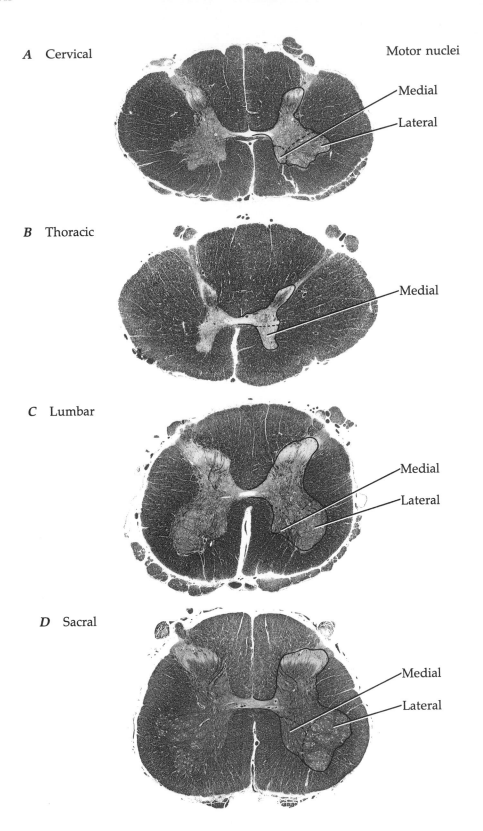

A Cervical

Motor nuclei

Medial

Lateral

B Thoracic

Medial

C Lumbar

Medial

Lateral

D Sacral

Medial

Lateral

Figure 9.16 Approximate locations of the medial and lateral motor nuclei are shown at four spinal cord levels: cervical *(A)*, thoracic *(B)*, lumbar *(C)*, and sacral *(D)*.

of the brain stem cranial nerve nuclei columns (Chapters 2 and 12). The longitudinal organization of the somatic and autonomic motor nuclei and the cranial nerve nuclei underscores the common architecture of the spinal cord and brain stem (see Chapter 2, section on spinal cord and brain stem development).

Spinal Cord Hemisection Produces Ipsilateral Motor Signs

In Chapter 5 we saw that spinal cord hemisection produces characteristic sensory deficits (below the level of the lesion): a loss of *tactile sense, vibration sense,* and *limb position sense* on the *ipsilateral side* and loss of *pain and temperature sense* on the *contralateral side*. These are the somatic sensory signs of the *Brown–Séquard syndrome*. Motor deficits are also a key feature of spinal cord hemisection. Interruption of the descending pathways releases motor neurons from their normal voluntary control. Initially, *flaccid paralysis* and *reduced myotactic reflexes* (spinal shock) occur in the limb innervated by motor neurons located caudal to the lesion. However, after a variable period of a few weeks, *spastic paralysis* develops, the *Babinski sign* emerges, and *myotactic reflexes become exaggerated*. These effects are expressed on the ipsilateral side because most descending motor pathways decussate in the brain stem.

Summary

There are six descending motor pathways that course in the white matter of the spinal cord (Figures 9.2 and 9.3): *lateral corticospinal tract, rubrospinal tract, ventral corticospinal tract, reticulospinal tract* (which is further subdivided into separate medullary and pontine components), *vestibulospinal tract* (which is subdivided into separate medial and lateral components), and *tectospinal tract* (Table 9.1). These pathways project directly on spinal motor neurons, through monosynaptic connections, and indirectly by synapsing first on segmental interneurons and propriospinal neurons.

The locations of the descending axons in the spinal cord provide insight into their functions (Figures 9.1 and 9.4). Those that control *limb muscles* descend in the *lateral column* of the spinal cord and terminate in the *lateral intermediate zone* and *lateral ventral horn* (Figures 9.2, 9.4, and 9.15). The *lateral corticospinal tract* and the *rubrospinal tract* are the two laterally descending pathways. In humans, the lateral corticospinal tract has more axons than the rubrospinal tract. The *primary motor cortex* (area 4), located on the precentral gyrus (Figures 9.5 and 9.6), and the *supplementary motor area* (area 6), which is located predominantly on the medial surface of the hemisphere, contribute most of the fibers of the lateral corticospinal tract. (The other major contributor to the lateral corticospinal tract is the parietal lobe.) Higher order motor cortical regions are located rostral to the primary motor cortex in cytoarchitectonic *area 6*. The descending projection neurons of the cortex are located in *layer V* (Figure 9.5B) and their axons descend through the *posterior limb of the internal capsule* (Figures 9.7 and 9.9), then along the ventral brain stem surface (Figures 9.10–9.14). The lateral corticospinal tract decussates in the ventral medulla in the *pyramidal decussation*, at the junction of the medulla and the spinal cord (Figure 9.14B). In the spinal cord, the lateral corticospinal tract courses in the dorsal portion of the *lateral column* (Figures 9.4, 9.15, and 9.16). The other laterally descending pathway, the *rubrospinal tract*, originates from the *magnocellular portion of the red nucleus* (Figure 9.10). The axons decussate in the midbrain and descend in the *dorsolateral portion of the brain stem and spinal cord* (Figures 9.2B and 9.4). The other division of the red nucleus, the *parvocellular* component, is part of a circuit that involves the cerebellum.

The remaining four pathways course in the medial portion of the spinal cord white matter, the *ventral column*. These medially descending pathways terminate in the medial ventral horn—where axial motor neurons are located—and the medial intermediate zone (Figures 9.3, 9.4, and 9.16). These pathways influence motor neurons bilaterally: either the axon of the descending projection neuron decussates in the spinal cord or its terminals synapse on interneurons and propriospinal neurons whose axons decussate. The *ventral corticospinal tract*, which originates mostly in the primary motor cortex and the supplementary motor area, descends in the brain stem along with the lateral corticospinal tract, but does not decussate in the medulla and courses in the ventral column of the spinal cord (Figures 9.3A and 9.4). It influences axial and girdle motor neurons bilaterally because many of these axons decussate in the ventral spinal cord commissure. The *reticulospinal tracts* (pontine and medullary) descend ipsilaterally for the entire length of the spinal cord and function in posture and automatic responses like locomotion. There are two vestibulospinal tracts. The *medial vestibulospinal tract* (also termed the *descending medial longitudinal fasciculus*) originates primarily from the *medial vestibular nucleus* (Figure 9.13) and descends bilaterally only as far as the cervical cord. This pathway is important in control of head position. The *lateral vestibulospinal tract*, important in maintaining balance, originates from the *lateral vestibular nucleus (Deiters' nucleus)* (Figure 9.13) and descends *ipsilaterally* to all levels of the spinal cord. The *tectospinal tract* originates from the deeper layers of the *superior colliculus* (Figure 9.10), decussates in the midbrain, and descends medially in the caudal brain stem and spinal cord. This path descends to the cervical spinal cord only and plays a key role in coordination of head and eye movements. ∎

References

Asanuma, H., Fernandes, H. J., Scheibel, M. E., and Scheibel, A. B. 1974. Characteristics of projections from the nucleus ventralis lateralis to the motor cortex in the cats: An anatomical and physiological study. Exp. Brain Res. 20:315–330.

Betz, V. 1874. Anatomischer Nachweis zweier Gehirncentra. Centralbl. Med. Wiss. 12:578–580, 595–599.

Carpenter, M. B., and Sutin, J. 1983. Human Neuroanatomy. Baltimore: Williams & Wilkins.

Crosby, E. C., Humphrey, T., and Lauer, E. W. 1962. Correlative Anatomy of the Nervous System. New York: Macmillan.

Freund, H.-J., and Hummelsheim, H. 1984. Premotor cortex in man: Evidence for innervation of proximal limb muscles. Exp. Brain Res. 53:479–482.

Kuypers, H. G. J. M., and Brinkman, J. 1970. Precentral projections to different parts of the spinal intermediate zone in the rhesus monkey. Brain Res. 24:151–188.

Muakkassa, K. F., and Strick, P. L. 1979. Frontal lobe inputs to primate motor cortex: Evidence for four somatotopically organized "premotor" areas. Brain Res. 177:176–182.

Murray, E. A., and Coulter, J. D. 1981. Organization of corticospinal neurons in the monkey. J. Comp. Neurol. 195:339–365.

Penfield, W., and Rasmussen, T. 1950. The Cerebral Cortex of Man: A Clinical Study of Localization of Function. New York: Macmillan.

Schell, G. R., and Strick, P. L. 1984. The origin of thalamic inputs to the arcuate premotor and supplementary motor areas. J. Neurosci. 4:539–560.

Sterling, P., Kuypers, H. G. J. M. 1967. Anatomical organization of the brachial spinal cord of the cat. III. The propriospinal connections. Brain Res. 4:419–443.

Selected Readings

Asanuma, H. 1981. The Pyramidal Tract. In Brooks, V. B. (ed.), Handbook of Physiology, Section I: The Nervous System, Vol. II, Motor Control. Bethesda, Md.: American Physiological Society, pp. 703–733.

Ghez, C. 1985. Introduction to the Motor Systems. In Kandel, E. R., and Schwartz, J. H. Principles of Neural Science. New York: Elsevier, pp. 429–442.

Ghez, C. 1985. Voluntary movement. In Kandel, E. R., and Schwartz, J. H. Principles of Neural Science. New York: Elsevier, pp. 487–501.

Jankowska, E., and Lundberg, A. 1981. Interneurons in the spinal cord. Trends in Neurosci. 4:230–233.

Kuypers, H. G. J. M. 1981. Anatomy of the Descending Pathways. In Brooks, V. B. (ed.), Handbook of Physiology, Section I: The Nervous System, Vol. II, Motor Control. Bethesda, Md.: American Physiological Society, pp. 597–666.

Lance, J. W., and McLeod, J. G. 1981. A Physiological Approach to Clinical Neurology. London: Butterworths.

Wiesendanger, M. 1981. Organization of secondary motor areas of cerebral cortex. In Brooks, V. B. (ed.), Handbook of Physiology, Section I: The Nervous System, Vol. II, Motor Control. Bethesda, Md.: American Physiological Society, pp. 1121–1147.

Wise, S. P. 1985. The primate premotor cortex: Past, present, and preparatory. Ann. Rev. Neurosci. 8:1–19.

The Cerebellum

10

The Cerebellum

Two major brain structures play a key role in movement by regulating the function of the descending motor pathways: the cerebellum and the basal ganglia. In this chapter we focus on the cerebellum, and in Chapter 11, the basal ganglia. Movements are not lost when the cerebellum is damaged; rather, movements that were once automatic and precise become uncoordinated and erratic. Important insights into the general role of the cerebellum in motor control can be gained through a consideration of its connections with other brain regions. The cerebellum receives input from virtually the entire central nervous system, including all of the sensory systems and cortical association areas, as well as diverse areas of the brain stem. Its output is focused on specific components of the motor system. The cerebellum provides the major input to the red nucleus and is one of the major sources of input (via the thalamus) to the primary motor cortex (area 4) and premotor cortex (lateral portion of area 6).

Because the three-dimensional organization of the cerebellum is so complex, rivaling that of the cerebral cortex, we consider the gross anatomy first and then its functional organization. Next the cytoarchitecture of the cerebellar cortex is discussed. Finally, sections through the spinal cord, brain stem, diencephalon, and cerebral hemisphere are examined to identify the locations of key components of the cerebellum and its associated afferent and efferent projections.

The Convoluted Surface of the Cerebellar Cortex Is Organized into Three Lobes

The cerebellum lies dorsal to the pons and medulla (Figure 10.1) and is covered by an outer cortex of gray matter containing neuronal cell bodies overlying the white matter, which contains predominantly myelinated axons (Figure 10.2A). Like the cerebral cortex, the cerebellar cortex is highly convoluted. These cerebellar convolutions, termed *folia*, are equivalent to the gyri of the cerebral cortex. Their function is to vastly increase the amount of cerebellar cortex that can be packed into the *posterior cranial fossa*, the cranial compartment in which the cerebellum is located. The cerebellar cortex contains a rich array of neuron types (see later), including Purkinje cells, one of the largest of central nervous system neurons, and granule cells, which nearly outnumber all other neurons in the central nervous system. Two shallow grooves running from rostral to caudal divide the cerebellar cortex into the *vermis*, located along the midline, and *two hemispheres* (Figures 10.1A and C).

The cerebellar cortex is organized into groups of folia, termed *lobules*. In a section through the vermis, the lobules appear to originate at the apex of the roof of the fourth ventricle and radiate like spokes on a wheel (Figures 10.2A). Anatomists recognize ten lobules. This nomenclature, which is difficult for students to master, is used largely by specialists studying the cerebellum. The cerebellar lobules are separated from one another by fissures. Two fissures are particularly deep and divide the various lobules into *three lobes* (Figures 10.1 and 10.2A). The first through the fifth lobules constitute the *anterior lobe*. The *primary fissure* separates

A

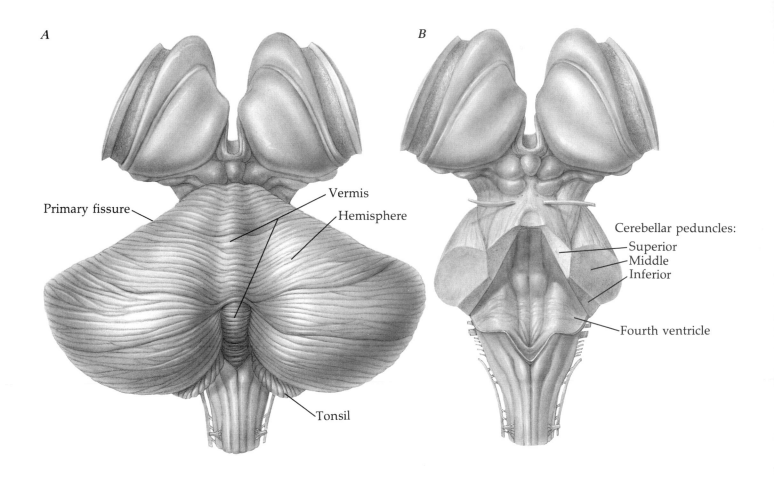

Primary fissure

Vermis

Hemisphere

Tonsil

B

Cerebellar peduncles:
Superior
Middle
Inferior

Fourth ventricle

C

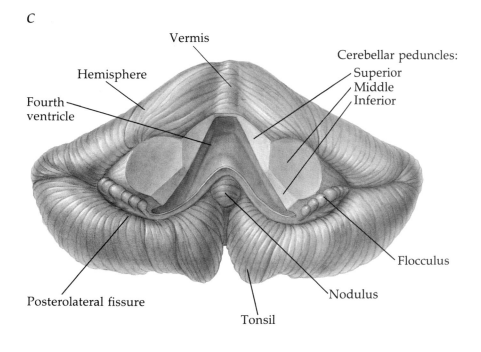

Vermis

Hemisphere

Fourth ventricle

Cerebellar peduncles:
Superior
Middle
Inferior

Flocculus

Nodulus

Posterolateral fissure

Tonsil

Figure 10.1 *A.* Dorsal view of the brain stem and cerebellum. *B.* The three cerebellar peduncles are revealed when the cerebellum is removed. *C.* The cerebellum, viewed from the ventral surface.

the anterior lobe from the *posterior lobe*, which contains the sixth through the ninth lobules. The anterior and posterior lobes collectively are important in the planning and control of *body movements*. The tenth lobule is the *flocculonodular lobe* and is separated from the posterior lobe by the *posterolateral fissure*. The nodulus is located on the midline (i.e., the vermis) and the flocculus, on either side. The flocculonodular lobe plays a key role in *maintaining balance and eye muscle control*.

Beneath the cerebellar cortex is *white matter*, which contains axons coursing to and from the cortex (Figure 10.2). The branching pattern of the white matter of the cerebellum inspired early anatomists to refer to it as the *arbor vitae* ("tree of life"); hence the name folia (leaves) rather than gyri is used to describe the convolutions of the cerebellar cortex. Embedded within the white matter of the cerebellum are four bilaterally paired nuclei, the *deep cerebellar nuclei*, shown in the schematic transverse section through the pons and cerebellum (Figure 10.2B): *fastigial nucleus*, *globose nucleus*, *emboliform nucleus*, and *dentate nucleus*. The globose and emboliform nuclei are collectively termed the *interposed nucleus*. The deep cerebellar nuclei are key elements in the neural circuit of the cerebellum (see later).

The cerebellum is attached to the brain stem by three *peduncles* (Figures 10.1B and C). Afferent axons projecting to the cerebellum and efferent axons exiting from the cerebellum course through the cerebellar peduncles: the *superior cerebellar peduncle* contains mostly *efferent axons*, the *middle cerebellar peduncle* contains *afferent axons*, and the *inferior cerebellar peduncle* contains predominantly *afferent axons*.[1] The different peduncles are distinguished in Figures 10.1B and C because each one has been given a different cut surface in the dissection. Three distinct peduncles would not be apparent had a single cut been made.

There Are Three Different Functional Divisions of the Cerebellar Cortex, All with a Similar Input–Output Organization

The cerebellar cortex has three functional divisions and the boundaries of these divisions correspond roughly with gross anatomical features (Figures 10.1 and 10.3). The *spinocerebellum* (1) receives somatic sensory information from the spinal cord and is important in guiding *limb movement* and *posture*. The spinocerebellum, corresponds to the *vermis* and paravermal cerebellar cortex, termed the *intermediate hemisphere*, of both the anterior and posterior lobes. The *cerebrocerebellum* (2) receives input from the *cerebral cortex* (via a relay in the pontine nuclei) and participates in the *planning of movement*. It is located lateral to the spinocerebellum in both the anterior and posterior lobes, regions termed the *lateral hemisphere*. The *vestibulocerebellum* (3) receives input from the *vestibular labyrinth* and functions in the *maintenance of balance* and the *control of head and eye movements*. This cerebellar division corresponds to the *flocculonodular lobe*.

Each functional division of the cerebellar cortex has a similar generalized pattern of afferent and efferent connections, but each division

---

[1] The cerebellar peduncles have an alternate nomenclature. The superior cerebellar peduncle is also called the brachium conjunctivum; the middle cerebellar peduncle, the brachium pontis; and the inferior cerebellar peduncle, the restiform body.

A

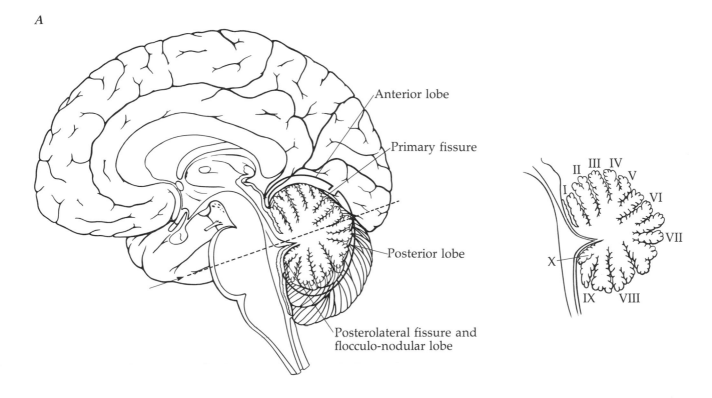

Anterior lobe

Primary fissure

Posterior lobe

Posterolateral fissure and
flocculo-nodular lobe

II III IV
V
I VI
VII
X
IX VIII

B

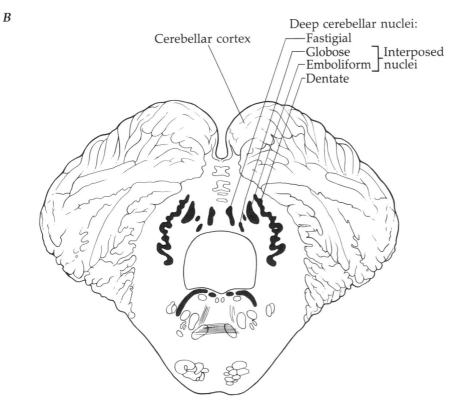

Cerebellar cortex

Deep cerebellar nuclei:
Fastigial
Globose ⎤ Interposed
Emboliform ⎦ nuclei
Dentate

Figure 10.2 *A.* Midsagittal cut
through the cerebellum. *B.* Schematic
transverse section through the pons
and cerebellum illustrating the
location of the deep cerebellar nuclei.

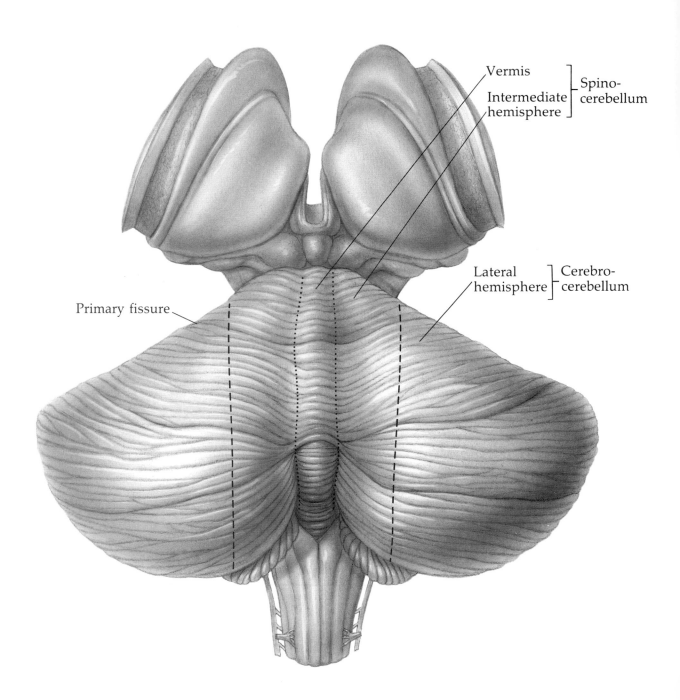

differs from the other with respect to the specific sources of input and the specific structures to which it projects. The basic organizational plan of the cerebellar functional divisions is shown in Figure 10.4. Input to the cerebellum is directed both to the cerebellar cortex and to the deep nuclei. The traditional view is that the axons of neurons projecting to the cerebellum terminate in both cerebellar cortex and deep nuclei (arrow marked

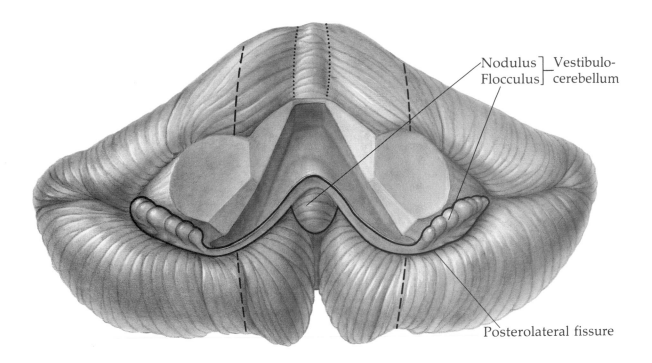

Nodulus ⎤ Vestibulo-
Flocculus ⎦ cerebellum

Posterolateral fissure

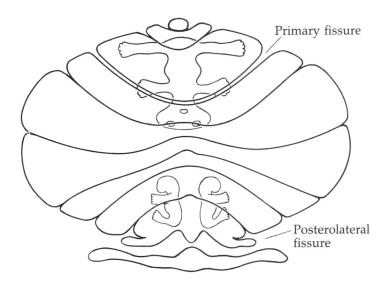

Primary fissure

Posterolateral
fissure

Figure 10.3   The three functional
divisions are shown in superior *(A)*
and inferior *(B)* views of the
cerebellum. Inset shows the
topographic organization of inputs to
the spinocerebellum. Somatic sensory
inputs are somatotopically organized.
Visual, auditory, and vestibular
inputs are directed predominantly to
the "head" areas.

b in Figure 10.4). Whereas this is the projection pattern for some sites (for
example, the inferior olivary nucleus, see later), recent anatomical studies
have demonstrated that many of the major sources of cerebellar input
terminate only in the cortex (arrow marked *a* in Figure 10.3). These new
findings will force a reevaluation of how neural circuits of the cerebellum
function. (We consider the intrinsic organization in a later section.)

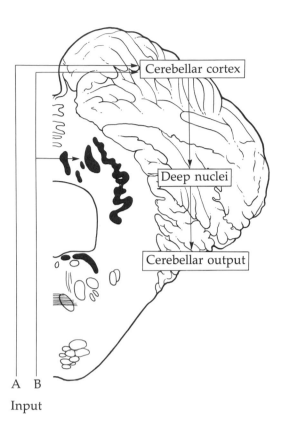

Figure 10.4 Key features of the input–output organization of the cerebellum.

The Vermis and the Intermediate Hemisphere Are the Anatomical Components of the Spinocerebellum

The *spinocerebellum* (Figures 10.5 and 10.6) is important in the control of body musculature. It is somatotopically organized, and the two anatomical portions of the spinocerebellum, the vermis and the intermediate hemisphere, control axial muscles and limb muscles, respectively (Figure 10.3 inset). This mediolateral somatotopic arrangement is reminiscent of the somatotopic organization of the ventral horn, where medial motor neurons innervate *axial muscles*, and those located laterally innervate *distal muscles* (Chapter 9).

The vermis receives somatic sensory information, originating largely from the trunk, via the *spinocerebellar tracts* (see later). Somatic sensory information from the head is transmitted to the vermis via the spinal nucleus of CN V. In addition, the vermis receives a direct projection from primary sensory neurons of the *vestibular labyrinth*, as well as *visual* and *auditory* input relayed by brain stem nuclei. The intermediate hemisphere receives somatic sensory information primarily from the limbs. This is the major input to the intermediate hemisphere, and it is transmitted from the spinal cord via the four spinocerebellar tracts: dorsal spinocerebellar tract, cuneocerebellar tract, ventral spinocerebellar tract, and rostral spinocerebellar tract. The *dorsal spinocerebellar tract* (Figure 10.5) transmits somatic sensory information from the leg and lower trunk. This tract originates in *Clarke's nucleus*, which receives input directly from large diameter primary afferent fibers that innervate muscle spindles (Table

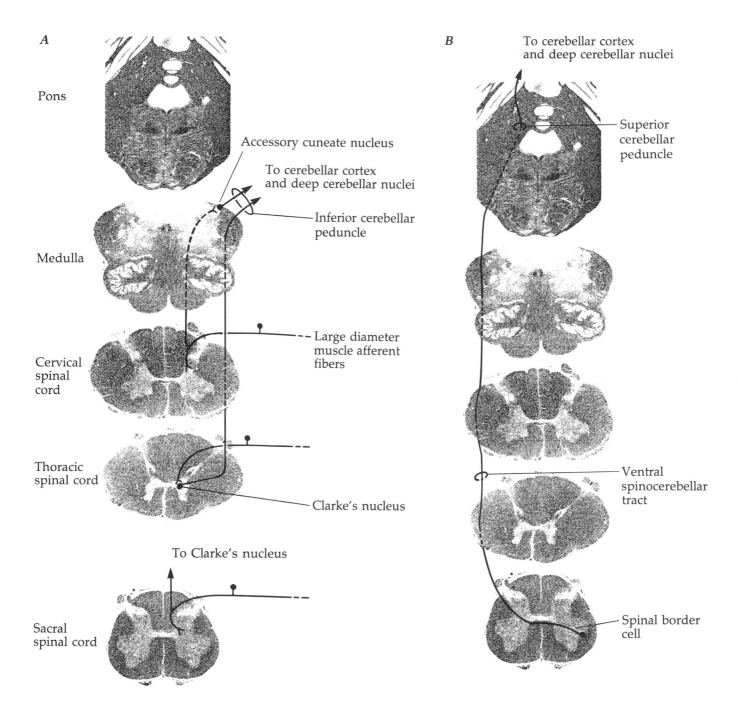

A

Pons

Accessory cuneate nucleus

To cerebellar cortex
and deep cerebellar nuclei

Inferior cerebellar
peduncle

Medulla

Large diameter
muscle afferent
fibers

Cervical
spinal
cord

Thoracic
spinal cord

Clarke's nucleus

To Clarke's nucleus

Sacral
spinal cord

B

To cerebellar cortex
and deep cerebellar nuclei

Superior
cerebellar
peduncle

Ventral
spinocerebellar
tract

Spinal border
cell

5.1). Neurons giving rise to the dorsal spinocerebellar tract send their axons into the *ipsilateral lateral column*. The *accessory cuneate nucleus*[2] is the functional equivalent of Clarke's nucleus for the upper limb. Afferent fibers course rostrally in the cuneate fascicle to synapse in the accessory cuneate nucleus. Both the dorsal spinocerebellar tract and the cuneocerebellar tract enter the cerebellum via the *ipsilateral inferior cerebellar pe-*

Figure 10.5 **A.** Spinocerebellar pathways relaying sensory feedback (dorsal spinocerebellar and cuneocerebellar tracts). **B.** Spinocerebellar pathways relaying information about the amount of activity in descending pathways (ventral spinocerebellar and rostral spinocerebellar tracts).

---

[2] At its caudal pole, the accessory cuneate nucleus merges with the cuneate nucleus. The accessory cuneate nucleus is also named the external cuneate nucleus and the lateral cuneate nucleus.

A

B

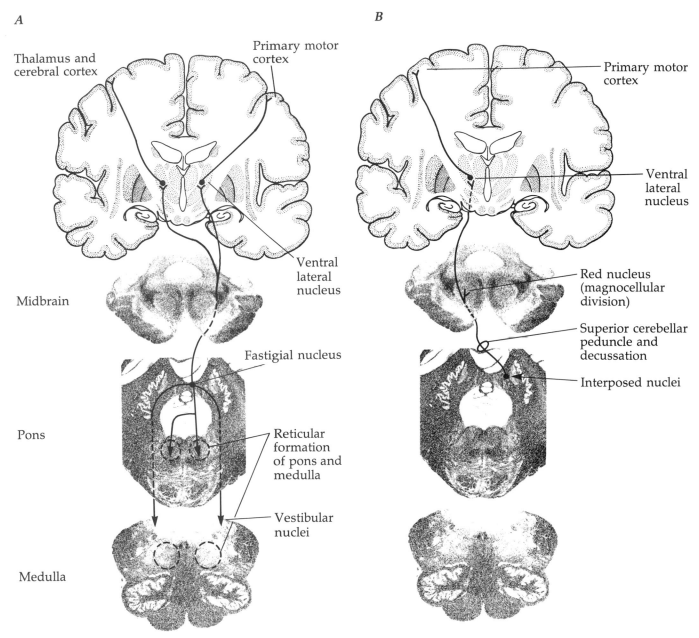

Thalamus and cerebral cortex

Primary motor cortex

Primary motor cortex

Ventral lateral nucleus

Midbrain

Ventral lateral nucleus

Red nucleus (magnocellular division)

Superior cerebellar peduncle and decussation

Fastigial nucleus

Interposed nuclei

Pons

Reticular formation of pons and medulla

Vestibular nuclei

Medulla

Figure 10.6 Efferent pathways from the vermis of the spinocerebellum *(A)* and the intermediate hemisphere *(B)*. Note that the ascending projection of the fastigial nucleus to the thalamus is small compared with the descending projection to the pons and medulla.

duncle. The pattern of termination of spinocerebellar input is somatotopic, forming the separate *homunculi* rostrally in the anterior lobe and caudally in the posterior lobe (Figure 10.3 inset).

The *ventral spinocerebellar* tract is a lower limb pathway; the *rostral spinocerebellar tract* is its upper limb equivalent. It is currently believed that these two pathways relay an *internal feedback signal* to the cerebellum, which reflects the amount of neural activity in descending motor pathways, rather than *sensory information* from the periphery. The ventral spinocerebellar tract (Figure 10.5B) originates from neurons predominantly in the intermediate zone. In contrast to the cells of origin of the dorsal spino- and cuneocerebellar tracts, the cells of origin of the ventral spinocerebellar tract are not confined to a discrete nucleus. These neurons are termed the *spinal border cells*. The axons decussate in the spinal cord and ascend in the ventral portion of the lateral column (Figure 10.5B). In the pons, the axons enter the cerebellum via the *superior cerebellar peduncle*. Once in the cerebellum, some axons decussate again and terminate in the ipsilateral cerebellum. This "double-crossed," contingent is smaller than the crossed group. The rostral spinocerebellar tract has an anatomical organization different from that of its lower limb equivalent: the rostral spinocerebellar tract is an *ipsilateral* pathway and enters the cerebellum via both the *inferior and the superior cerebellar peduncles*.[3]

The two components of the spinocerebellum project to two deep cerebellar nuclei: the vermis projects to the *fastigial nucleus* and the intermediate hemisphere projects to the *interposed nuclei*. The deep nuclei, in turn, influence motor neurons primarily through their projections onto the descending systems (Figure 10.6). The fastigial nucleus projects to nuclei that give rise to the brain stem motor pathways that descend in the *medial spinal cord*, the reticulospinal and vestibulospinal tracts. The fastigial nucleus also has a small ascending projection, via a thalamic relay in the ventral lateral nucleus, to the cells of origin of the ventral corticospinal tract. The interposed nuclei project to the *lateral descending systems*, the magnocellular component of the red nucleus, which gives rise to the rubrospinal tract and, via the ventral lateral nucleus, to the portions of the motor area of the frontal lobe that give rise to the lateral corticospinal tract.

The Lateral Hemisphere Corresponds to the Cerebrocerebellum

There is no gross anatomical boundary between the spinocerebellum and the *cerebrocerebellum* (Figure 10.3), which is located in the most lateral portion of the cerebellar hemisphere. The cerebrocerebellum is involved in the planning of movement and is interconnected with the *cerebral cortex*. The afferent and efferent connections of the cerebrocerebellum are illustrated in Figure 10.7. The major input to the cerebrocerebellum is from the *contralateral cerebral cortex*: this is not a direct projection, but one that is relayed by the *pontine nuclei* and the *middle cerebellar peduncle*. The efferent projection from the cerebrocerebellum is to the *dentate nucleus*, which in turn sends its axons to two main sites. The first is the ventral lateral nucleus, the motor relay nucleus of the thalamus. The second site is the *red nucleus*; however, it projects to the *parvocellular* portion of the red nucleus, not the magnocellular portion. Whereas the magnocellular

---

[3] The spinocerebellar pathways are direct pathways from the spinal cord to the cerebellum: the axon of a neuron in the spinal cord terminates in the cerebellum. In addition, there exist indirect routes from the spinal cord. These pathways synapse in the reticular formation and the inferior olivary nuclear complex, adding an additional neuron to the circuit.

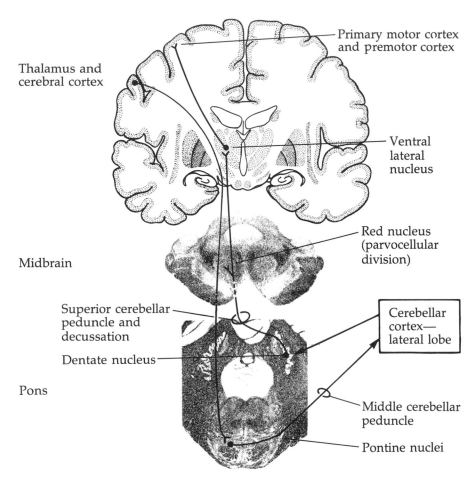

Thalamus and
cerebral cortex

Primary motor cortex
and premotor cortex

Ventral
lateral
nucleus

Red nucleus
(parvocellular
division)

Midbrain

Superior cerebellar
peduncle and
decussation

Dentate nucleus

Cerebellar
cortex—
lateral lobe

Pons

Middle cerebellar
peduncle

Pontine nuclei

Figure 10.7 Afferent and efferent connections of the cerebrocerebellum. Note that the major input to the pontine nuclei is from the entire cerebral cortex although input from only a single site is shown.

portion of the red nucleus gives rise to the rubrospinal tract (Chapter 9), the parvocellular division projects to the ipsilateral *inferior olivary nucleus*, a major source of input to the cerebellum.

The Flocculonodular Lobe Corresponds to the Vestibulocerebellum

The *vestibulocerebellum* (Figure 10.3) is important in maintaining balance and control of eye muscles. This cerebellar division receives afferent input from *primary vestibular afferents* and secondary vestibular neurons in the *vestibular nuclei*. In fact, the vestibular afferents are the only primary sensory neurons that project directly to the cerebellum. Unlike the spinocerebellum and the cerebrocerebellum, which project to the deep cerebellar nuclei, the vestibulocerebellum projects both to the fastigial nucleus as well as the medial, inferior, and superior *vestibular nuclei* (Figure 10.8).[4] These vestibular nuclei give rise to the medial vestibulospinal tract

---

[4] Purkinje cells in certain restricted portions of the vermis of the spinocerebellum also project to the lateral vestibular nucleus.

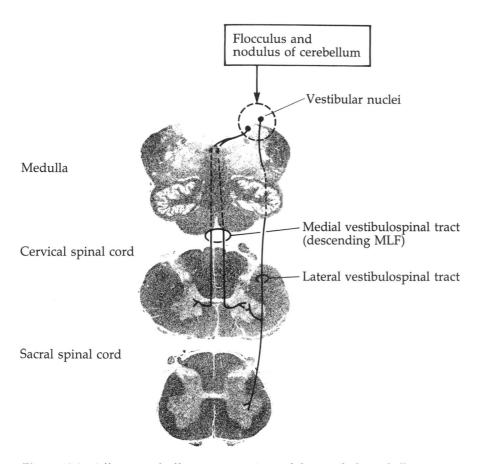

Flocculus and
nodulus of cerebellum

Vestibular nuclei

Medulla

Cervical spinal cord

Medial vestibulospinal tract
(descending MLF)

Lateral vestibulospinal tract

Sacral spinal cord

Figure 10.8 Afferent and efferent connections of the vestibulocerebellum.

as well as fibers in the medial longitudinal fasciculus. The vestibular nuclei are anatomically similar to the deep cerebellar nuclei (see later).

In the remaining sections the regional anatomy of cerebellum and associated nuclei and tracts is examined. First, the histology of the cerebellar cortex is explored. The cellular constituents and synaptic connections of the cerebellum are among the best understood of the central nervous system. Then cuts through key levels illustrating locations of the cerebellar peduncles, afferent and efferent pathways, and deep cerebellar nuclei are examined.

The Intrinsic Circuitry of the Cerebellar Cortex Is Similar for the Different Functional Divisions

The cerebellar cortex consists of three layers (Figure 10.9), progressing from its external surface inward: the *molecular layer*, the *Purkinje layer*, and the *granular layer*, which is adjacent to the white matter. There are five types of neurons in the cerebellar cortex, and they have a different laminar distribution (Table 10.1): (1) Purkinje cell, (2) granule cell, (3) basket cell, (4) stellate cell, and (5) Golgi cell. The cellular organization of the cerebellar cortex is considered in a stepwise fashion in Figures 10.10A–C, beginning with the Purkinje cell and its excitatory inputs.

A

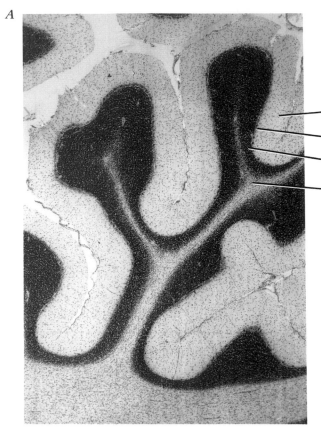

Molecular layer

Purkinje layer

Granular layer

White matter

Figure 10.9 Nissl-stained section through the cerebellar cortex. *A.* Low-power view. *B.* High-power view. (Photograph by Al Lamme, Department of Pathology, Columbia University.)

B

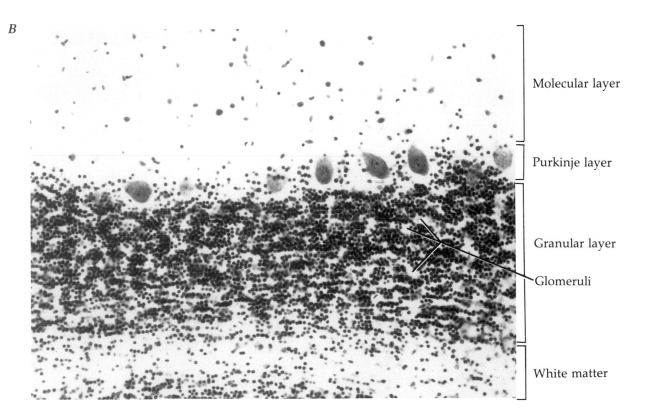

Molecular layer

Purkinje layer

Granular layer

Glomeruli

White matter

Table 10.1   Cerebellar Cortex Neurons

Cell Type	Laminar Distribution	Postsynaptic Action	Postsynaptic Target
Projection neuron			
Purkinje	Purkinje	Inhibitory	Neurons of deep nuclei, vestibular nuclei
Interneurons			
Granule	Granular	Excitatory	Purkinje, stellate, basket, and Golgi cells
Basket	Molecular	Inhibitory	Purkinje cells
Stellate	Molecular	Inhibitory	Purkinje cells
Golgi	Granular	Inhibitory	Granule cells

The Purkinje layer contains only one type of cell, the *Purkinje cell*. This is the only type of neuron whose axon projects from the cerebellar cortex (Figures 10.10 and 10.11). Purkinje cells receive inputs from the two major cerebellar afferents: climbing fibers and mossy fibers. *Climbing fibers* originate entirely from the *inferior olivary nuclear complex* (Figure 10.13) and reach all parts of the cerebellum, including both the cerebellar cortex and the deep nuclei. There is a remarkable degree of specificity of the connections of Purkinje cells and climbing fibers: *each Purkinje cell receives input from a single climbing fiber*, which will make contact with no more than ten other Purkinje cells. An individual climbing fiber makes multiple synapses with the Purkinje cell, forming one of the strongest excitatory connections in the central nervous system. *Mossy fibers* provide the second major input to the Purkinje cell, although these fibers do not make monosynaptic connections like those of the climbing fiber. The cell bodies of mossy fibers are located primarily in the spinal cord (Figure 10.12) and two brain stem nuclear groups, pontine nuclei (Figures 10.14 and 10.15), and nuclei of the reticular formation. Axon collaterals of mossy fibers were previously thought to synapse on neurons of the deep nuclei. However, recent studies suggest that mossy fibers from major brain stem nuclei, in particular the pontine nuclei, synapse only in the cerebellar cortex. In the cerebellar cortex, mossy fibers synapse on *granule cells*, which are excitatory interneurons in the granular layer (Figure 10.10A). The granule cell axon ascends through the Purkinje layer into the molecular layer, where it bifurcates to form the *parallel fibers*, which synapse on Purkinje cells and cerebellar interneurons (Figure 10.10B). One parallel fiber will synapse with thousands of Purkinje cells, and each Purkinje cell receives synapses from thousands of parallel fibers. Unlike the climbing fiber, which makes multiple synaptic contacts with the Purkinje cell, the parallel fiber makes only a few synapses with each Purkinje cell. This paucity of parallel fiber synaptic contacts on the Purkinje cell is a reflection of the orientation of Purkinje cell dendrites in relation to the parallel fibers. Briefly, the Purkinje cell dendritic tree (Figures 10.10 and 10.11) is planar and oriented orthogonal to the long axis of the folium in which it is located (much like coins stacked on top of one another). The parallel fiber courses at a right angle to the dendritic plane of the Purkinje cell

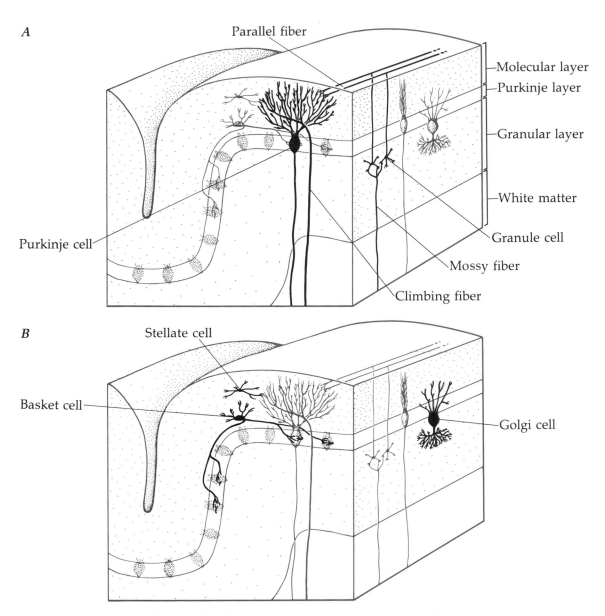

Figure 10.10 The circuitry of the cerebellar cortex is illustrated in a stepwise fashion. *A.* Two major excitatory inputs to Purkinje cells, climbing fibers and mossy fibers–parallel fibers. *B.* Inhibitory interneurons.

(i.e., parallel to the long axis of the folium) and, therefore, makes only a few contacts with a single Purkinje cell as the axon passes through the dendritic tree. As a consequence of these differences in the number of synaptic contacts, the strength of parallel fiber input to a Purkinje cell is much less than that of climbing fiber input. It has been suggested that the efficacy of parallel fiber input onto a given Purkinje cell is increased immediately after Purkinje cell activation by a climbing fiber. Purkinje cells, the projection neurons of the cerebellar cortex, synapse on cells of the deep cerebellar nuclei and vestibular nuclei.

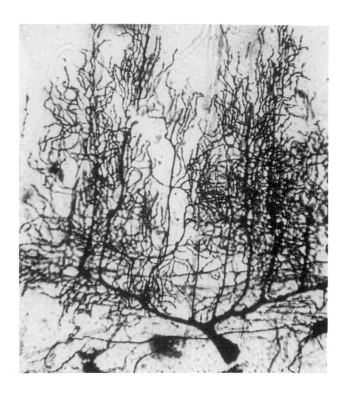

Figure 10.11 Golgi-stained section of the cerebellar cortex showing a Purkinje cell.

The Purkinje cell is inhibited by two groups of interneurons (Figure 10.10B): *stellate cells*, located in the outer portion of the molecular layer, and *basket cells*, located close to the border between the molecular and Purkinje layers. Both of these neurons receive their predominant input from the parallel fibers. The locations of the synaptic terminals of the basket and stellate cells have important functional significance. The basket cell synapse is located on the Purkinje cell body, forming a dense mesh-work, or "basket," of inhibitory synaptic contacts. The basket cell synapse is one of the strongest inhibitory synapses in the central nervous system because of its close proximity to the spike initiation zone, at the axon hillock of the Purkinje cell. In contrast, the stellate cell synapse is located on the distal dendrites, far from the axon hillock, and hence the degree of inhibition it produces on Purkinje cells is much less than that of the basket cell. As we see in Figure 10.10, the basket cell axon is oriented at a right angle to the folium; therefore, only Purkinje cells located in a band on either side of the basket cell are contacted.

The *Golgi cell* (Figure 10.10B) is the interneuron that inhibits the granule cell. This inhibitory synapse is made in the granular layer, in a complex structure termed the *cerebellar glomerulus*. The cerebellar glomerulus consists of two presynaptic elements, the *mossy fiber terminal* and the *Golgi cell axon*,[5] and one main postsynaptic element, the *granule cell dendrite*. Synaptic glomeruli ensure specificity of connections because this entire synaptic complex is contained within a *glial capsule*. The mossy fiber

---

[5] The mossy fiber terminal is also termed the mossy fiber rosette because of the configuration of its enlarged terminal.

terminals are located in the clear zones seen under high power in the Nissl-stained section of the cerebellar cortex (Figure 10.9B).

If we now take an inventory of the synaptic action of the interneurons of the cerebellar cortex (Table 10.1) we see that all but the granule cell are inhibitory. Interestingly, even the projection neuron of the cerebellar cortex, the Purkinje cell, is inhibitory. It is thought that the direct excitatory synaptic connection on deep cerebellar nuclei of the mossy fibers from the spinal cord and climbing fibers on neurons of the deep cerebellar nuclei (Figure 10.4) contributes to a high level of background neuronal activity which is then "sculpted" by the inhibitory action of the Purkinje cell.

In the remaining portions of the chapter we considered sections through the spinal cord, brain stem, and diencephalon for the purpose of examining locations of pathways projecting to the cerebellum, components of the cerebellum itself, and its associated efferent projections. We begin with the spinal cord and the spinocerebellar tracts, which bring somatic sensory information to the cerebellum that is important for the control of movement. Then we consider sections through the medulla and pons which cut through important nuclei that project to the cerebellum as well as the four deep cerebellar nuclei. Finally, we examine a series of sections through the rostral pons, midbrain, and diencephalon to follow cerebellar efferent paths.

Sections through the Spinal Cord and Medulla Reveal the Nuclei and Pathways That Relay Somatic Sensory Information to the Cerebellum

Clarke's nucleus and the accessory cuneate nucleus are the principal nuclei that relay somatic sensory information to the spinocerebellum. *Clarke's nucleus* (Figure 10.12) is located in the *medial portion* of the intermediate zone of the spinal cord gray matter (lamina VII). Clarke's nucleus

Figure 10.12 Myelin-stained transverse section through the lumbar spinal cord.

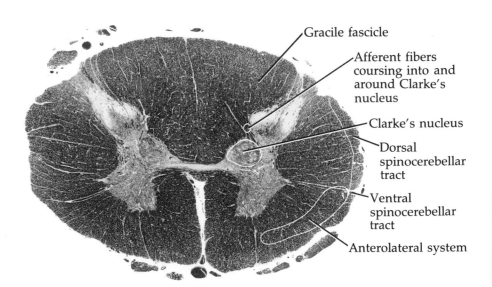

Gracile fascicle

Afferent fibers coursing into and around Clarke's nucleus

Clarke's nucleus

Dorsal spinocerebellar tract

Ventral spinocerebellar tract

Anterolateral system

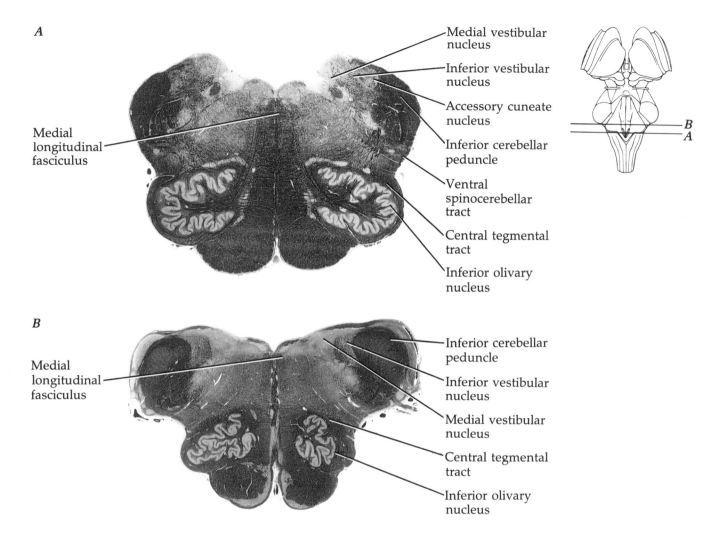

A

Medial longitudinal fasciculus

Medial vestibular nucleus

Inferior vestibular nucleus

Accessory cuneate nucleus

Inferior cerebellar peduncle

Ventral spinocerebellar tract

Central tegmental tract

Inferior olivary nucleus

B

Medial longitudinal fasciculus

Inferior cerebellar peduncle

Inferior vestibular nucleus

Medial vestibular nucleus

Central tegmental tract

Inferior olivary nucleus

B
A

Figure 10.13 Myelin-stained transverse sections through the medulla through the accessory cuneate nucleus *(A)* and more rostrally *(B)*.

forms a column with a limited rostrocaudal distribution.[6] In the human, Clarke's nucleus spans the *eighth cervical segment (C8)* to approximately the *second lumbar segment* (L2). It is curious that most of Clarke's nucleus is located caudal to the cervical enlargement and rostral to the lumbo-sacral enlargement. The functional significance of this is unclear. The large-diameter afferent fibers that synapse in Clarke's nucleus course medially around the cap of the dorsal horn and through the ipsilateral dorsal column en route to their termination site. In Figure 10.12 some of the axons can be seen following this trajectory. Afferent fibers arriving over dorsal roots caudal to the second lumbar segment first ascend in the *gracile fascicle* and then leave the white matter to terminate in Clarke's nucleus. Clarke's nucleus gives rise to the dorsal spinocerebellar tract, which ascends in the outermost portion of the lateral column (lateral to the corticospinal and rubrospinal tracts). The location of the other pathway from the lower limb, the ventral spinocerebellar tract, is also shown in Figure 10.12 in relation to the ascending fibers of the anterolateral system. The ventral spinocerebellar tract originates from the spinal border cells.

---

[6] Two other names for Clarke's nucleus are Clarke's column and nucleus dorsalis.

The Vestibulocerebellum Receives Input from Primary and Secondary Vestibular Neurons

In the cervical spinal cord and caudal medulla, the spatial relationship between the locations of the dorsal spinocerebellar tract and the ventral spinocerebellar tract is maintained. More rostrally in the medulla, the dorsal spinocerebellar tract enters the cerebellum via the *inferior cerebellar peduncle* (Figure 10.13). At this level the accessory cuneate nucleus can be identified (Figure 10.13A). It receives input from the *cuneate fascicle* and, like the dorsal spinocerebellar tract, projects to the cerebellum via the *inferior cerebellar peduncle*. In contrast, the ventral spinocerebellar tract continues to ascend within the brain stem and enters the cerebellum via the *superior cerebellar peduncle* (Figure 10.15).

In addition to afferent information from the spinal cord, there are three major groups of brain stem nuclei that project to the cerebellum: the *inferior olivary nucleus,*[7] the *vestibular nuclei,* and the *pontine nuclei.* Two of these nuclei, the inferior olivary nucleus and the vestibular nuclei, can be seen in the transverse sections through the medulla shown in Figure 10.13. The inferior olivary nucleus, from which the *climbing fibers* originate, is large and forms an elevation on the ventral surface of the medulla termed the *olive.* The vestibular nuclei are located in the rostral medulla and caudal pons (Figures 10.13 and 10.14). Purkinje cells of the flocculonodular lobe send their axons primarily to the vestibular nuclei, rather than to the deep cerebellar nuclei, as do Purkinje cells in other regions of the cerebellum. (Exceptions exist and some Purkinje cells of the flocculonodular lobe project their axons to the fastigial nucleus.) The vestibular nuclei and deep cerebellar nuclei share two similarities in the sources of afferent input. First, both of these groups of nuclei receive a projection from the inferior olivary nucleus. Other than the cerebellar cortex, the only other major structure to which the inferior olivary nucleus projects is the deep cerebellar nuclei. Second, neurons in both the vestibular nuclei and the deep cerebellar nuclei are monosynaptically inhibited by Purkinje cells. The vestibular nuclei may serve as the anatomical equivalent of the deep cerebellar nuclei of the vestibulocerebellum. The vestibular nuclei (Figure 10.13) give rise to the vestibulospinal tracts (Chapter 9) and also contribute to the *medial longitudinal fasciculus* (Figures 10.13–10.17), which plays a key role in eye muscle control (Chapter 13). Thus, the vestibulocerebellum has direct control of head and eye position via its influence on the vestibular nuclei.

The Pontine Nuclei Provide the Major Input to the Cerebrocerebellum

The pontine nuclei (Figures 10.14 and 10.15) relay input from the cerebral cortex to the cerebrocerebellum. The densest projections from the cerebral cortex to the pontine nuclei derive from four regions, from rostral to caudal: (1) *premotor cortex* and *supplementary motor area (area 6),* (2) *primary motor cortex (area 4),* (3) *primary somatic sensory cortex* (areas 1,2,

---

[7] The inferior olivary nucleus (or nuclear complex) is a collection of three nuclei: the principal olivary nucleus, the dorsal accessory olivary nucleus, and the medial accessory olivary nucleus.

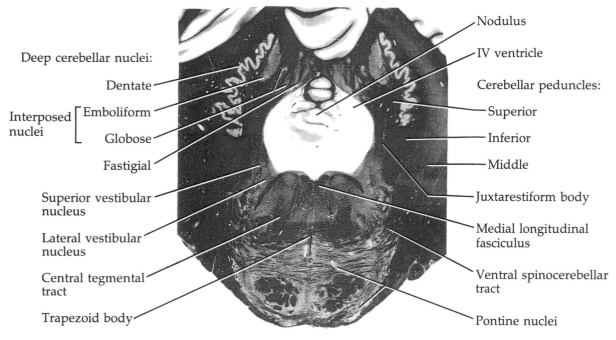

Deep cerebellar nuclei:

Dentate

Interposed nuclei [Emboliform

Globose

Fastigial

Superior vestibular nucleus

Lateral vestibular nucleus

Central tegmental tract

Trapezoid body

Nodulus

IV ventricle

Cerebellar peduncles:

Superior

Inferior

Middle

Juxtarestiform body

Medial longitudinal fasciculus

Ventral spinocerebellar tract

Pontine nuclei

Figure 10.14 Myelin-stained transverse section through the caudal pons and deep cerebellar nuclei.

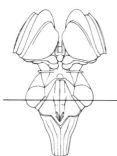

and 3), and (4) *higher-order somatic sensory cortex (area 5)*. Corticopontine neurons are located in layer V of the cerebral cortex, the same layer that gives rise to the corticospinal and corticobulbar neurons (Figure 9.5B), and the descending axons course within the internal capsule and basis pedunculi (see later). The axons of neurons of the pontine nuclei decussate in the pons and enter the cerebellum via the *middle cerebellar peduncle* (Figures 10.14 and 10.15). (The auditory decussation [trapezoid body] is located dorsal to the decussating pontine nucleus axons [Figure 10.14].)

The Deep Cerebellar Nuclei Are Located within the White Matter

The deep cerebellar nuclei can be identified in the transverse section through the pons and cerebellum shown in Figure 10.14, from medial to lateral: fastigial, globose, emboliform, and dentate nuclei. (The globose and emboliform nuclei collectively are termed the interposed nuclei.) The efferent projections of the deep nuclei course through the inferior and superior cerebellar peduncles. (The middle cerebellar peduncle carries afferent information to the cerebellum.) The major projection of the fastigial nucleus is to the pons and medulla, via a "descending" projection that courses in the inferior cerebellar peduncle. These axons are segregated within the peduncle to form the *juxtarestiform body* (Figure 10.14). The "ascending" projections from the four deep nuclei course in the *superior cerebellar peduncle* (Figure 10.15). In Figure 10.15A, the superior cerebellar peduncle is dorsal to the pons and, farther rostrally (Figure 10.15B), it is located within the pontine *tegmentum*.

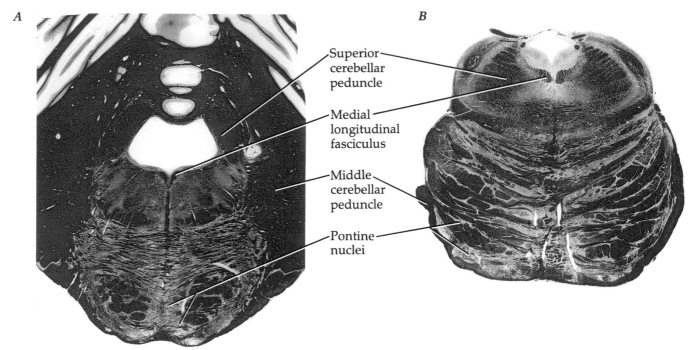

A

B

Superior
cerebellar
peduncle

Medial
longitudinal
fasciculus

Middle
cerebellar
peduncle

Pontine
nuclei

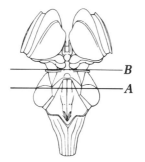

B

A

Figure 10.15   Myelin-stained transverse sections through the pons, rostral to the deep cerebellar nuclei **(A)** and farther rostrally (isthmus) in the pons **(B)**.

The Superior Cerebellar Peduncle Decussates in the Caudal Midbrain

Each of the deep cerebellar nuclei has a projection that courses in the superior cerebellar peduncle (Figure 10.15). At the level shown in Figure 10.15A, the axons are located ipsilateral to the cells of origin in the deep cerebellar nuclei. The *decussation* of the superior cerebellar peduncle occurs in the caudal midbrain, at the level of the inferior colliculus (Figure 10.16A). (Actually, a small contingent of decussating axons can be seen in Figure 10.15B.) The ascending axons of the interposed nuclei synapse in the *magnocellular* portion of the red nucleus. The rubrospinal tract originates from this division of the red nucleus. Neurons of the dentate nucleus synapse in the parvocellular portion of the red nucleus (Figure 10.16B). In humans the parvocellular division is much larger than the magnocellular division. Neurons of the parvocellular division of the red nucleus send their axons to the ipsilateral inferior olivary nucleus via the *central tegmental tract* (Figures 10.13 and 10.14). The ascending projection from the dentate nucleus to the red nucleus can be traced in the section shown in Figure 10.17. This section was cut obliquely, along the long axis of the superior cerebellar peduncle. The paths taken by the axons of dentate nucleus neurons are schematically illustrated.

The ventral surface of the midbrain is the basis pedunculi, where the descending corticopontine projection courses. The corticopontine projection from the frontal lobe is located in the medial basis pedunculi, whereas the projection from the parietal, temporal, and occipital lobes

A

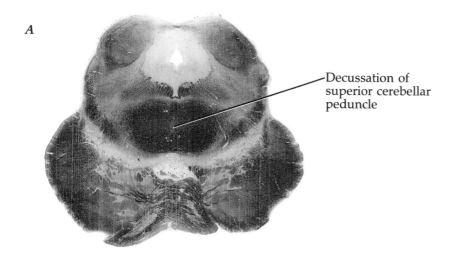

Decussation of
superior cerebellar
peduncle

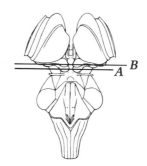

B

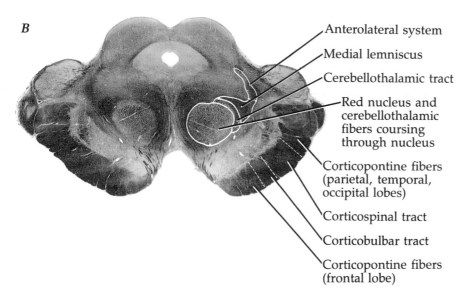

Anterolateral system

Medial lemniscus

Cerebellothalamic tract

Red nucleus and
cerebellothalamic
fibers coursing
through nucleus

Corticopontine fibers
(parietal, temporal,
occipital lobes)

Corticospinal tract

Corticobulbar tract

Corticopontine fibers
(frontal lobe)

Figure 10.16 Myelin-stained
transverse sections through the
caudal *(A)* and the rostral *(B)*
midbrain. The organization of the
fibers in the basis pedunculi is
shown in part B.

descends laterally. The corticospinal and corticobulbar fibers (Chapter 9)
are interposed between these two contingents of corticopontine fibers.

The Ventral Lateral Nucleus Relays Cerebellar Output to the Premotor and Primary Motor Cortices

Each of the deep cerebellar nuclei has an ascending projection that
synapses in the ventral lateral nucleus of the thalamus. However, the
projection from the dentate nucleus is much denser than that of the interposed nuclei. The ascending projection of the fastigial is the lightest
of the deep nuclei. This projection, termed the cerebellothalamic tract,
courses directly through the red nucleus (Figure 10.17) as well as forms
a dense ring of myelinated fibers around it (Figure 10.16B). The ventral
lateral nucleus (Figure 10.18) is difficult to identify. One clue that makes
identification easier is the presence of the thalamic fasciculus. This band

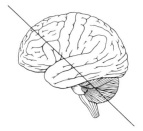

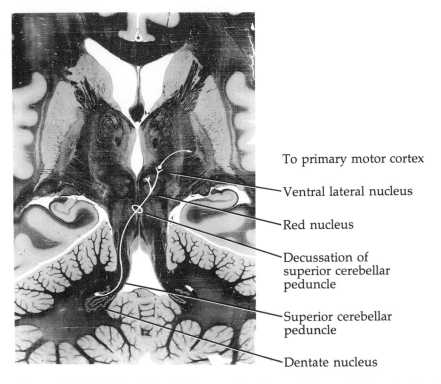

To primary motor cortex

Ventral lateral nucleus

Red nucleus

Decussation of
superior cerebellar
peduncle

Superior cerebellar
peduncle

Dentate nucleus

Figure 10.17   Myelin-stained oblique section through the cerebellum, brain stem, and cerebral hemispheres. The path of the cerebellothalamic tract from the dentate nucleus to the ventral lateral nucleus and the path to the red nucleus are shown.

Figure 10.18   Myelin-stained coronal section through the ventral lateral nucleus.

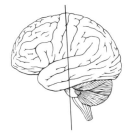

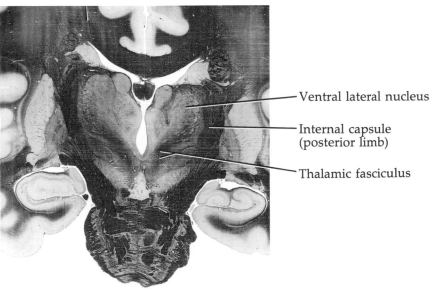

Ventral lateral nucleus

Internal capsule
(posterior limb)

Thalamic fasciculus

of myelinated fibers contains axons of the cerebellothalamic tract as well as from components of the basal ganglia (see Chapter 11).

The ventral lateral nucleus is one of the relay nuclei of the lateral thalamus (see Figure 10.17). It is located rostral to the ventral posterior nucleus,[8] the somatic sensory relay nucleus. The ventral lateral nucleus, similar to the ventral posterior nucleus, is somatotopically organized. The projections from the medial and lateral parts of the spinocerebellum, the vermis and intermediate lobe, project via the fastigial and interposed nuclei to separate regions of the ventral lateral nucleus. These thalamic regions, in turn, send their axons to the axial and limb portions of the motor cortex representation, respectively. The projection from the ventral lateral nucleus is focused principally on two motor regions of the frontal lobe: *primary motor cortex, area 4*, and *premotor cortex*, the lateral portion of *area 6* (see Chapter 9). The primary motor cortex contributes axons to the lateral and ventral corticospinal tracts. While the lateral corticospinal tract is a crossed pathway, the ventral corticospinal tract descends ipsilaterally but has bilateral terminations in the spinal cord gray matter.

Damage to the Cerebellum Produces Neurological Signs on the Same Side as the Lesion

There are three classic signs of cerebellar damage: ataxia, nystagmus, and tremor. *Ataxia* is inaccuracy in the speed, force, and distance of movement. In reaching for an object, the arm overshoots or undershoots the target. Ataxia of gait produces staggering and lurching. *Nystagmus* is a rhythmic involuntary oscillation of the eyes. *Tremor* is involuntary oscillation of the limbs or trunk. Cerebellar tremor is characteristically present when the patient is trying to perform an accurate reaching movement, such as touching the examiner's finger or bringing a forkful of food to the mouth. Ataxia and nystagmus typically occur after damage to cerebellar inputs, such as the spinocerebellar tracts or the inferior cerebellar peduncle (see later). In contrast, tremor is more often a consequence of damage to cerebellar output pathways, such as the superior cerebellar peduncle. Combinations of signs occur with damage to the cerebellum itself depending on the site and size of the lesion.

Knowledge of the anatomy of the motor system is crucial for understanding why cerebellar damage typically produces *ipsilateral motor signs*. A discrete cerebellar lesion produces neurological signs on the side ipsilateral to the lesion, because the cerebellar efferent projections are crossed as are the descending pathways, the targets of cerebellar action. The combined decussations result in a system of connections that is "doubly crossed" (Figure 10.19). Damage to cerebellar input from the spinal cord also produces ipsilateral signs because the principal spinocerebellar pathway, the dorsal spinocerebellar tract, ascends ipsilaterally. Occlusion of the *posterior inferior cerebellar artery* produces infarction of the *inferior cerebellar peduncle*, also resulting in ipsilateral signs. Two key signs related

---

[8] In the Rhesus monkey, the ventral lateral nucleus includes the most rostral portion of the ventral posterior lateral nucleus (the oral part—VPLo), a portion that is located rostral to the part of the ventral posterior nucleus that projects to the primary somatic sensory cortex (the caudal part—VPLc), as well as additional subdivisions. The ventrolateral nucleus (including VPLo) is cytoarchitectonically distinct from the VPLc.

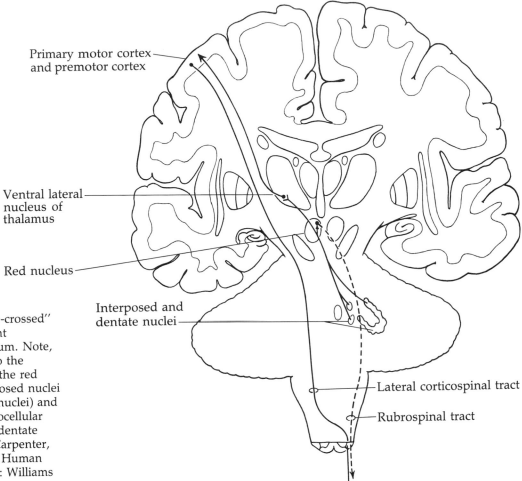

Primary motor cortex
and premotor cortex

Ventral lateral
nucleus of
thalamus

Red nucleus

Interposed and
dentate nuclei

Lateral corticospinal tract

Rubrospinal tract

Figure 10.19 The "double-crossed" arrangement of the efferent projections of the cerebellum. Note, the cerebellar projection to the magnocellular division of the red nucleus is from the interposed nuclei (globose and emboliform nuclei) and the projection to the parvocellular division originates in the dentate nucleus. (Adapted from Carpenter, M. B., and Sutin, J. 1983. Human Neuroanatomy. Baltimore: Williams & Wilkins.)

to infarction of the peduncle are nystagmus (also a consequence of damage to the vestibular nuclei) and ataxia. These are the cerebellar signs associated with the *lateral medullary*, or *Wallenberg's*, syndrome. Somatic sensory deficits are also present with posterior inferior cerebellar artery occlusion because infarction of the dorsolateral medulla interrupts ascending fibers of the anteriolateral system (Chapter 5) as well as the trigeminal spinal tract and nucleus (Chapter 12). Damage to the decussation of the superior cerebellar peduncle produces bilateral signs.

Summary

The cerebellum (Figure 10.1) participates in the control of movement through projections to the lateral and medial descending pathways. The cerebellar cortex overlies the white matter (Figure 10.2). The cerebellar surface contains numerous *folia*, which are grouped into three *lobes* (Figures 10.1 and 10.2): *anterior lobe, posterior lobe*, and *flocculonodular lobe* (Figure 10.2). Embedded within the white matter of the cerebellum are four bilaterally paired deep nuclei, from medial to lateral (Figure 10.2B): *fastigial nucleus, globose nucleus, emboliform nucleus*, and *dentate nucleus*. The globose and emboliform nuclei are collectively termed the *interposed nuclei*.

The cerebellar cortex consists of three cell layers, from the cerebellar surface to the white matter (Figure 10.9): *molecular, Purkinje*, and *granular* layers. Five neuron classes are found in the cerebellar cortex (Table 10.1, Figure 10.10): (1) *Purkinje cell* (Figure 10.11), the *projection neuron* of the cerebellum—which is *inhibitory*, (2) *granule cell*, the only *excitatory interneuron* in the cerebellum, (3) *basket cell*, (4) *stellate cell*, and (5) *Golgi cell*. The basket cell, the stellate cell, and the Golgi cell are the *three inhibitory interneurons*. Two principal classes of afferent fibers reach the cerebellum: *climbing fibers* (Figure 10.10), which are the axons of neurons of the *inferior olivary nuclei* (Figure 10.13), and *mossy fibers*, which originate from numerous sources, including the *pontine nuclei* (Figure 10.11–10.16), *reticular formation nuclei, vestibular nuclei* (Figures 10.13 and 10.14), and *spinal cord* (Figure 10.12). The climbing fiber input is directed to both the deep cerebellar nuclei and the cerebellar cortex (Figure 10.4), whereas mossy fiber input is directed predominantly to the cerebellar cortex (Figure 10.4). The *climbing fibers make monosynaptic connections with the Pukinje cells*; the *mossy fibers synapse on granule cells*, which in turn synapse on Purkinje cells via their *parallel fibers*. The Purkinje cells project from the cerebellar cortex to the deep nuclei (Figure 10.10) and the vestibular nuclei (Figures 10.13 and 10.14).

The cerebellum is divided into three functional regions (Figure 10.3). The vestibulocerebellum (1) is important in balance and eye muscle control and corresponds anatomically to the *flocculonodular lobe* (Figures 10.1C and 10.8). It receives input from the *vestibular nuclei* and *primary vestibular afferents* and projects back to the vestibular nuclei via the *inferior cerebellar peduncle* (Figure 10.13).

The *spinocerebellum* (2) (Figures 10.5 and 10.6), which is important in posture and limb movement, is subdivided into two regions that also have functional counterparts: the medial *vermis* subserves control of axial and girdle muscles, and the *intermediate hemisphere* controls *limb muscles*. The principal input to the spinocerebellum originates from the spinal cord. The *dorsal spinocerebellar tract* (Figure 10.5A) and the *ventral spinocerebellar tract* (Figure 10.5B) are the *lower limb pathways* and the *cuneocerebellar tract* (Figure 10.5A) and the *rostral spinocerebellar tract* (Figure 10.5B) are the *upper limb* homologues, respectively. Purkinje cells of the vermis project to the *fastigial nucleus* (Figure 10.14) which influences *medial descending pathways*: the reticulospinal, vestibulospinal, and ventral corticospinal tracts (Figure 10.17). The projection to the lower brain stem is via the *inferior cerebellar peduncle* (Figure 10.15), and the thalamic projection is via the *superior cerebellar peduncle* (Figures 10.16 and 10.17). The *intermediate hemisphere* projects to the interposed nuclei, which in turn influence the *lateral descending pathways*: the rubrospinal and lateral corticospinal tracts. All projections from the spinocerebellum course through the superior cerebellar peduncle. The *cerebrocerebellum* (3) (Figure 10.7) corresponds anatomically to the *lateral hemisphere*, and it plays a role in planning movements. The cerebral cortex projects to the *pontine nuclei* (Figures 10.14 and 10.15), which provide the main input to the cerebrocerebellum. Purkinje cells of this functional division project to the dentate nucleus (Figure 10.14). From there, dentate neurons project to the contralateral *parvocellular red nucleus* (Figure 10.16B) and the *ventral lateral nucleus* of the thalamus (Figure 10.18), both via the *superior cerebellar peduncle*. The principal projection of the ventral lateral nucleus is to the *primary motor cortex* (area 4) and the *premotor cortex* (lateral area 6). ■

References

Angevine, J. B., Jr., Mancall, E. L., and Yakovlev, P. I. 1961. The Human Cerebellum: An Atlas of Gross Topography in Serial Sections. Boston: Little, Brown.

Carpenter, M. B., and Sutin, J. 1983. Human Neuroanatomy. Baltimore: Williams & Wilkins.

Dietrichs, E., and Walberg, F. 1987. Cerebellar nuclear afferents—where do they originate? Anat. Embryol. 177:165–172.

Heimer, L. 1983. The Human Brain and Spinal Cord. New York: Springer-Verlag.

Schell, G. R., and Strick, P. L. 1984. The origin of thalamic inputs to the arcuate premotor and supplementary motor areas. J. Neurosci. 4:539–560.

Rexed, B. 1952. The cytoarchitectonic organization of the spinal cord in the cat. J. Comp. Neurol. 96:415–495.

Selected Readings

Brodal, A. 1981. Neurological Anatomy. New York: Oxford University Press.

Brooks, V. B. 1986. The neural basis of motor control. New York: Oxford University Press.

Brooks, V. B., and Thatch, W. T. 1981. Cerebellar Control of Posture and Movement. In Brooks, V. B. (ed.), Handbook of Physiology, Section I: The Nervous System, Vol. II, Motor Control. Bethesda, Md.: American Physiological Society, pp. 877–946.

Eccles, J. C., Ito, M., and Szentágothai, J. 1967. The Cerebellum as a Neuronal Machine. New York: Springer-Verlag.

Ghez, C. 1985. The Cerebellum. In Kandel, E. R., and Schwartz, J. H. Principles of Neural Science. New York: Elsevier, pp. 502–521.

Ito, M. 1984. The Cerebellum and Neural Control. New York: Raven Press.

The Basal Ganglia

11

The Basal Ganglia

The basal ganglia are a collection of subcortical nuclei that develop from the telencephalon and diencephalon. Traditionally, the basal ganglia were viewed as motor control structures, a view based largely on the most overt symptoms of basal ganglia disease. A rather simple anatomy was envisioned. Receiving input from wide regions of the cerebral cortex, the basal ganglia were thought to funnel their output through the thalamus to the primary motor cortex. Modern anatomical approaches have cast serious doubt on this simplistic view of the connections of the basal ganglia. Rather than focusing their output on the primary motor cortex, the basal ganglia actually influence the frontal lobe *rostral* to the motor cortex. Whereas a portion of this region is thought to participate in the planning of movement (Chapter 9), most of this region is prefrontal association cortex. The prefrontal association cortex plays a key role in such functions as organizing goal-directed behaviors and complex thought and reasoning. Indeed, careful neurological assessment of patients with Parkinson's disease—a disorder involving the basal ganglia—reveals that they have cognitive deficits as well as deficits in controlling movement.

In this chapter the constituents of the basal ganglia and their three-dimensional organization are considered first. Then their functional organization is surveyed. Finally, we examine a series of slices through the cerebral hemisphere and brain stem, tracing regional anatomy of the diencephalon and telencephalon with an emphasis on the basal ganglia.

Separate Components of Basal Ganglia Process Incoming Information and Mediate the Output

To understand the general organization of the basal ganglia we must first take an inventory of the various components. The nomenclature of the basal ganglia is more complex than that of other regions of the brain. Moreover, recent developments pinpointing basal ganglia connections and potential functions are at odds with the earlier taxonomy. Table 11.1 lists the components of the basal ganglia. On the basis of their connections, the various components can be divided into three categories: (1) *input nuclei*, which receive afferent connections from brain regions other than the basal ganglia; (2) *output nuclei*, which have efferent projections that leave the basal ganglia; and (3) *intrinsic nuclei*, which receive input from and project to the input and output nuclei.

The general organization of the basal ganglia from input to output is shown in Figure 11.1. The four lobes of the cerebral cortex—the frontal, parietal, occipital, and temporal lobes—are the major sources of input to the basal ganglia. However, only the frontal lobe is the recipient of its output. The *input* side of the basal ganglia, receiving afferent projections from primarily the cerebral cortex, is the *striatum*, and it consists of three nuclei: *caudate nucleus*, *putamen*, and *nucleus accumbens*. It should be recalled (Chapter 2) that the striatum has a complex three-dimensional configuration (Figure 11.2). The putamen is shaped like a disk when viewed from its lateral surface and it is joined with the caudate nucleus at its rostral pole. Ventrally, the caudate nucleus, putamen, and nucleus ac-

Table 11.1 Components of the Basal Ganglia

Input nuclei (striatum)[a]	1. Caudate nucleus
	2. Putamen[b]
	3. Nucleus accumbens
Output nuclei	1. Substantia nigra pars reticulata
	2. Globus pallidus—internal segment[b]
	3. Ventral pallidum
Intrinsic nuclei	1. Globus pallidus—external segment[b]
	2. Subthalamic nucleus
	3. Substantia nigra pars compacta
	4. Ventral tegmental area

 [a] The striatum is also termed the *neostriatum*.
 [b] The putamen and the internal and external segments of the globus pallidus together are also termed the *lenticular nucleus* because their form is similar to that of a lens.

cumbens are joined. The nucleus accumbens is not shown in Figure 11.2 because it is located medial to the putamen. The caudate nucleus has a C-shape, which is a consequence of the extensive development of the cerebral cortex (Chapter 2). Although it is one continuous structure, separate names are given to three portions of the caudate nucleus: head, body, and tail (Figure 11.2).

There are three nuclei on the *output* side of the basal ganglia (Table 11.1, Figure 11.1): the *internal segment of the globus pallidus*, the *ventral pallidum*, and the *substantia nigra pars reticulata*. The output nuclei send their axons primarily to thalamic nuclei that, in turn, project to different areas of the frontal lobe.

There are four intrinsic nuclei of the basal ganglia (Table 11.1) and their connections are closely related to the input and output nuclei just outlined: *external segment of the globus pallidus, subthalamic nucleus, sub-*

Figure 11.1 Block diagram illustrating the general features of the input–output organization of the basal ganglia. Note that the input nuclei of the basal ganglia receive their major projections from the entire cerebral cortex but only the frontal lobe is the recipient of the output of the basal ganglia, relayed via the thalamus.

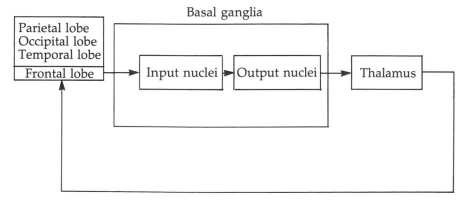

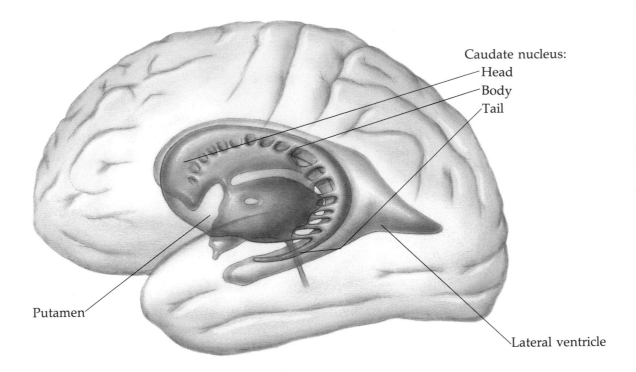

Caudate nucleus:
Head
Body
Tail

Putamen

Lateral ventricle

stantia nigra pars compacta, and *ventral tegmental area*. The external segment of the globus pallidus and the subthalamic nucleus are part of a basal ganglia circuit that receives input from other basal ganglia nuclei and, in turn, projects back. The substantia nigra pars compacta is an anatomical division separate from the *pars reticulata*. Like the two divisions of the red nucleus (Chapter 9), the two divisions of the substantia nigra are adjacent, but have strikingly *different anatomical connections* (see later). The substantia nigra pars compacta and the ventral tegmental area contain *dopaminergic neurons that project to the striatum.*

Various Components of the Basal Ganglia Are Separated by Axons of the Internal Capsule

Learning the numerous components and subdivisions of the basal ganglia poses a problem to the neuroanatomy student. One way to try to understand this nomenclature is to recall that the basal ganglia develop beneath the cerebral cortex. Axons coursing to and from the cortex have divided many of the major divisions of the basal ganglia. As we saw in Chapter 2, the *caudate nucleus* and *putamen* develop from a common pool of immature neurons in the floor of the lateral ventricle. During development they become incompletely separated by axons of the *internal capsule*. Nevertheless, their cytoarchitecture and histochemistry are similar, thereby suggesting that they represent a single nuclear region. The nucleus accumbens also develops from the common pool of immature neurons that give rise to the caudate nucleus and putamen. The nucleus accumbens is also contiguous with both the caudate nucleus and the putamen. The internal segment of the globus pallidus and the substantia nigra pars reticulata also have a similar cytoarchitecture and histochemistry. Here too, the internal capsule separates these two structures (see Figure 11.13).

There Are Parallel Circuits through the Basal Ganglia

The basal ganglia receive input from virtually the entire cerebral cortex but project, via a relay in the thalamus, only to portions of the frontal lobe located rostral to the motor cortex. Numerous anatomical "loops" have been identified from separate cortical regions, through different components of the input and output nuclei, and back through thalamic nuclei to separate areas of the frontal lobe. There are four principal loops and each is thought to mediate a different set of functions. The *motor* (1) and *oculomotor* (2) loops play important roles in the control of body musculature and extraocular muscles, respectively. The functions of the *association* (3) and *limbic* (4) loops are not as clearly characterized. The association loop may subserve such functions as spatial memory and evaluation of the effectiveness of behavior, and the limbic loop may subserve emotions and their visceral consequences. The key features of the connections of the four loops are illustrated in Figure 11.3: part A shows the components of the loops and part B presents the separate sites in the frontal lobe that are the targets of the loops. There are four important points concerning the general organization of these neural circuits passing through the basal ganglia. First, even though each of the loops originates from numerous cortical regions, these regions have similar general functions. For example, the frontal eye field and the posterior parietal association cortex provide the major input to the oculomotor loop. The frontal eye field is the region of the frontal lobe where electrical stimulation produces conjugate eye movements; the posterior parietal association cortex may process visual information that is critical for controlling the speed and direction of eye movements. Second, each loop passes through different basal ganglia and thalamic nuclei (or *separate portions* of the same nucleus). Third, the "cortical" targets of all loops are separate portions of the frontal lobe rostral to the primary motor cortex. These regions are illustrated in Figure 11.3B. The fourth important point is that the anatomical organization of the limbic loop is clearly different from that of the motor, oculomotor, and association loops. The limbic loop selectively passes through the *ventral striatum* (Figure 11.3D), which includes the nucleus accumbens, together with ventromedial portions of the caudate nucleus and putamen. (The olfactory tubercle—see Figure 11.7— is also considered to be a part of the ventral striatum. The precise boundary between structures on the basal surface of the forebrain that participate in olfaction and emotions is not clearly understood.)

A   **1.**   Sensory-motor loop

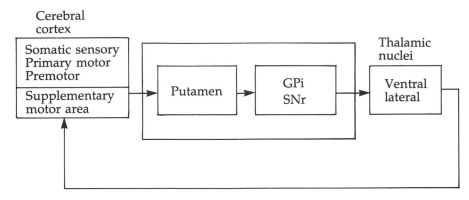

2.   Oculomotor loop

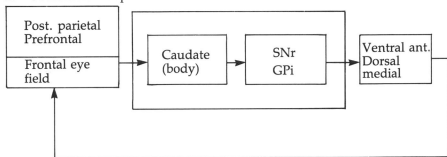

3.   Association loop

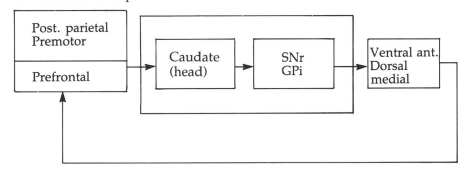

4.   Limbic loop

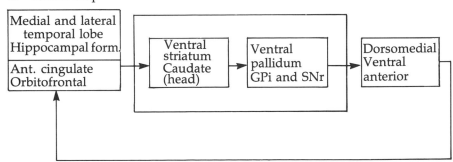

B

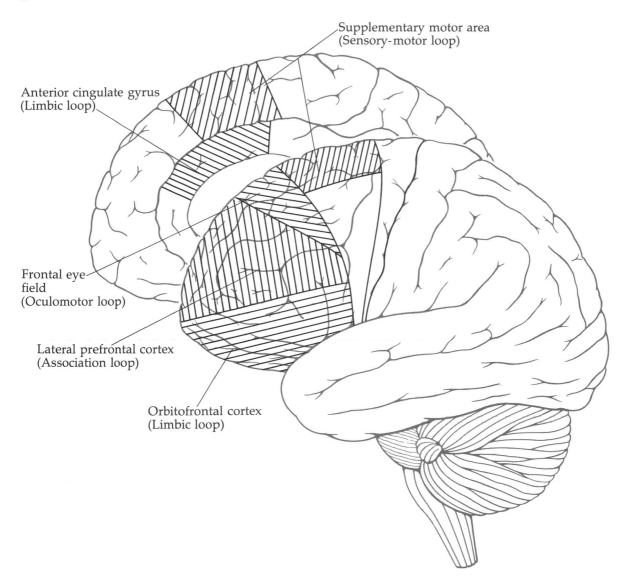

Supplementary motor area
(Sensory-motor loop)

Anterior cingulate gyrus
(Limbic loop)

Frontal eye
field
(Oculomotor loop)

Lateral prefrontal cortex
(Association loop)

Orbitofrontal cortex
(Limbic loop)

Figure 11.3 There are four principal input–output loops through the basal ganglia. *A.* Block diagrams illustrating the general organization of the four main loops through the basal ganglia. (1) Sensory-motor loop, (2) oculomotor loop, (3) association loop, and (4) limbic loop. (Abbreviations: GPi, globus pallidus internal segment; SNr, substantia nigra pars reticulata.) *B.* Lateral and medial views of cerebral cortex, illustrating the approximate location of the "target" regions in the frontal lobe. (Adapted from Alexander, G., DeLong, M. R., and Strick, P. L. 1986. Parallel organization of functionally segregated circuits linking basal ganglia and cortex. Ann. Rev. Neurosci. 9:357–381.)

The Connections of the Substantia Nigra Pars Compacta and the Subthalamic Nucleus Are Clinically Important

The intrinsic nuclei of the basal ganglia (Table 11.1) form subsidiary circuits that are thought to modify transmission of information through the four principal loops just described. The *substantia nigra pars compacta* provides the *dopaminergic* input to the caudate nucleus and putamen (Figure 11.4, right). In *Parkinson's disease*, a motor disorder characterized by tremor, rigidity, and bradykinesia (slowing of movement), the dopaminergic neurons of the pars compacta are destroyed and striatal dopamine is profoundly reduced. Replacement therapy using L-*dopa*, a precursor to dopamine, leads to a dramatic improvement of symptoms. Similar to the caudate nucleus and putamen, the nucleus accumbens receives a dopaminergic projection from the midbrain (Figure 11.4, right), however, to a greater extent from the region medial to the substantia nigra pars compacta, termed the *ventral tegmental area*. The *dorsal raphe nucleus* gives rise to a serotonergic projection to the striatum; however, the clinical significance of this second neurotransmitter-specific projection is not yet known. A second system of interconnections within the basal ganglia involves the *subthalamic nucleus* and the *external segment of the globus pallidus* (Figure 11.4, left). These two intrinsic nuclei are part of a "side loop": the subthalamic nucleus receives input from the external segment of the globus pallidus and projects to *both segments of the globus pallidus* and to the *substantia nigra pars reticulata*. The ventral pallidum also has reciprocal connections with the subthalamic nucleus (not shown in Figure 11.4). Thus, the subthalamic nucleus can modulate the function of all the output nuclei of the basal ganglia. A remarkable clinical disturbance, termed *hemiballism*, occurs after lesion of the subthalamic nucleus. As its name suggests, the stricken patient makes uncontrollable *ballistic* (flinging) movements of the contralateral limbs. The subthalamic nucleus is somatotopically organized; as a consequence, either the upper limb or the lower limb may be affected after a small lesion.

In the following sections the regional anatomy of the diencephalon and telencephalon is examined, with the focus on basal ganglia. Initially, a horizontal slice through the cerebral hemisphere is considered and then serial coronal slices. It is useful to start with a horizontal slice because it permits visualization of the components of the internal capsule, which form major subcortical landmarks. In addition to learning the regional anatomy of the basal ganglia, a secondary objective of examination of serial coronal sections is synthesis of an overall view of the regional anatomy of the *deep structures of the cerebral hemisphere*. This second objective will be completed when we consider the hypothalamus (Chapter 14) and the limbic system (Chapter 15).

The Anterior Limb of the Internal Capsule Separates the Head of the Caudate Nucleus from the Putamen

The dominant feature of the horizontal section (Figure 11.5) is the presence of the *internal capsule*. A three-dimensional view of the internal capsule is illustrated in Figure 11.6, where structures lateral to the internal capsule (including the putamen and the globus pallidus) have been re-

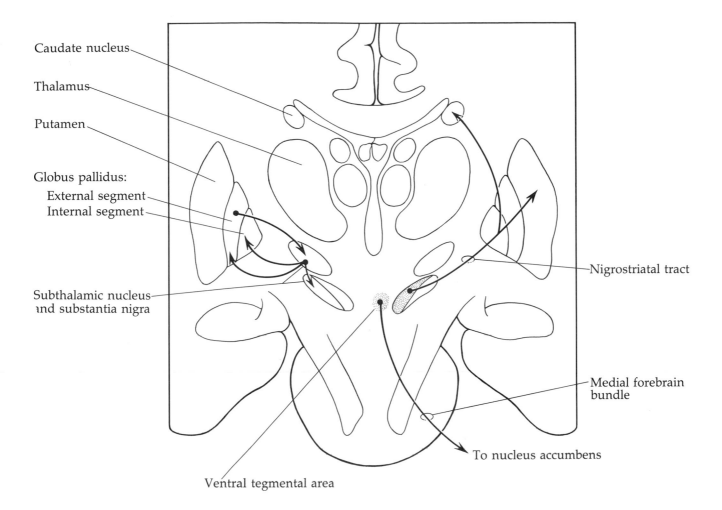

Caudate nucleus

Thalamus

Putamen

Globus pallidus:
 External segment
 Internal segment

Subthalamic nucleus
and substantia nigra

Ventral tegmental area

Nigrostriatal tract

Medial forebrain
bundle

To nucleus accumbens

moved. The internal capsule contains ascending thalamocortical fibers and descending fibers that terminate in the basal ganglia, brain stem, and spinal cord. There are three main segments of the internal capsule (Chapter 3) and they separate components of the basal ganglia. The three segments of the internal capsule are: the *anterior limb*, the *posterior limb*, and the *genu*, which connects the two limbs (Figures 11.5 and 11.6). In horizontal sections, the internal capsule has an arrowhead shape with the genu pointing toward the midline (Figure 11.5). In addition to the three main segments of the internal capsule, there are the retrolenticular and sublenticular portions (Figure 11.6). Their names derive from their locations with respect to the lenticular nucleus, which is the putamen and globus pallidus. The anterior limb separates the *head of the caudate nucleus from the putamen* (Figure 11.5). This limb contains axons projecting to and from the frontal lobe, excluding the primary motor cortex and higher order motor areas. The posterior limb separates the *putamen* and globus pallidus from the *thalamus* and *body of the caudate nucleus* (Figure 11.5). The posterior limb contains the corticospinal tract as well as the projections to and from the somatic sensory areas in the parietal lobe. The genu contains the corticobulbar tract and descending corticoreticular fibers.

Figure 11.4 Schematic of the connections of the intrinsic basal ganglia nuclei. (Left) The subthalamic nucleus and external segment of the globus pallidus; (right) the midbrain dopaminergic system, which includes the substantia nigra pars compacta (shaded) and the ventral tegmental area.

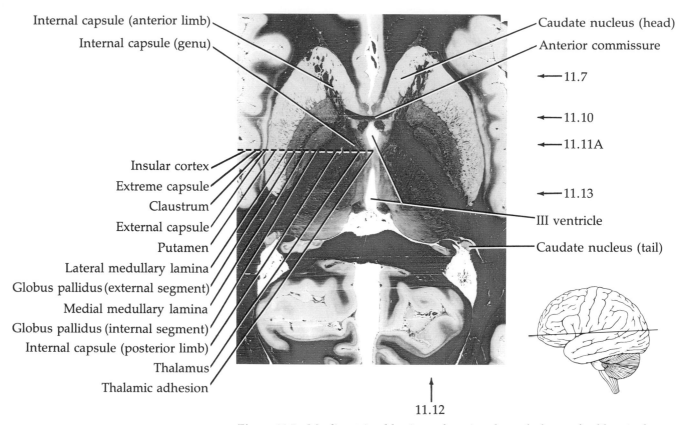

Internal capsule (anterior limb)
Internal capsule (genu)

Caudate nucleus (head)
Anterior commissure

←11.7

←11.10

←11.11A

←11.13

Insular cortex
Extreme capsule
Claustrum
External capsule
Putamen
Lateral medullary lamina
Globus pallidus (external segment)
Medial medullary lamina
Globus pallidus (internal segment)
Internal capsule (posterior limb)
Thalamus
Thalamic adhesion

III ventricle
Caudate nucleus (tail)

11.12

Figure 11.5 Myelin-stained horizontal section through the cerebral hemispheres. The locations of sections illustrated in Figures 11.7, 11.10, 11.11A, 11.12, and 11.13 are indicated.

Examination of the horizontal section in Figure 11.5 also provides an opportunity to review the locations of major telencephalic and diencephalic structures. A useful framework for examining regional anatomy is provided by identification of the various structures, beginning at the lateral margin of the cerebral cortex and proceeding toward the midline (Figure 11.5, dashed line):

1. *Insular cortex.* Contains part of the cortical representation for taste.
2. *Extreme capsule.* Thin lamina of white matter that contains corticocortical association fibers.
3. *Claustrum.* Thin sheet of neurons that are reciprocally and topographically connected with the cerebral cortex.
4. *External capsule.* Thin sheet of white matter that contains corticocortical association fibers.
5. *Putamen.* A component of the striatum.
6. *Lateral medullary lamina.* Axons that separate the putamen from the external segment of the globus pallidus.
7. *External segment of the globus pallidus.* Projects to the subthalamic nucleus.
8. *Medial medullary lamina.* Separates the external and internal segments of the globus pallidus.

Retrolenticular and
sublenticular portions

Posterior limb

Genu

Anterior limb

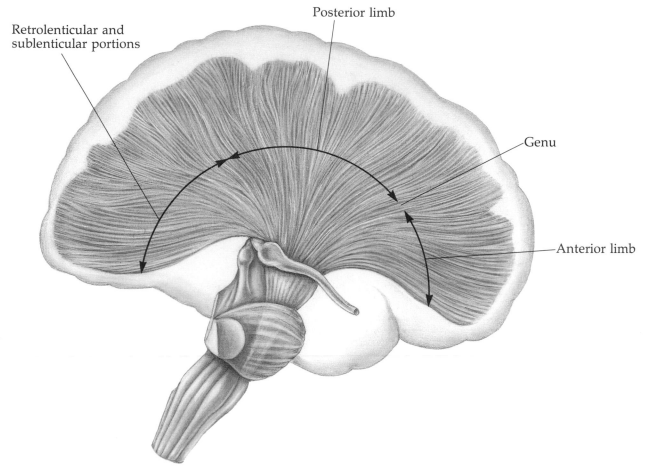

Figure 11.6 A three-dimensional view of the internal capsule. (Adapted from Carpenter, M. B., and Sutin, J. 1983. Human Neuroanatomy. Baltimore: Williams & Wilkins.)

9. *Internal segment of the globus pallidus.* Projects to the thalamus.
10. *Posterior limb of the internal capsule.* Contains descending corticospinal axons as well as other descending fibers and ascending thalamocortical fibers.
11. *Thalamus.* Contains the principal sensory and motor relay nuclei for the cerebral cortex.
12. *Thalamic adhesion*[1] (spanning the third ventricle). A small portion of the thalamus that physically adheres to its counterpart on the contralateral side.

A feature of the complex three-dimensional structure of the caudate nucleus can be identified in Figure 11.5. Because the caudate nucleus has a C-shaped configuration, it can be seen in two separate locations in this section. The head of the caudate nucleus is located rostrally and the tail of the caudate nucleus is located caudally. In certain coronal sections (see later), the caudate nucleus is also seen in two locations (dorsally and ventrally).

[1] Another name for the thalamic adhesion is the massa intermedia.

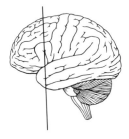

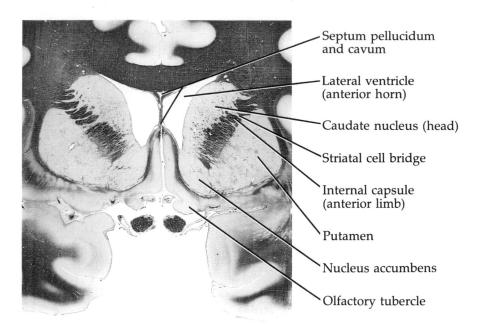

Septum pellucidum and cavum

Lateral ventricle (anterior horn)

Caudate nucleus (head)

Striatal cell bridge

Internal capsule (anterior limb)

Putamen

Nucleus accumbens

Olfactory tubercle

Figure 11.7 Myelin-stained coronal section through the head of the caudate nucleus.

Cell Bridges Link the Caudate Nucleus and the Putamen

A coronal slice through the anterior limb of the internal capsule (Figure 11.7) reveals the three components of the striatum: (1) caudate nucleus (at this level, the head of the caudate nucleus), (2) putamen, and (3) nucleus accumbens. Although the internal capsule courses between the caudate nucleus and the putamen, *striatal cell bridges* connect the two structures. The cell bridges are a reminder that, in the developing brain (Chapter 2), axons coursing to and from the cortex divide the group of immature neurons in the floor of the lateral ventricle that give rise to the striatum. The *nucleus accumbens*, which is cytoarchitecturally and histochemically similar to the caudate nucleus and putamen, is located ventromedially. (The nucleus accumbens is formally termed *nucleus accumbens septi*, which literally means "leaning against the septum.") The *septum pellucidum* (Figure 11.7) is a thin connective tissue membrane that separates the anterior horn and body of the lateral ventricles of the two cerebral hemispheres (Chapter 1).[2] The *ventral striatum*, in many species, is formed by the nucleus accumbens and the olfactory tubercle (Figure 11.7).

The head of the caudate nucleus bulges into the anterior horn of the lateral ventricle and serves as an important radiological landmark. The head of the caudate nucleus can be seen in the MRI scan of a normal individual (Figure 11.8). This scan is of a slice of the cerebral hemisphere that is similar in location and orientation to that of the myelin-stained section shown in Figure 11.7. In patients with Huntington's disease, a hereditary neurological disease caused by a single gene mutation, there is a loss of a single class of neurons in the caudate nucleus. In these patients, the characteristic bulge of the head of the caudate nucleus into

---

[2] There are two membranes, one on each side of the cerebral hemisphere. The space between the membranes is the cavum of the septum pellucidum. There is a normal variation among individuals in the size of the cavum of the septum pellucidum.

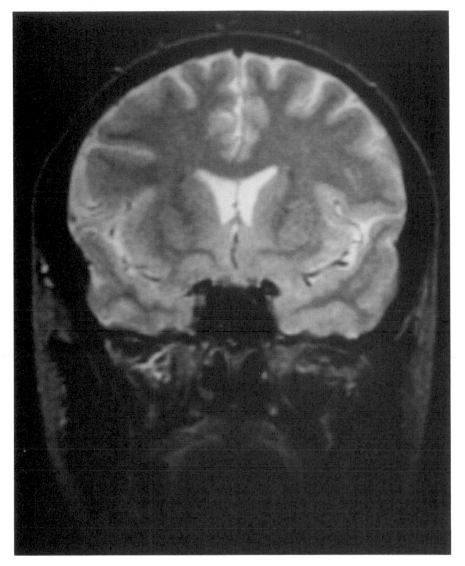

Figure 11.8 Magnetic resonance image of a brain slice through the head of the caudate nucleus in normal individual, plane of section similar to that of Figure 11.7. (Courtesy of Dr. Neal Rutledge, University of Texas at Austin.)

the lateral ventricle is absent (Figure 11.9). Huntington's disease causes dementia as well as *chorea*, a disorder characterized by involuntary rapid and random movements of the limbs and trunk.

The External Segment of the Globus Pallidus and the Ventral Pallidum Are Separated by the Anterior Commissure

The external segment of the globus pallidus, as we saw earlier, is an intrinsic basal ganglia nucleus that sends its axons to the subthalamic nucleus and the ventral pallidum is the output nucleus for the limbic loop. The external segment of the globus pallidus and the ventral palli-

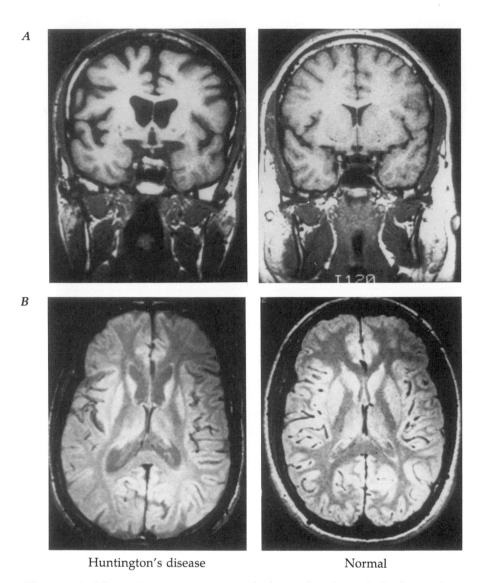

Huntington's disease   Normal

Figure 11.9 Magnetic resonance image of a brain slice through the head of the caudate nucleus of a Huntington's patient. Note that the head of the caudate nucleus is smaller in the Huntington's patient compared with normal. The imaging planes and locations of the MRI scans in *A* and *B* are similar to the planes of section and locations of the myelin-stained sections in Figures 11.7 and 11.5 respectively (Courtesy of Dr. Susan Folstein, Department of Psychiatry, Johns Hopkins Medical School.)

dum are separated by the *anterior commissure* (Figure 11.10). The anterior commissure, like the corpus callosum, interconnects regions of the cerebral cortex of either hemisphere. Unlike the corpus callosum, which connects wide regions of the frontal, parietal, occipital, and posterior temporal lobes, the anterior commissure interconnects very restricted regions, parts of the *anterior temporal lobes* (Chapter 15), *amygdaloid nuclear complex*, and *olfactory structures* (Chapter 8).

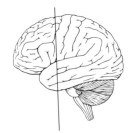

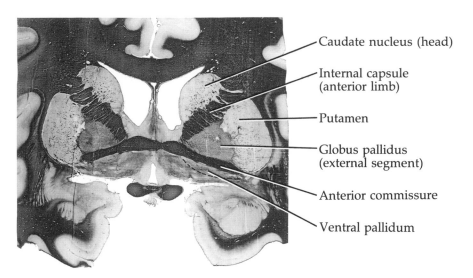

Caudate nucleus (head)

Internal capsule
(anterior limb)

Putamen

Globus pallidus
(external segment)

Anterior commissure

Ventral pallidum

Figure 11.10 Myelin-stained coronal section through the external segment of the globus pallidus.

The Internal Segment of the Globus Pallidus Projects to the Thalamus via the Ansa Lenticularis and the Lenticular Fasciculus

In Figure 11.11A, a coronal section, we see the two laminae that separate components of the basal ganglia. The *lateral medullary lamina* (1) separates the *external segment of the globus pallidus* from the *putamen*. The *medial medullary lamina* (2) separates the internal and external segments of the globus pallidus. Often a third lamina is observed, the *accessory medullary lamina* which divides the internal segment. As we saw earlier, neurons of the internal segment of the globus pallidus project their axons to the thalamus. These axons course in two anatomically separate pathways: the *ansa lenticularis* and the *lenticular fasciculus*. The internal capsule is a barrier for fibers of the ansa lenticularis: they course around it to reach the thalamus. The ansa lenticularis can be seen in Figures 11.11A and B (the section in part B is cut obliquely). The axons of the lenticular fasciculus course directly through the internal capsule, but these axons are not clearly visualized until they collect medial to the internal capsule (Figure 11.11). A parasagittal section through the internal segment of the globus pallidus is presented in Figure 11.12. The posterior limb of the internal capsule separates the globus pallidus from the thalamus (and substantia nigra pars reticulata). The accessory medullary lamina separates neurons that course through the two different projection paths. The ansa lenticularis originates predominantly from neurons located in the lateral part of the internal segment (i.e., lateral to the accessory medullary lamina), whereas the lenticular fascicularis originates from neurons located medially. This is another example of the topographic precision of the anatomical organization of the nervous system. The ansa lenticularis and lenticular fasciculus converge and join fibers of the cerebellothalamic tract to form the *thalamic fasciculus* before entering the ventral anterior and ventral lateral nuclei (Figure 11.11B). There is an alternate nomen-

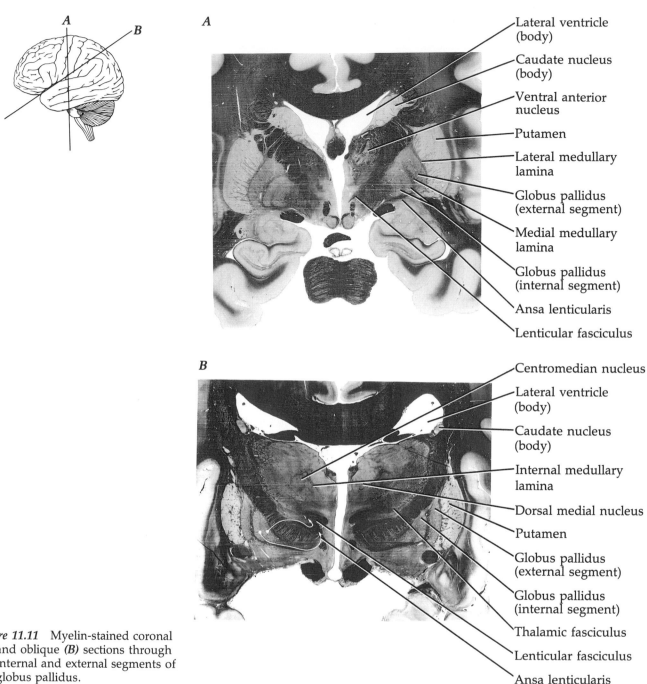

A
- Lateral ventricle (body)
- Caudate nucleus (body)
- Ventral anterior nucleus
- Putamen
- Lateral medullary lamina
- Globus pallidus (external segment)
- Medial medullary lamina
- Globus pallidus (internal segment)
- Ansa lenticularis
- Lenticular fasciculus

B
- Centromedian nucleus
- Lateral ventricle (body)
- Caudate nucleus (body)
- Internal medullary lamina
- Dorsal medial nucleus
- Putamen
- Globus pallidus (external segment)
- Globus pallidus (internal segment)
- Thalamic fasciculus
- Lenticular fasciculus
- Ansa lenticularis

Figure 11.11 Myelin-stained coronal *(A)* and oblique *(B)* sections through the internal and external segments of the globus pallidus.

clature for lenticular and thalamic fasciculi that is still sometimes used. The lenticular fasciculus is also termed *Forel's field H2* and the thalamic fasciculus, *Forel's field H1*. A third Forel field termed *H* is the region ventromedial to field H1 and is continuous with the tegmentum of the midbrain.

The three thalamic nuclei to which the output nuclei of the basal ganglia project can be identified in Figures 11.11–11.13. The *dorsal medial*

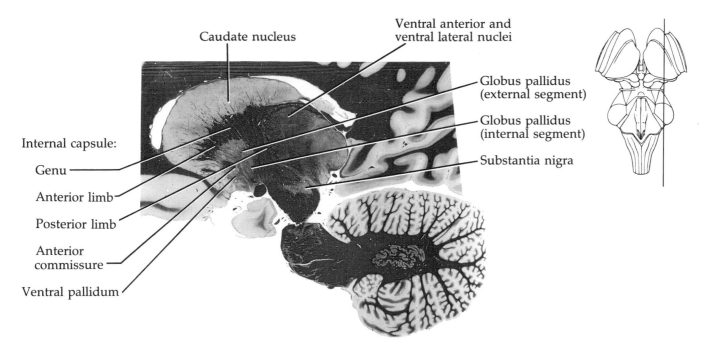

Caudate nucleus

Ventral anterior and
ventral lateral nuclei

Globus pallidus
(external segment)

Globus pallidus
(internal segment)

Substantia nigra

Internal capsule:

Genu

Anterior limb

Posterior limb

Anterior
commissure

Ventral pallidum

nucleus (also shown in Figure 11.13) is located medial to the internal medullary lamina of the thalamus, and the *ventral lateral* and *ventral anterior nuclei* are located lateral to the lamina. Another thalamic nucleus is anatomically related to the basal ganglia, the *centromedian nucleus* (Figure 11.11B), which is an *intralaminar nucleus* (Chapter 3). The major projection of this intralaminar nucleus is to the striatum; the function of this projection is not known. The intralaminar nuclei also project to wide regions of the cerebral cortex. For this reason, the intralaminar nuclei are considered to be diffuse-projecting (and not relay) thalamic nuclei. The cortical projections are believed to play a role in *arousal*.

Figure 11.12 Myelin-stained parasagittal section through the globus pallidus.

Figure 11.13 Myelin-stained coronal section through the thalamus and subthalamic region.

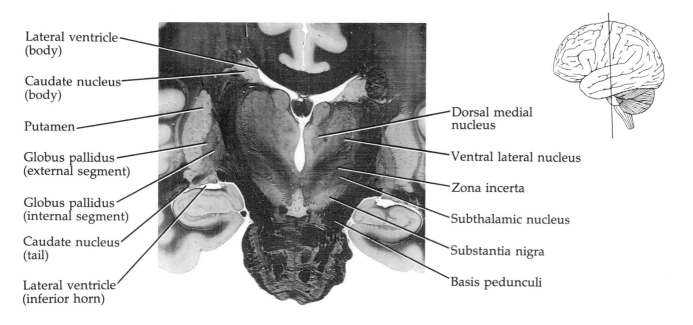

Lateral ventricle
(body)

Caudate nucleus
(body)

Putamen

Globus pallidus
(external segment)

Globus pallidus
(internal segment)

Caudate nucleus
(tail)

Lateral ventricle
(inferior horn)

Dorsal medial
nucleus

Ventral lateral nucleus

Zona incerta

Subthalamic nucleus

Substantia nigra

Basis pedunculi

The *subthalamic nucleus* is seen on the coronal section in Figure 11.13, dorsal to the substantia nigra and ventral to the thalamus. Little is known of the function of the *zona incerta*, a nuclear region that is interposed between the subthalamic nucleus and the thalamus. The zona incerta receives projections from a variety of sources, including the spinal cord and cerebellum.

The Substantia Nigra Contains Two Anatomical Divisions

The substantia nigra *pars compacta* is located dorsally and contains the dopaminergic neurons; the substantia nigra *pars reticulata* is adjacent to the basis pedunculi. The differences in the histochemistry of the two divisions of the substantia nigra are discussed in the next section. In the coronal section through the rostral portion of the substantia nigra (Figure 11.13), we see that it is interposed between the subthalamic nucleus and the basis pedunculi. The transverse sections through the rostral and caudal midbrain (Figure 11.14) reveal the substantia nigra dorsal to the base of the midbrain in both sections. The substantia nigra is the largest nuclear

Figure 11.14 Myelin-stained transverse sections through the superior colliculus *(A)* and the inferior colliculus *(B)*.

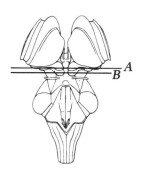

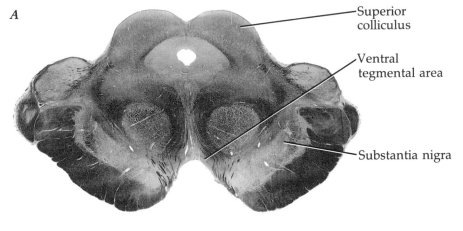

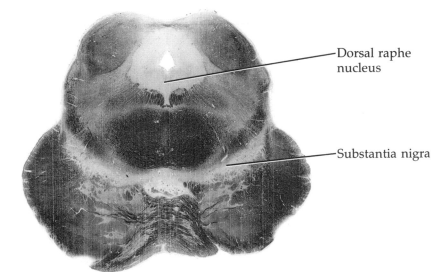

structure in the midbrain. As a consequence of its large size, vascular injury rarely disrupts substantia nigra function and the symptoms of Parkinson's disease do not typically occur. The ventral tegmental area is located dorsomedial to the substantia nigra, beneath the floor of the interpeduncular fossa (Figure 11.14A). Dopaminergic neurons in the ventral tegmental area send their axons to the nucleus accumbens via the medial forebrain bundle (Chapters 14 and 15). The serotonergic projection to the striatum originates from the dorsal raphe nucleus (Figure 11.14B). The substantia nigra pars reticulata also projects to the superior colliculus (Figure 11.14A). In Rhesus monkeys, this projection has been shown to play a role in controlling saccadic eye movements to remembered visual targets.

Histochemistry of the Basal Ganglia

Biochemical methods and immunohistochemical staining techniques have identified a diversity of neurotransmitters and neuromodulatory agents in the basal ganglia (Figure 11.15). In this section, we briefly survey the histochemistry of the striatum, globus pallidus, and substantia nigra.

The similarity of the histochemistry of the three components of the striatum is demonstrated in Figure 11.16. In Figure 11.16A, tissue has been stained to show the distribution of the enzyme *acetylcholinesterase*, which is thought to parallel the distribution of the neurotransmitter *acetylcholine*. Acetylcholine is located in striatal interneurons and is an important neurotransmitter in the function of *local neuronal circuits*. Acetylcholinesterase in the striatum is confined to a "matrix" of tissue surrounding small "patches" with lower acetylcholinesterase concentration. This patch and matrix appearance also characterizes the localization of other neurotransmitters (for example, enkephalin, Figure 11.16B) and even the distribution of cortical axon terminals. An important research goal is determination of the functional significance of the discontinuous distribution of neurotransmitters and axon terminals in the striatum.

Figure 11.15 The neurotransmitters of the basal ganglia (boldface labels) are shown in relation to the organization of the principal and subsidiary basal ganglia circuits. (Abbreviations: GABA, gamma aminobutyric acid; GP, globus pallidus; SNr, substantia nigra pars reticulata; SNc, substantia nigra pars compacta.) (Adapted from Haber, S. N. 1986. Neurotransmitters in the human and nonhuman primate basal ganglia. Human Neurobiol. 5:159–168.)

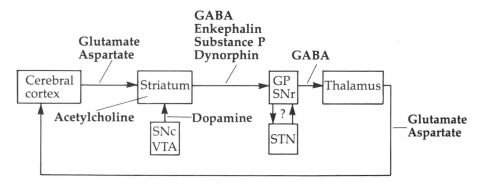

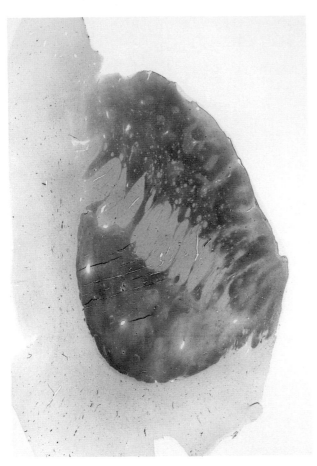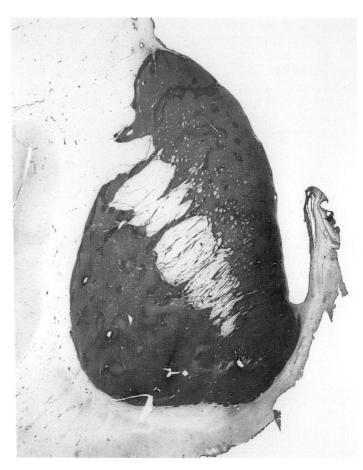

Figure 11.16 Histochemical localization of acetylcholinesterase *(A)* and enkephalin *(B)* in the human striatum. (Courtesy of Dr. Suzanne Haber, University of Rochester School of Medicine.)

In contrast to the various components of the striatum which have a similar histochemistry, the histochemistry of the internal segment of the globus pallidus is different from that of the external segment. The neuropeptides *substance P* and *enkephalin*, for example, have different distributions in the globus pallidus (Figure 11.17). Enkephalin is restricted largely to the *external segment* of the globus pallidus, whereas *substance P* is in greater abundance in the *internal segment* of the globus pallidus. The source of pallidal substance P and enkephalin is the striatum. Striatal projection neurons that have different pallidal projections may utilize different neurotransmitters.

Neurons in the two divisions of the substantia nigra use different chemical transmitters, in addition to having different sets of connections. The pars compacta of the substantia nigra contains dopaminergic neurons, whereas neurons in the pars reticulata contain the inhibitory neurotransmitter γ-aminobutyric acid (GABA). The term *substantia nigra* derives from the presence of neurons in the pars compacta that contain the pigment *neuromelanin*, a polymer of the catecholamine precursor dihydroxyphenylalanine (or Dopa). Not surprisingly, neuromelanin is not present in the substantia nigra pars compacta of Parkinson's patients.

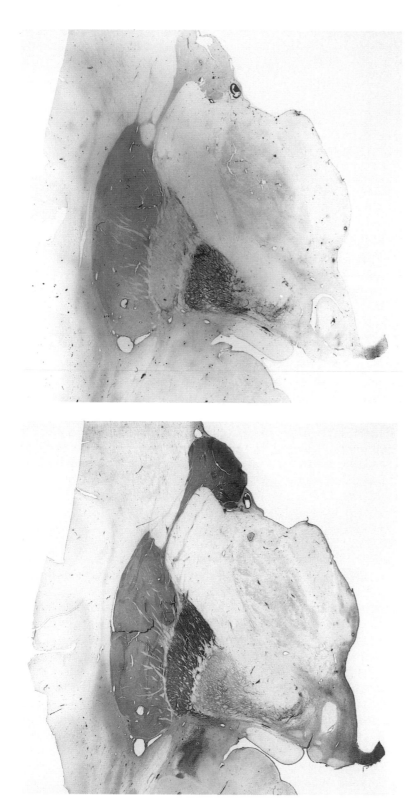

Figure 11.17 Histochemical localization of substance P-like immunoreactivity *(A)* and enkephalin-like immunoreactivity *(B)* in the human globus pallidus. (Courtesy of Dr. Suzanne Haber, University of Rochester School of Medicine.)

The neurotoxin 1-methyl-4-phenyl-1,2,3,6-tetrahydropyridine (MPTP), a contaminant of a certain kind of synthetic heroin, kills the dopaminergic neurons of the pars compacta and produces a permanent clinical syndrome in humans exposed to this toxin that is remarkably similar to Parkinson's disease.

The Vascular Supply of the Basal Ganglia Is Provided by the Middle Cerebral Artery

As described in Chapter 4, the vascular supply to the deep structures of the cerebral hemisphere—*thalamus, basal ganglia,* and *internal capsule*—is provided by branches of the internal carotid artery and the three cerebral arteries. Most of the striatum is supplied by perforating branches of the middle cerebral artery, termed the *lenticulostriate arteries* (see Figures 4.6 and 4.7). However, regions located rostromedially are supplied by perforating branches of the anterior cerebral artery. Most of the globus pallidus is supplied by the *anterior choroidal artery*, which is a branch of the internal carotid artery.

Summary

The basal ganglia contain numerous component nuclei (Table 11.1, Figures 11.2 and 11.15) that can be divided into three groups based on their connections. The *input nuclei* (1) include the *caudate nucleus*, the *putamen*, and the *nucleus accumbens* (Figure 11.7) and collectively are termed the *striatum*. The *output nuclei* (2) include the *internal segment* of the *globus pallidus* (Figure 11.11), the *ventral pallidum* (Figures 11.10 and 11.17), and the *substantia nigra pars reticulata* (Figure 11.14). The *intrinsic nuclei* (3) include the *external segment* of the *globus pallidus* (Figures 11.10 and 11.17), the *subthalamic nucleus* (Figure 11.13), the *substantia nigra pars compacta* (Figure 11.14), and the *ventral tegmental area* (Figure 11.14A).

The basic input–output pathway through the basal ganglia links wide regions of the cerebral cortex with, in sequence, the input nuclei of the basal ganglia (striatum), the output nuclei, the thalamus, and a portion of the frontal lobe rostral to the motor cortex (Figure 11.1). There are four principal functional "loops" through the basal ganglia (Figure 11.3). The *motor* (1) and *oculomotor* (2) loops play important roles in the control of body musculature and extraocular muscles; the *association* (3) loop may subserve such functions as spatial memory and evaluation of the effectiveness of behavior, and the *limbic* (4) loop may subserve emotions and their visceral consequences. The *motor, oculomotor,* and *association* loops begin in the *somatic sensory, motor,* and *association areas* of the cerebral cortex and pass through the *caudate nucleus* and *putamen* (Figures 11.2 and 11.7). The output nuclei of these loops are the *internal segment of the globus pallidus* (Figure 11.11) and the *substantia nigra pars reticulata* (Figures 11.13 and 11.14). They, in turn, synapse in the *ventral lateral, ventral anterior,* and *dorsomedial nuclei* of the thalamus (Figures 11.11B and 11.13). There are two pathways by which the internal segment of the globus pallidus projects to the thalamus: the *ansa lenticularis* and the *lenticular fasciculus* (Figures 11.11B and 11.12). However, components of the various loops synapse on neurons that are located in different nuclei or different portions of the same nuclei. The *limbic* loop begins in *association cortical* areas. The *ventral striatum* is the principal input nucleus of the limbic loop; the output and thalamic nuclei of the limbic loop are the *ventral pallidum* and the *dorsomedial nucleus*. The cortical targets of the four loops are (Figure 11.3B) *supplementary motor area* for the motor loop, *frontal eye field* for the oculomotor loop, *prefrontal association cortex* for the association loop, and *anterior cingulate gyrus* (and *orbitofrontal gyri*) for the limbic loop.

The intrinsic nuclei have interconnections with the input and output nuclei. Dopaminergic (Figure 11.15) neurons of the *substantia nigra pars compacta* project to the *caudate nucleus* and *putamen*; dopaminergic neurons of the *ventral tegmental area* project to the *nucleus accumbens* (Figure 11.4). The *external segment of the globus pallidus* projects to the *subthalamic nucleus* which projects to both the *internal and external segments of the globus pallidus*, the *substantia nigra pars reticulata*, and the *ventral pallidum* (Figure 11.4). ■

References

Gusella, J. F., Wexler, N. S., Conneally, P. M., et al. 1983. A polymorphic DNA marker genetically linked to Huntington's disease. Nature 306:234–238.

Haber, S. N., Groenewegen, H. J., Grove, E. A., et al. 1985. Efferent connections of the ventral pallidum: Evidence of a dual striato-pallidofugal pathway. J. Comp. Neurol. 235:322–335.

Haber, S. N., and Watson, S. J. 1985. The comparative distribution of enkephalin, dynorphin and substance P in the human globus pallidus and basal forebrain. Neurosci. 4:1011–1024.

Jones, E. G., and Leavitt, R. Y. 1974. Retrograde axonal transport and the demonstration of non-specific projections to the cerebral cortex and striatum from thalamic intralaminar nuclei in the rat, cat and monkey. J. Comp. Neurol. 154:349–378.

Poirier, L. J., Giguère, M., and Marchand, R. 1983. Comparative morphology of the substantia nigra and ventral tegmental area in the monkey, cat and rat. Brain Res. Bull. 11:371–397.

Selemon, L. D., and Goldman-Rakic, P. S. 1985. Longitudinal topography and interdigitation of corticostriatal projections in the rhesus monkey. J. Neurosci. 5:776–794.

Schell, G. R., and Strick, P. L. 1984. The origin of thalamic inputs to the arcuate premotor and supplementary motor areas. J. Neurosci. 4:539–560.

Yeterian, E. H., and Van Hoesen, G. W. 1978. Cortico-striate projections in the rhesus monkey: The organization of certain cortico-caudate connections. Brain Res. 139:43–63.

Selected Readings

Alexander, G. E., DeLong, M. R., and Strick, P. L. 1986. Parallel organization of functionally segregated circuits linking basal ganglia and cortex. Ann. Rev. Neurosci. 9:357–381.

Carpenter, M. 1981. Anatomy of the Corpus Striatum and Brain Stem Integrating Systems. In Brooks, V. B. (ed.), Handbook of Physiology, Section I: The Nervous System, Vol. II, Motor Control. Bethesda, Md.: American Physiological Society, pp. 947–995.

Côté, L., and Crutcher, M. D. 1985. Motor functions of the basal ganglia and diseases of transmitter metabolism. In Kandel, E. R., and Schwartz, J. H. Principles of Neural Science. New York: Elsevier, pp. 523–535.

DeLong, M. R., and Georgopoulos, A. P. 1981. Motor function of the basal ganglia. In Brooks, V. B. (ed.), Handbook of Physiology, Section I: The Nervous System, Vol. II, Motor Control. Bethesda, Md.: American Physiological Society, pp. 1017–1061.

Gunilla, R., Öberg, E., and Divac, I. 1981. Commentary: The basal ganglia and the control of movement. Levels of motor planning, cognition and the control of movement. Trends in Neurosci. 4:122–125.

Haber, S. N. 1986. Neurotransmitters in the human and nonhuman primate basal ganglia. Human Neurobiol. 5:159–168.

Heimer, L., Switzer, R. D., and Van Hoesen, G. W. 1982. Ventral striatum and ventral pallidum. Trends in Neurosci. 5:83–87.

General Organization of the Cranial Nerve Nuclei and the Trigeminal System

12

Cranial Nerve Nuclei

The study of the neuroanatomy of sensation and motor control of cranial structures has traditionally been separate from that of the limbs and body axis. This is because the head is innervated by the cranial nerves, whereas the limbs and trunk are innervated by the spinal nerves. There are, however, similarities in the functional organization of the cranial and spinal nerves, as well as similarities in the organization of the components of the central nervous system with which they are directly connected. Sensory axons in cranial nerves synapse in sensory cranial nerve nuclei. This is similar to sensory axons in spinal nerves, which synapse on neurons of the dorsal horn of the spinal cord and the dorsal column nuclei. The motor cranial nerve nuclei, like the motor nuclei of the ventral horn, contain the motor neurons whose axons project to the periphery. Extending this parallel between brain stem nuclei and spinal cord gray matter further, the autonomic cranial nerve nuclei are analogous to autonomic nuclei of the intermediate zone of the spinal cord, which contains autonomic preganglionic neurons.

In this chapter and the next, the principles of organization of the brain stem cranial nerve nuclei are considered. These are the nuclei that subserve cranial sensory and motor function. We examine both the columnar organization of the cranial nerve nuclei, a topic introduced in Chapter 2 when the development of the central nervous system was considered, and the regional anatomy of the brain stem. In earlier chapters, cranial nerve sensory function was considered when we examined the anatomical substrates of perception. The study of cranial nerve sensory function is completed in this chapter by examination of the trigeminal system, which mediates somatic sensation from the face and head. Before the trigeminal system is considered, the cranial nerves and the columnar organization of the cranial nerve nuclei are examined. In the next chapter the motor functions of the cranial nerves are examined.

A Review of the 12 Cranial Nerves

In contrast to the spinal nerves, which number approximately 31 pairs, there are only 12 pairs of cranial nerves (Figure 12.1). The cranial nerves are listed in Table 12.1, along with the foramina through which they pass to the periphery and key features of their functional organization. The first two cranial nerves—olfactory (I) and optic (II)—are purely sensory nerves and enter the *telencephalon* and *diencephalon* directly. It should be recalled that the optic nerve contains the axons of retinal ganglion cells (Chapter 6). Because the retina develops from the diencephalon, the optic nerve is actually a displaced central nervous system pathway and not a peripheral nerve. The other 10 cranial nerves enter and leave the *brain stem*. The oculomotor (III) and trochlear (IV) nerves, which are motor nerves, exit from the midbrain. There are four cranial nerves of the pons. The trigeminal (V) nerve is located at the middle of the pons. It is termed a *mixed nerve* because it subserves both sensory and motor functions. Three cranial nerves are located at the pontomedullary junction: the abducens (VI) nerve, which is a motor nerve; the facial (VII) nerve, a mixed nerve; and the vestibulocochlear (VIII) nerve, a sensory nerve. There are four cranial nerves of the medulla. The glossopharyngeal

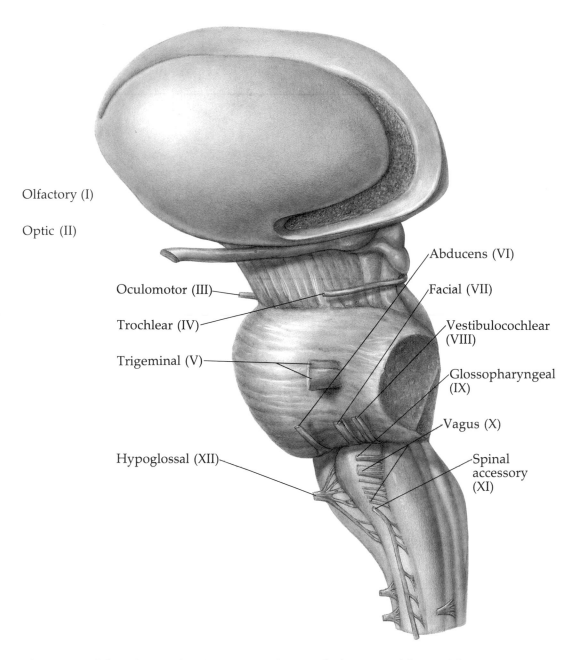

Olfactory (I)

Optic (II)

Oculomotor (III)

Trochlear (IV)

Trigeminal (V)

Hypoglossal (XII)

Abducens (VI)

Facial (VII)

Vestibulocochlear (VIII)

Glossopharyngeal (IX)

Vagus (X)

Spinal accessory (XI)

Figure 12.1 A lateral view of the brain stem, showing the locations of the cranial nerves. Note that the olfactory nerve (I) enters the olfactory bulb and the optic nerve (II) (which is actually a displaced central nervous system pathway) enters the diencephalon.

Table 12.1

Cranial Nerve and Root	Function	Cranial Foramina	Peripheral Sensory Ganglia	CNS Nucleus	Peripheral Autonomic Ganglia	Peripheral Structure Innervated
I Olfactory	SVA	Cribriform plate	—	Olfactory bulb		Olfactory receptors of olfactory epithelium
II Optic	SSA	Optic	—	Lateral geniculate nucleus		Retina (ganglion cells)
III Oculomotor	GSE	Superior orbital fissure		Oculomotor		Medial, superior, inferior rectus, inferior oblique, and levator palpebrae muscles
	GVE			Edinger–Westphal	Ciliary	Constrictor muscles of iris; ciliary muscle
IV Trochlear	GSE	Superior orbital fissure		Trochlear		Superior oblique muscle
V Trigeminal	GSA	Superior orbital fissure (Ophthalmic) Rotundum (Maxillary)	Semilunar	Spinal nucleus, main sensory nucleus, mesencephalic nucleus of CN V		Skin and mucous membranes of the head, muscle receptors, meninges
	SVE	Ovale (Mandibular)		Motor nucleus of CN V		Jaw muscles, tensor tympani and tensor palati
VI Abducens	GSE	Superior orbital fissure		Abducens		Lateral rectus muscle
VII Intermediate	SVA	Internal auditory meatus	Geniculate	Solitary nucleus		Taste (anterior two thirds of tongue), palate
	GSA GVE	Internal auditory meatus	Geniculate	Spinal nucleus of CN V Superior salivatory	Pterygopalatine submandibular	Skin of external ear Lacrimal glands, glands of nasal mucosa, salivary glands
Facial	SVE	Internal auditory meatus		Facial		Muscles of facial expression, digastric (posterior belly), and stapedius

Nerve	Component	Exit	Ganglion	Nucleus		Peripheral distribution
VIII Vestibulocochlear	SSA	Internal auditory meatus	Spiral	Cochlear		Hair cells in organ of Corti
	SSA		Vestibular	Vestibular		Hair cells in vestibular labyrinth
IX Glossopharyngeal	GSA	Jugular	Superior	Spinal nucleus of CN V		Skin of external ear
	GVA		Petrosal (inferior)	Solitary nucleus (caudal)		Mucous membranes in pharyngeal region, middle ear, carotid body, and sinus
	SVA		Petrosal	Solitary nucleus (rostral)		Taste (posterior one third of tongue)
	GVE			Inferior salivatory nucleus	Otic	Parotid gland
	SVE			Ambiguus (rostral)		Striated muscle of pharynx
X Vagus	GSA	Jugular	Jugular (superior)	Spinal nucleus of CN V		Skin of external ear, meninges
	GVA		Nodose (inferior)	Solitary nucleus (caudal)		Larynx, trachea, gut, aortic arch receptors
	SVA		Nodose (inferior)	Solitary nucleus (rostral)		Taste buds (posterior oral cavity, larynx)
	GVE			Dorsal motor nucleus of CN X	Peripheral autonomic	Gut (to splenic flexure of colon), respiratory structures, heart
	SVE			Ambiguus (middle region)		Striated muscles of palate, pharynx, and larynx
XI Spinal accessory	SVE	Jugular		Ambiguus (caudal), Accessory nucleus, pyramidal decussation to C5		[Aberrant vagus branches] sternocleidomastoid and portion of trapezius muscles
XII Hypoglossal	GSE	Hypoglossal		Hypoglossal		Intrinsic muscles of tongue, hyoglossus, genioglossus, and styloglossus muscles

(IX) and the vagus (X) nerves are both mixed nerves, whereas the spinal accessory (XI) and the hypoglossal (XII) nerves subserve motor function.

Many of the cranial nerves actually contain multiple roots or anatomically distinct subdivisions. The trigeminal nerve contains separate sensory and motor roots. This separation of sensory and motor axons is reminiscent of the segregation of function in the dorsal and ventral spinal roots. The facial nerve contains two roots, a large root consisting of the axons of motor neurons that innervate skeletal muscle, and a smaller root that contains primary afferent fibers and the axons of parasympathetic preganglionic neurons. The smaller root is termed the *intermediate nerve*. As noted in Chapter 7, the vestibulocochlear nerve contains two separate roots which innervate the vestibular labyrinth and the cochlea. The four medullary cranial nerves each contain numerous roots that leave from different rostrocaudal locations. It is not clearly understood whether roots that are associated with a single cranial nerve, but exit from different medullary locations, contain axons that subserve different sensory or motor functions.

In general, the peripheral organization of sensory (afferent) fibers in cranial nerves is similar to that of spinal nerves: the cell body of the primary sensory neuron gives off two processes; one innervates peripheral structures and transduces stimulus energy, and the other synapses on structures in the central nervous system. (The term *primary sensory neuron* is generally reserved for the cell in the circuit that has its cell body located in a peripheral sensory ganglion.) The peripheral sensory ganglia, in which the cell bodies of primary sensory neurons of the different cranial nerves are located, are listed in Table 12.1. However, two important differences exist between primary sensory neurons in spinal and cranial nerves: (1) primary sensory neurons in cranial nerves are often associated with a separate *receptor cell* that transduces stimulus energy, and (2) primary sensory neurons in cranial nerves have either a *pseudounipolar* or a *bipolar morphology* (Figure 12.2).

The peripheral organization of the sensory cranial nerves becomes easier to understand if we first distinguish the sensory innervation of the skin and mucous membranes (tactile, thermal, and pain senses) from the innervation of other structures. The skin and mucous membranes of the head, like those of the limbs and trunk, are innervated by primary sensory neurons that have a *pseudounipolar* morphology. Their cell bodies are located in *peripheral sensory ganglia*, and only the *distal portion* of the primary afferent fiber is sensitive to stimulus energy. Stretch receptors in jaw muscles are innervated by pseudounipolar primary sensory neurons. These neurons mediate *jaw proprioception*. However, the cell bodies of these stretch receptors are located in the central nervous system. The primary sensory neurons of the *olfactory system* (Chapter 8), which innervate the olfactory epithelium, have a chemosensitive distal terminal and a proximal portion that transmits the information to the central nervous system. However, these neurons have a *bipolar* morphology, and their total length is less than 1 cm (Figure 12.2). The remaining sensory modalities—taste, vision, audition, and balance—use at least two separate cells to transduce stimulus energy (receptor cell) and to transmit information, encoded in the form of action potentials, to the central nervous system.

The structures innervated by the motor fibers of cranial nerves, like

Modality	Receptor	Peripheral nerve	CNS	Actual size

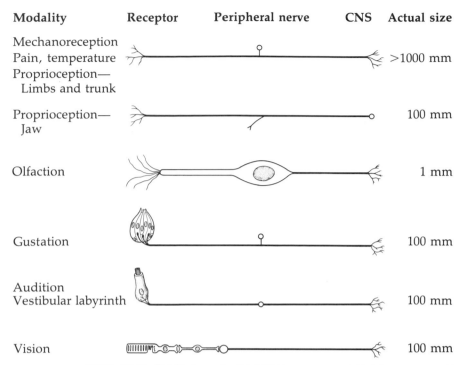

Mechanoreception
Pain, temperature — >1000 mm

Proprioception—
  Limbs and trunk

Proprioception—
  Jaw — 100 mm

Olfaction — 1 mm

Gustation — 100 mm

Audition
Vestibular labyrinth — 100 mm

Vision — 100 mm

Figure 12.2 Schematic illustration of morphology of primary sensory neurons, the location of cell bodies, and the approximate differences in actual sizes. Note that primary sensory neurons in the spinal cord have a pseudounipolar morphology, whereas, in cranial nerves, their morphology is more complex. The primary sensory neuron for jaw proprioception is further distinguished because its cell body is located in the central nervous system.

motor fibers in spinal nerves, include striated muscle and autonomic postganglionic neurons. In contrast to striated muscle of the limbs and trunk, which develop from body somites, cranial striated muscle develops either from cranial somites (somatic) or the branchial arches (visceral). The extraocular muscles and the tongue muscles are of somatic origin. The muscles of visceral origin include mastication, facial expression, laryngeal, palatal, and two neck muscles.

Seven functional categories of cranial nerve fibers are recognized on the basis of whether the individual axons innervate *sensory* (*afferent*) or *motor structures* and whether those structures develop from the *somites* or the *viscera*. Four of these categories are shared by the cranial nerves and the spinal nerves:

1. *General somatic afferents* subserve somatic sensations, including tactile sense, vibration sense, pain and temperature senses, and jaw (and limb) proprioception.
2. *General visceral afferents* mediate visceral sensations and chemoreception from body organs.
3. *General somatic motor* fibers are the axons of motor neurons that innervate striated muscle that develops from the somites.
4. *General visceral motor* fibers are the axons of autonomic preganglionic neurons.

However, because cranial nerves are more complex than spinal nerves, there are three additional categories:

5. *Special somatic afferents* subserve vision (Chapter 6) and audition and balance (Chapter 7).
6. *Special visceral afferents* mediate taste and smell (Chapter 8).
7. *Special visceral motor* fibers are the axons of motor neurons that innervate striated muscle that develops from the branchial arches.

The Cranial Nerve Nuclei Are Organized into Columns

The primary sensory neurons in cranial nerves that enter the brain stem synapse in *sensory cranial nerve nuclei;* the cell bodies of motor axons in cranial nerves are located in *motor cranial nerve nuclei.* Each cranial nerve nucleus subserves a single sensory or motor function. This is in contrast with many of the cranial nerves themselves, which contain a mixture of axons that have different functions (Table 12.1).[1] As there are seven functional categories of cranial nerves, there are also seven categories of cranial nerve nuclei. Nuclei of each of these categories are organized into discontinuous *columns that extend rostrocaudally through the brain stem* (Figures 12.3 and 12.4). However, there are only six columns because two of the functional categories of sensory cranial nerve axons synapse on neurons in separate rostrocaudal locations in a single column (see later). There is a systematic relationship between the function subserved by neurons in one of these columns and a column's location with respect to the midline (Figures 12.3 and 12.4). Knowledge of the approximate locations of these nuclear columns greatly simplifies the study of the cranial nerve nuclei and the regional anatomy of the brain stem.

Cell bodies of the three categories of motor axons in the cranial nerves are arranged in three separate columns of motor nuclei: general somatic motor column, special visceral motor column, and general visceral motor column. The *general somatic motor* column is located close to the midline in the midbrain, pons, and medulla. Nuclei in this column contain the cell bodies of motor neurons that innervate somatic striated muscle: the extraocular muscles and the tongue muscles. The *special visceral motor* column also contains motor neurons. It is located in the pons and medulla but it is displaced from the ventricular floor. This column contains motor neurons that innervate visceral striated muscle which are derived from the branchial arches: muscles of mastication, muscles of facial expression, laryngeal, palatal, and two neck muscles. The *general visceral motor* column is located in the floor of the fourth ventricle in the pons and medulla and ventral to the cerebral aqueduct in the rostral midbrain. This column contains parasympathetic preganglionic neurons.

The four categories of sensory, or afferent, axons in the cranial nerves synapse in three separate columns of sensory nuclei: combined special and general visceral afferent column, special somatic afferent col-

---

[1] The distal portions of specific autonomic components of the oculomotor, facial, and glossopharyngeal nerves actually leave these nerves and course with the trigeminal nerve. This switch in the peripheral course of the axons from one cranial nerve to the other occurs in peripheral plexes and is similar to the mixing of sensory and motor axons from the spinal cord.

A

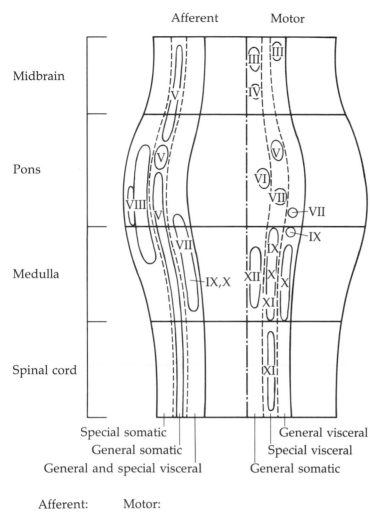

Afferent   Motor

Midbrain

Pons

Medulla

Spinal cord

Special somatic
General somatic
General and special visceral

General visceral
Special visceral
General somatic

B

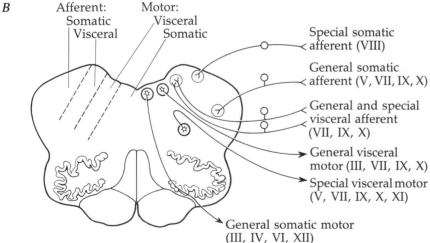

Afferent:
Somatic
  Visceral

Motor:
Visceral
  Somatic

Special somatic
afferent (VIII)

General somatic
afferent (V, VII, IX, X)

General and special
visceral afferent
(VII, IX, X)

General visceral
motor (III, VII, IX, X)

Special visceral motor
(V, VII, IX, X, XI)

General somatic motor
(III, IV, VI, XII)

Figure 12.3 *A.* Schematic dorsal view of brain stem, showing that the cranial nerve nuclei are organized into discontinuous columns. *B.* Schematic cross section through the medulla, showing the locations of cranial nerve nuclear columns. (*A.* Adapted from Nieuwenhuys, R., Voogd, J., and van Huijzen, Chr. 1988. The Human Central Nervous System, A Synopsis and Atlas, Third Edition. Berlin: Springer-Verlag. *B.* Adapted from Kandel, E. R. and Schwartz, J. H. 1985. Principles of Neural Science. New York: Elsevier.)

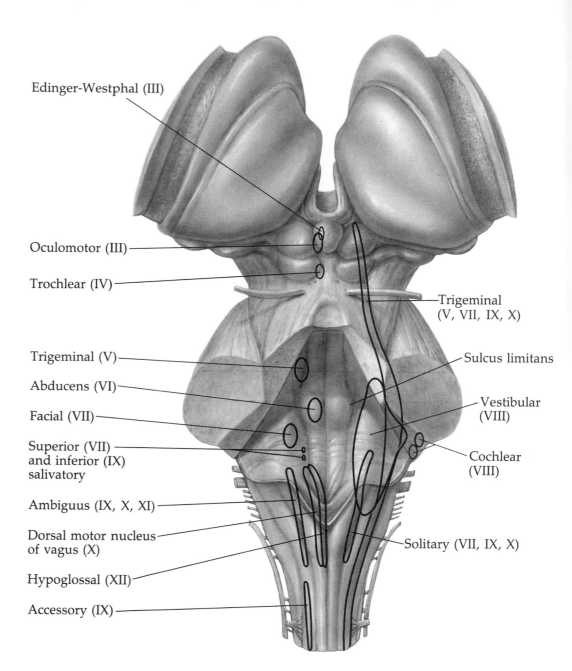

Edinger-Westphal (III)

Oculomotor (III)

Trochlear (IV)

Trigeminal (V, VII, IX, X)

Trigeminal (V)

Abducens (VI)

Facial (VII)

Superior (VII) and inferior (IX) salivatory

Ambiguus (IX, X, XI)

Dorsal motor nucleus of vagus (X)

Hypoglossal (XII)

Accessory (IX)

Sulcus limitans

Vestibular (VIII)

Cochlear (VIII)

Solitary (VII, IX, X)

Figure 12.4 Dorsal view of the brain stem, indicating the locations of the cranial nerve nuclei.

umn, and general somatic afferent column. These columns of sensory nuclei are separated from the columns of motor nuclei by the *sulcus limitans*, which separated the alar and basal plates in the embryonic brain and spinal cord (Chapter 2). The single *visceral afferent* column has a special visceral component subserving taste that is located rostral to the general visceral component, which subserves aspects of visceral sensation and processing of chemical stimuli. This column corresponds to a single nucleus, the *solitary nucleus* (Chapter 8), and it is located in the medulla beneath the floor of the fourth ventricle. The *special somatic afferent* column is located in the pons and medulla and consists of the *vestibular* and *cochlear nuclei* (Chapter 7). The *general somatic afferent* column is located from the rostral spinal cord to the midbrain. This column consists of the three trigeminal sensory nuclei—the *spinal nucleus* of CN V, the *main sensory nucleus* of CN V, and the *mesencephalic nucleus* of CN V—and mediates somatic sensation of cranial structures.

The remaining portions of this chapter are devoted to the trigeminal system,which mediates tactile, pain and thermal sensations of the head as well as jaw proprioception. The functions of the trigeminal system are comparable to those of the spinal nerves and the ascending spinal cord pathways, which were considered in Chapter 5. For each somatic sensory modality, we consider initially the general organization of the pathways mediating these functions. Then the organization of the different trigeminal sensory systems is approached from a regional perspective as we examine sections through the brain stem and thalamus.

Trigeminal System

Separate Trigeminal Pathways Mediate Tactile Sensation, Pain and Temperature Senses, and Jaw Proprioception

Somatic sensation of the head and oral cavity is carried by four cranial nerves. The *trigeminal nerve* (1) innervates most of the head and oral cavity. The *facial* (2), the *glossopharyngeal* (3), and the *vagus* (4) nerves innervate certain areas of the skin about the external ear, pharynx, nasal cavity and sinuses, and middle ear. The meninges are innervated by the trigeminal and vagus nerves. The axons of these nerves mediating somatic sensations are of the general somatic afferent category. It should be recalled that facial, glossopharyngeal, and vagus nerves also contain visceral afferent fibers that mediate taste and chemoreception (Chapter 8). Because of the modest overall contribution of facial, glossopharyngeal, and vagus nerves to facial somatic sensation, we focus primarily on the trigeminal nerve.

There are functional differences among individual afferent fibers in the trigeminal nerve, just as there are differences among afferent fibers in spinal nerves. Tactile sensation and jaw proprioception are mediated by the largest diameter fibers, which are myelinated. Pain and temperature senses are mediated collectively by the smaller diameter myelinated fibers and unmyelinated fibers. These functional differences set the stage for the organization of three anatomically and functionally separate trigeminal ascending systems (Figures 12.5 and 12.6): a system important for discriminative tactile sensation, a system important in pain and temperature senses, and a system important in proprioception of the jaw.

The Main Sensory Nucleus of Cranial Nerve V Mediates Tactile Sensation

Large-diameter axons of the trigeminal nerve, which mediate tactile sense, enter the ventral pons and course to the dorsal portion. Here, most afferent fibers emit a short ascending branch and a longer descending

A

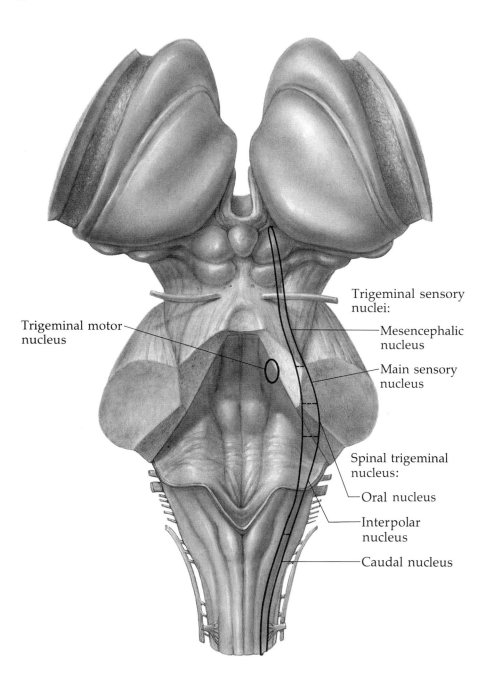

Trigeminal motor nucleus

Trigeminal sensory nuclei:

Mesencephalic nucleus

Main sensory nucleus

Spinal trigeminal nucleus:

Oral nucleus

Interpolar nucleus

Caudal nucleus

branch (Figure 12.5). The ascending branch terminates in the *main* (or *principal*) *sensory nucleus of the trigeminal nerve*. The longer branch descends in the *spinal tract of the trigeminal nerve* (see later). The majority of neurons in the main sensory nucleus give rise to axons that decussate in the pons

B

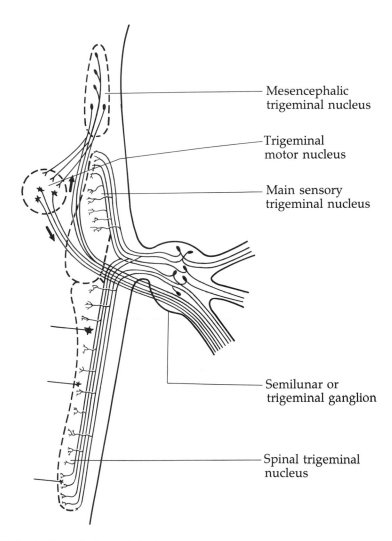

Mesencephalic
trigeminal nucleus

Trigeminal
motor nucleus

Main sensory
trigeminal nucleus

Semilunar or
trigeminal ganglion

Spinal trigeminal
nucleus

Figure 12.5   A. Dorsal view of the brain stem without cerebellum indicates the locations of the trigeminal nuclei. *B.* Neuronal and synaptic organization of the trigeminal nuclei. (Arrows indicate directions of information flow for jaw jerk reflex. Sensory information from jaw proprioceptors is transmitted to trigeminal motor neurons in the trigeminal motor nucleus.) (Adapted from Cajal, S. Ramon y. 1909, 1911. Histologie du système nerveux de l'homme et des vertébres. 2 vols. Paris: Maloine.)

and ascend dorsomedial to fibers from the dorsal column nuclei in the medial lemniscus. The ascending second-order trigeminal fibers, which are collectively termed the *trigeminal lemniscus*, synapse in the medial division of the ventral posterior nucleus of the thalamus, the *ventral pos-*

Figure 12.6 General organization of the ascending trigeminal pathways for *(A)* tactile sensation and *(B)* pain and temperature senses.
C. Mesencephalic trigeminal nucleus and primary afferent fibers for proprioception.

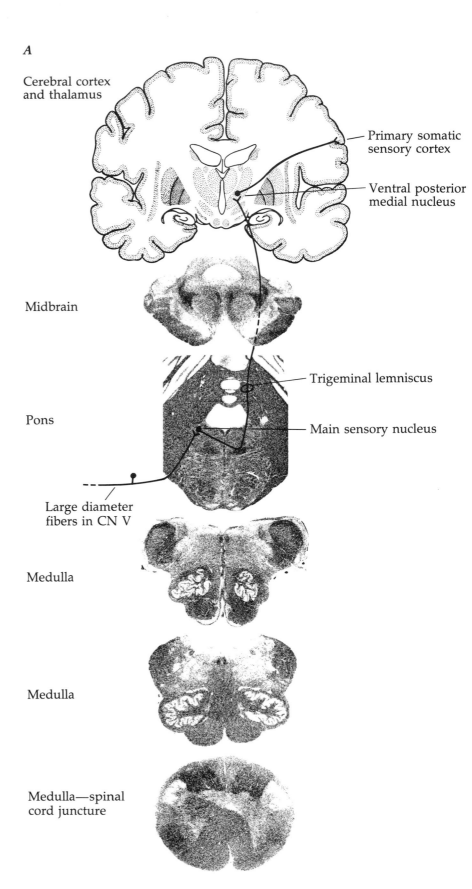

A

Cerebral cortex and thalamus

Primary somatic sensory cortex

Ventral posterior medial nucleus

Midbrain

Trigeminal lemniscus

Pons

Main sensory nucleus

Large diameter fibers in CN V

Medulla

Medulla

Medulla—spinal cord juncture

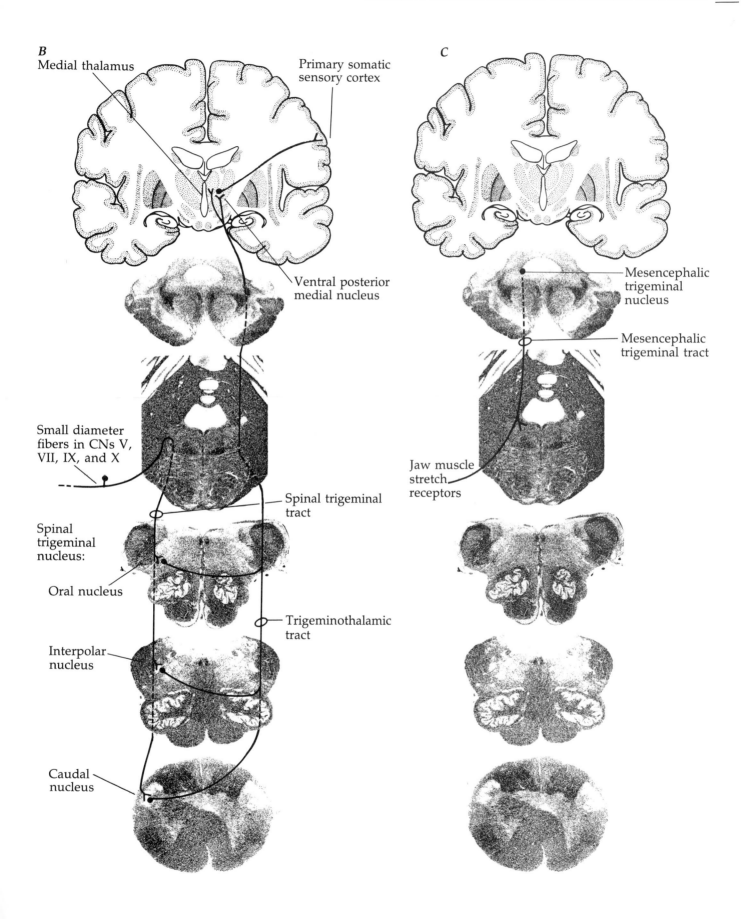

B

Medial thalamus

Primary somatic sensory cortex

C

Ventral posterior medial nucleus

Mesencephalic trigeminal nucleus

Mesencephalic trigeminal tract

Small diameter fibers in CNs V, VII, IX, and X

Jaw muscle stretch receptors

Spinal trigeminal tract

Spinal trigeminal nucleus:

Oral nucleus

Trigeminothalamic tract

Interpolar nucleus

Caudal nucleus

terior medial nucleus (Figure 12.6A). From the ventral posterior medial nucleus, the axons of thalamic neurons project, via the posterior limb of the internal capsule, to the *primary somatic sensory cortex*. This cortical area is located in the postcentral gyrus. This is the principal pathway for tactile perception on the face and is analogous to the dorsal column–medial lemniscal system. The ascending and descending axons of the primary sensory neurons are analogous to the dorsal column axons, and the main sensory nucleus of CN V is functionally similar to the dorsal column nuclei. The *secondary somatic sensory cortex*, which is located in the parietal operculum and posterior insular cortex (Chapter 5), receives its major input from the primary somatic sensory cortex. A second smaller ascending pathway originates from neurons in the dorsal portion of the main sensory nucleus. This pathway ascends ipsilaterally through the dorsal tegmentum of the brain stem and, like the ventral path, terminates in the ventral posterior medial nucleus. The ventral pathway (in the trigeminal lemniscus), which is *crossed* and ascends with the medial lemniscus, mediates tactile sensation from the face and head. By contrast, the dorsal pathway ascends *ipsilaterally* in the central tegmental tract and may process mechanical stimuli from the teeth and soft tissues of the oral cavity.

The Spinal Nucleus of Cranial Nerve V Mediates Pain and Temperature Senses

Small-diameter myelinated and unmyelinated fibers enter the pons and descend in the spinal tract of the trigeminal nerve (CN V) (Figure 12.5). These branches terminate in the *spinal nucleus of CN V* (also termed the spinal trigeminal nucleus).[2] Few small-diameter axons ascend in the spinal tract of CN V. Large-diameter fibers also descend in this tract to terminate in the spinal nucleus of CN V. However, the large- and small-diameter afferent fibers have different patterns of termination in the spinal nucleus (see later).

The spinal nucleus of CN V has a rostrocaudal anatomical and functional organization (Figure 12.6B) with three components: (1) *oral nucleus*, (2) *interpolar nucleus*, and (3) *caudal nucleus*. The functions of the caudal nucleus are similar to those of the dorsal horn of the spinal cord, with which it is continuous, but the caudal nucleus mediates *facial* sensation. Like the dorsal horn, the caudal nucleus plays an important role in *pain* and *temperature* senses, including dental pain, and a lesser role in tactile sensation. The functions of the interpolar and oral nuclei are less well defined compared with those of the caudal nucleus. They may be important in reflexes. For example, interneurons for the *jaw-opening reflex*, the reflex opening of the mouth in response to tactile stimulation of oral and perioral structures, are located in the interpolar and oral nuclei. The interpolar nucleus may also function in mediating dental pain, especially its caudal portion, which is continuous with the caudal nucleus.

---

[2] Many components of the trigeminal system have names that are not well suited to their locations. The spinal tract and nucleus of CN V are actually located in the pons, medulla, and spinal cord and receive input from other cranial nerves in addition to the trigeminal nerve. Another component of the trigeminal system, the mesencephalic tract and nucleus of CN V, is located in the pons and midbrain.

An ascending trigeminal pathway, important principally for facial and dental pain, originates from the spinal trigeminal nucleus, especially the caudal and interpolar nuclei and terminates in the thalamus (Figure 12.6B). The organization of this path is similar to that of the spinothalamic tract (Chapter 5): the ascending *trigeminothalamic tract*[3] is predominantly crossed and ascends with fibers of the *anterolateral system*. Subcomponents terminate in two locations in the thalamus: ventral posterior medial nucleus and intralaminar nuclei. The projection to the *ventral posterior medial nucleus* is thought to mediate discriminative aspects of pain and temperature senses, for example, stimulus localization. In contrast, the projection to the *intralaminar nuclei* is thought to participate in the affective and motivational aspects of facial pain and temperature senses. A further parallel between the trigeminal and spinal ascending systems is that the ventral posterior medial nucleus projects to the facial representation of the primary somatic sensory cortex, in the lateral portion of the *postcentral gyrus*.

The Mesencephalic Nucleus of Cranial Nerve V Contains the Cell Bodies of Muscle Stretch Receptors

The trigeminal nerve innervates stretch receptors that are located in the muscles of mastication. These receptors are unusual because their cell bodies are located in the central nervous system, in the *mesencephalic trigeminal nucleus* (Figures 12.5 and 12.6C). In contrast, the cell bodies of the other trigeminal afferent fibers lie in the trigeminal ganglion.[4] The axons that bring sensory information from the periphery ascend to the mesencephalic nucleus of CN V in close association with the ventricular system, in the *mesencephalic tract of CN V*. These primary afferent fibers have a pseudounipolar morphology and, therefore, are similar to their counterparts in the dorsal root ganglia and the trigeminal ganglion. The other branch of these primary sensory neurons projects to various sites in the brain, sites important for motor control and proprioception of the jaw. For example, the projection to the motor nucleus of CN V is important for mediating jaw reflexes, including the monosynaptic jaw closure—or *jaw jerk*—reflex, which is analogous to the knee jerk reflex (Figure 12.5).

In the remaining sections, the regional anatomical organization of the trigeminal system is examined. We begin with the peripheral nerve roots and the areas they innervate. Then, in sequence, the distribution and terminations in the spinal trigeminal tract and nuclei are examined. Finally, we consider the ascending trigeminal pathways through the rostral brain stem, to the thalamus, and then the cerebral cortex. As we examine brain stem sections serially, we review the locations of the other cranial nerve sensory nuclei: the vestibular and cochlear nuclei and the solitary nucleus.

---

[3] The trigeminothalamic tract is also termed the quintothalamic tract.

[4] The trigeminal nerve also innervates stretch receptors in the extraocular muscles, but it is thought that these afferent fibers have their somata located in the trigeminal ganglion, and their axons course within the ophthalmic division of the trigeminal nerve.

The Trigeminal System Is Somatotopically Organized

The trigeminal nerve consists of three sensory roots and one motor root. The sensory roots are analogous to the dorsal spinal roots, and the motor root is analogous to a ventral spinal root. The analogy is a functional one only because the trigeminal roots are not located dorsal and ventral to one another. The motor root innervates the muscles of mastication and will be discussed in the next chapter. The sensory roots contain the primary afferent fibers whose cell bodies are located in the trigeminal ganglion and the trigeminal mesencephalic nucleus. The sensory fibers are of the general somatic afferent class. Each root innervates the skin and mucous membranes of separate regions of the head: the *ophthalmic division*, the *maxillary division*, and the *mandibular division* (Figure 12.7A). Unlike dorsal roots of adjacent spinal cord segments, where the dermatomes overlap extensively, the trigeminal dermatomes (i.e., the area of skin innervated by a single trigeminal sensory nerve division) overlap very little. Thus, a peripheral anesthetic region is more likely to occur after damage to one trigeminal division than after damage of a single dorsal root. After entering the pons, the fibers of each division occupy a discrete rostrocaudal-oriented slice in the spinal tract of CN V (Figure 12.7B). The organization is that of an inverted figure of a face: the mandibular division is located dorsal, the ophthalmic division is located ventral, and the maxillary division is interposed.

In addition to the trigeminal nerve, the *intermediate* (a branch of the *facial nerve*), *glossopharyngeal*, and *vagus nerves* innervate the skin and mucous membranes of the head. The skin of the ear and the external auditory meatus are innervated by the intermediate and vagus nerves (Figure 12.7A). The glossopharyngeal nerve innervates the posterior one third of the tongue and portions of the oral cavity, the nasal cavity and sinuses, and the middle ear. (The dura is innervated by trigeminal and vagus nerves.) The cell bodies of the primary afferent fibers that subserve somatic sensation lie in the *superior ganglia* of the glossopharyngeal and vagus nerves and the *geniculate ganglion* of the facial nerve; their central processes join the spinal trigeminal tract and terminate in the spinal trigeminal nucleus (Figure 12.7B). The cell bodies of vagal and glossopharyngeal afferent fibers that subserve visceral sensations (taste and chemoreception) are located in the *inferior ganglia* of both nerves (Chapter 8). This is another example of the anatomical segregation of functionally dissimilar neural elements.

The Key Components of the Trigeminal System Are Present at Different Levels of the Brain Stem

The three trigeminal nuclei are located at different levels of the brainstem and subserve different functions. The *spinal trigeminal nucleus* (1) is important in facial pain and is located principally in the medulla and the caudal pons. The *main trigeminal sensory nucleus* (2) mediates facial tactile sense and is located in the pons. The *mesencephalic trigeminal nucleus* (3) mediates proprioception from the jaw, and is located in the rostral pons and midbrain.

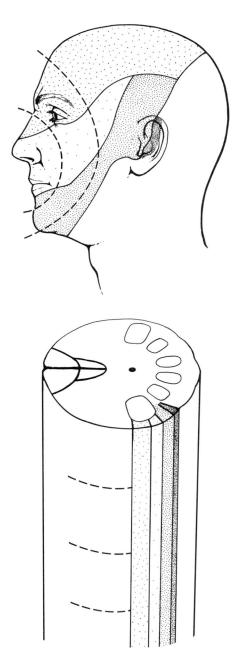

Figure 12.7 Somatotopic organization of the trigeminal system. The peripheral innervation territories of the three divisions of the trigeminal nerve and the intermediate and vagus nerves are illustrated on top. The organization of the spinal trigeminal tract in relation to the three trigeminal nerve divisions and the intermediate, glossopharyngeal, and vagus nerves is shown below for the portion of the medulla that includes the caudal nucleus. *A, B,* and *C* correspond to the "onion-skin" pattern of representation of trigeminal afferents in the caudal nucleus. Regions marked A (located rostral), B, and C (located caudal), correspond to the concentric zones on the face indicated in *A*. (Adapted from Brodal, A. 1981. Neurological Anatomy. New York: Oxford University Press.)

The Spinal Nucleus of Cranial Nerve V Is the Rostral Extension of the Spinal Cord Dorsal Horn

The dorsal horn extends rostrally into the medulla as the spinal trigeminal nucleus. We can understand this point by first recalling that the developing spinal cord and brain stem contain two zones of developing neurons, the alar and basal plates, that form rostrocaudal-oriented columns of cells from the spinal cord to the midbrain. In the spinal cord these cells form the dorsal and ventral horns. The extension of the alar plate in the caudal medulla is accompanied by a further subdivision, as the central nervous system matures into the *dorsal column nuclei* and the *spinal trigeminal nucleus* of CN V. There are three subdivisions of the spinal trigeminal nucleus, from caudal to rostral: caudal nucleus, interpolar nucleus, and oral nucleus. The caudal nucleus and the dorsal horn of the spinal cord have three key similarities: (1) morphology and lamination, (2) laminar distribution of afferent fiber terminals, and (3) laminar distribution of projection neurons. By comparing sections of the spinal cord and the caudal medulla, the similarity in morphology of the dorsal horn and the caudal nucleus can be seen (Figure 12.8). In fact, the caudal nucleus is sometimes called the *medullary dorsal horn* because it has a laminar organization that is similar to that of the spinal cord dorsal horn. Lamina I, the outermost, is equivalent to the marginal zone of the dorsal horn, lamina II is equivalent to the substantia gelatinosa, and laminae III and IV, termed the magnocellular nucleus in the trigeminal system, are equivalent to the nucleus proprius. Laminae V and VI of the spinal cord (base of dorsal horn) extend rostrally into the base of the spinal nucleus of CN V. The portion of the spinal tract of CN V overlying lamina I of the spinal nucleus is the rostral extension of the zone of Lissauer. The portion ventral to lamina VI forms part of the reticular formation and is continuous with the intermediate zone of the spinal cord.

Important insights into the function of the spinal nucleus of CN V have been obtained from a neurosurgical procedure in which the spinal tract of CN V is transected. This procedure, rarely done at present, produces selective disruption of facial pain and temperature senses with little effect on tactile perception. If the tract is transected near the border between the caudal and interpolar nuclei, facial pain and temperature senses over the entire face are disrupted. Transection of the tract near its caudal border with the cervical spinal cord spares pain and temperature senses over the perioral region and nose. This clinical finding indicates that there is a rostrocaudal somatotopic organization in the spinal trigeminal tract in addition to a mediolateral organization (Figure 12.7). Trigeminal fibers that innervate the portion of the head adjacent to the cervical spinal cord representation (Figure 12.7B) terminate more caudally in the caudal nucleus, whereas fibers that innervate the oral cavity, perioral face, and nose terminate more rostrally. Thus, proceeding rostrally from the cervical spinal cord, neurons of the spinal dorsal horn process somatic sensory information from the arm, neck, and occiput. Neurons of the caudal nucleus at the spinal cord–medulla border process somatic sensory information from the posterior face and ear. Farther rostrally, the neurons process information from the perioral region, nose, and oral cavity. This organization is termed "onion-skin" because of the concentric-ring con-

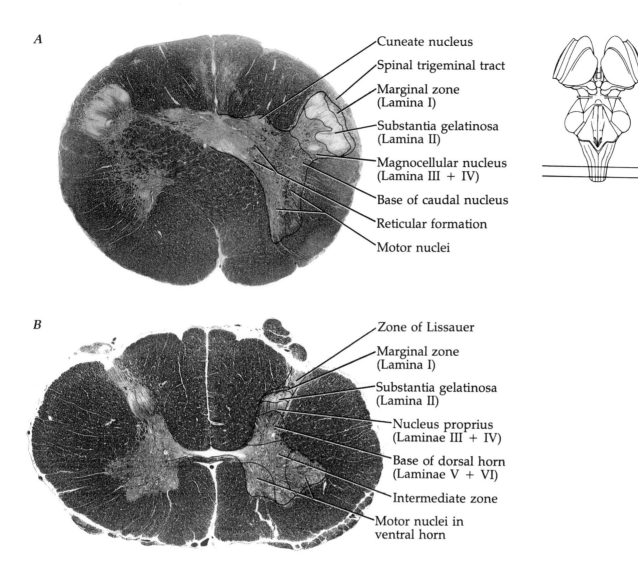

A

Cuneate nucleus

Spinal trigeminal tract

Marginal zone
(Lamina I)

Substantia gelatinosa
(Lamina II)

Magnocellular nucleus
(Lamina III + IV)

Base of caudal nucleus

Reticular formation

Motor nuclei

B

Zone of Lissauer

Marginal zone
(Lamina I)

Substantia gelatinosa
(Lamina II)

Nucleus proprius
(Laminae III + IV)

Base of dorsal horn
(Laminae V + VI)

Intermediate zone

Motor nuclei in
ventral horn

Figure 12.8 The spinal cord dorsal horn and the caudal nucleus have a similar organization. Myelin-stained transverse sections through the caudal nucleus— the level of pyramidal decussation *(A)*—and the cervical spinal cord *(B)*.

figuration of the peripheral fields processed at a given level by the medullary dorsal horn.

The second similarity between the spinal dorsal horn and the caudal nucleus is the pattern of termination of primary afferent fibers. Like the afferent fiber termination pattern in the dorsal horn of the spinal cord, afferent fibers of different diameters terminate in different laminae of the caudal nucleus. Whereas small-diameter trigeminal afferent fibers terminate in laminae I and II, large-diameter fibers terminate primarily in laminae III through VI. The third similarity between the dorsal horn of the spinal cord and the caudal nucleus is the laminar distribution of ascending projection neurons. The ascending pathway for facial pain is the trigeminothalamic tract and the ascending projection neurons are principally located in laminae I and V. These neurons project primarily to the

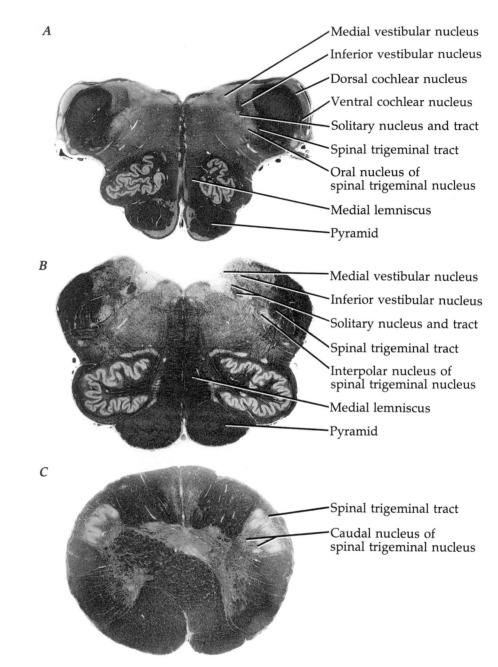

A

Medial vestibular nucleus
Inferior vestibular nucleus
Dorsal cochlear nucleus
Ventral cochlear nucleus
Solitary nucleus and tract
Spinal trigeminal tract
Oral nucleus of
spinal trigeminal nucleus
Medial lemniscus
Pyramid

B

Medial vestibular nucleus
Inferior vestibular nucleus
Solitary nucleus and tract
Spinal trigeminal tract
Interpolar nucleus of
spinal trigeminal nucleus
Medial lemniscus
Pyramid

C

Spinal trigeminal tract
Caudal nucleus of
spinal trigeminal nucleus

Figure 12.9 Myelin-stained transverse sections through the three divisions of the spinal trigeminal nucleus: oral nucleus *(A)*, interpolar nucleus *(B)*, and caudal nucleus *(C)*.

contralateral thalamus. Cells that project to other brain stem sites, such as the reticular formation, have a broader laminar distribution. The projection to the reticular formation also has a larger ipsilateral component.

The three subdivisions of the spinal trigeminal nucleus—caudal, interpolar, and oral nuclei—are shown in Figure 12.9. The section shown in Figure 12.8A is duplicated in Figure 12.9C to facilitate comparison of the configurations of the three subdivisions of the spinal nucleus. Although the boundaries between the subdivisions are not precise, the different components of the trigeminal spinal nuclear complex can be identified with respect to brain stem landmarks (see Figure 12.5A). The caudal nucleus extends from approximately the first or second cervical segment of the spinal cord to the medullary level at which the central canal "opens" to form the fourth ventricle. The interpolar nucleus extends from the rostral boundary of the caudal nucleus to the rostral medulla. Finally, the oral nucleus extends from the rostral boundary of the interpolar nucleus to the level at which the trigeminal nerve enters the pons. The other cranial nerve sensory nuclei—solitary nucleus, vestibular nuclei, and cochlear nuclei—are also labeled in Figure 12.9.

Occlusion of the Posterior Inferior Cerebellar Artery Interrupts Pain and Temperature Senses on the Same Side of the Face and on the Opposite Side of the Body

As we saw in earlier chapters, the posterior inferior cerebellar artery provides the arterial supply to the dorsolateral portion of the medulla (Figure 12.10) and caudal pons. Occlusion of this artery produces a complex set of sensory and motor deficits (the *lateral medullary syndrome* or *Wallenberg's syndrome*). One sign of this syndrome is loss of pain and temperature senses on the contralateral side of the body (Chapter 5). Pain and temperature senses are affected because axons of the anterolateral system ascend in the *lateral medulla*. The distribution of the sensory deficit is on the contralateral body because fibers of the anterolateral system decussate in the spinal cord. Occlusion of the posterior inferior cerebellar artery also produces deficits in pain and temperature senses of the face because the neurons that mediate these senses, the descending primary afferent fibers in the spinal tract of CN V and the neurons in the spinal nucleus of CN V, are also located in the lateral medulla. The facial sensory deficits are on the side ipsilateral to the occlusion because the primary afferent fibers and projection neurons are destroyed before they decus-

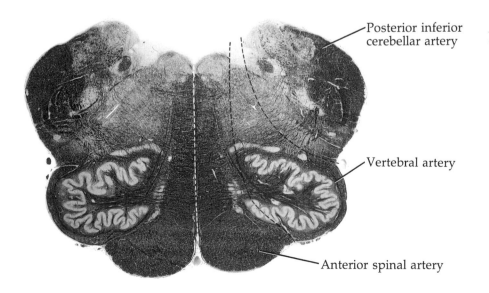

Posterior inferior cerebellar artery

Vertebral artery

Anterior spinal artery

Figure 12.10 The arterial supply of the medulla.

sate.[5] Motor deficits are also an important part of the symptoms of the lateral medullary syndrome because the vestibular nuclei and the inferior cerebellar peduncle are located in the dorsolateral medulla. These symptoms were considered in Chapter 10 and will be examined further in Chapter 13.

The major cause of a posterior inferior cerebellar artery stroke is occlusion of the *vertebral artery*. The posterior inferior cerebellar artery is an *end-artery with little collateral flow* from other vessels into the territory it serves. As a consequence, the dorsolateral region of the medulla and caudal pons is infarcted (Figure 12.10). The reason why the medial region of the medulla and caudal pons does not become infarcted is that there is collateral flow into the territories of the vertebral and spinal arteries.

The Main Sensory Nucleus of Cranial Nerve V Is the Trigeminal Equivalent of the Dorsal Column Nuclei

Rostral to the oral nucleus is the *main trigeminal sensory nucleus* (Figure 12.11). This component of the trigeminal nuclear complex subserves tactile sensation of the face and head, including mechanosensation from the teeth. Neurons located primarily in the ventral two thirds of this nucleus give rise to axons that *decussate* and ascend to the *ventral posterior medial nucleus* of the thalamus. Their axons are located in the *trigeminal lemniscus*. The main trigeminal sensory nucleus may be the trigeminal equivalent of the dorsal column nuclei because (1) both structures project to the contralateral ventral posterior nucleus (but to different subdivisions), and (2) both structures subserve tactile sensation. The trigeminal lemniscus at brain stem levels caudal to the main sensory nucleus contains axons from neurons in the spinal nucleus of CN V. This contingent, which may be analogous to the group of dorsal column axons that originate from dorsal horn neurons (Chapter 5), joins with the ascending fibers from the main sensory nucleus in the rostral pons.

The dorsal one third of the main sensory nucleus receives mechanoreceptive information from the soft tissues of the oral cavity and the teeth. Neurons from this portion of the main sensory nucleus give rise to an *ipsilateral pathway* that ascends in the *central tegmental tract* (Figure 12.11) and terminates in the ipsilateral ventral posterior medial nucleus of the thalamus. It is interesting that a lesion of the central tegmental tract produces a motor disturbance involving *palatal muscles* and no obvious sensory impairment. This clinical finding may provide insight into the function of the dorsal portion of the main sensory nucleus. It may play a more important role in cranial motor control than in mechanosensation.

The Mesencephalic Nucleus and Tract of Cranial Nerve V Course in Parallel with the Cerebral Aqueduct

The mesencephalic trigeminal nucleus is located in the lateral portion of the floor of the fourth ventricle and the periaqueductal gray; the mesencephalic trigeminal tract is located lateral to the nucleus. The mes-

---

[5] The decussation of the axons of ascending projection neurons in the spinal trigeminal nucleus (as well as the main sensory nucleus) occurs rostral to their cell bodies, similar to the anterolateral system of the spinal cord (see Figure 5.8).

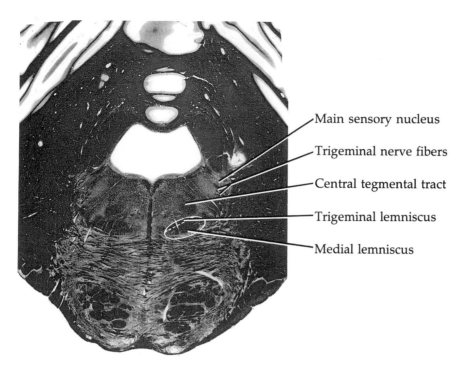

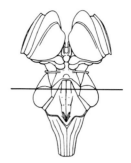

Main sensory nucleus

Trigeminal nerve fibers

Central tegmental tract

Trigeminal lemniscus

Medial lemniscus

Figure 12.11 Myelin-stained transverse section through the pons at the level of the main sensory nucleus and the trigeminal motor nucleus.

encephalic tract can be identified because its axons are myelinated (Figure 12.12). Both the mesencephalic nucleus and tract are present from the level of the main trigeminal sensory and motor nuclei in the pons to the superior colliculus in the midbrain. However, the tract can be easily identified only in the midbrain. The mesencephalic nucleus is equivalent to a peripheral sensory ganglion because cell bodies of primary afferent neurons are located there. After ascending to the mesencephalic trigeminal nucleus, the other axon branch of the primary sensory neurons projects

Figure 12.12 Myelin-stained transverse section through the rostral midbrain.

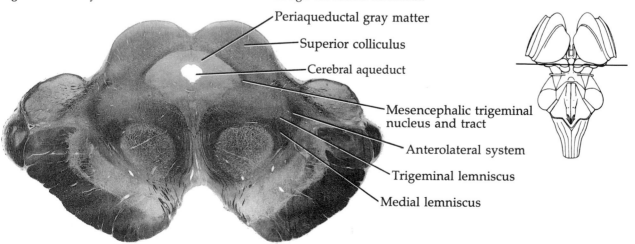

Periaqueductal gray matter

Superior colliculus

Cerebral aqueduct

Mesencephalic trigeminal nucleus and tract

Anterolateral system

Trigeminal lemniscus

Medial lemniscus

back down to the trigeminal motor nucleus, as well as to the reticular formation (see Figures 12.5 and 12.6C). At the midbrain level shown in Figure 12.12, the medial and trigeminal lemnisci have migrated laterally; however, the ascending trigeminal fibers are located dorsomedial. The trigeminal lemniscus terminates in the *medial* division of the ventral posterior nucleus (see later).

The Ventral Posterior Nucleus Contains Separate Divisions That Mediate Somatic Sensation of the Face and Body

The ventral posterior nucleus contains two principal divisions that mediate somatic sensation (Chapter 5). The ventral posterior lateral nucleus mediates somatic sensation from the limbs and trunk, and the *ventral posterior medial nucleus* (Figure 12.13) processes somatic sensation from the head. The ventral posterior medial nucleus is further subdivided into a lateral *magnocellular* and a medial *parvocellular* division. It is the magnocellular division that receives the projection from the trigeminal lemniscus. Although most of the magnocellular portion is difficult to distinguish from the ventral posterior lateral nucleus, the *parvocellular* portion, which mediates taste (Chapter 8), has a characteristic pale appearance in myelin-stained sections (Figure 12.13). Once the parvocellular portion is identified, the position of the magnocellular portion can be inferred. The second

Figure 12.13 Myelin-stained coronal section through the ventral posterior nucleus of the thalamus. The magnocellular and parvocellular portions of the medial division (ventral posterior medial nucleus) are the trigeminal and taste relay nuclei, whereas the lateral division (ventral posterior lateral nucleus) is the relay nucleus for the medial lemniscus (i.e., spinal sensory input).

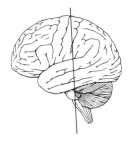

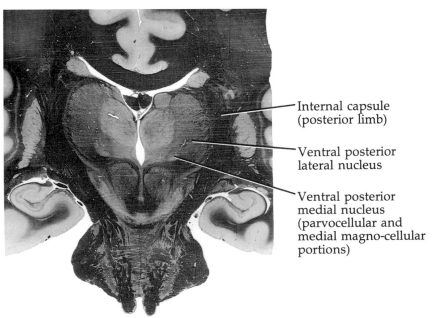

Internal capsule (posterior limb)

Ventral posterior lateral nucleus

Ventral posterior medial nucleus (parvocellular and medial magno-cellular portions)

major site receiving trigeminal input is the intralaminar nuclei. In contrast to the ventral posterior medial nucleus, which is a thalamic sensory relay nucleus that projects to a restricted portion of the postcentral gyrus (see later), the intralaminar nuclei have a diffuse projection pattern.

The Ventral Posterior Medial Nucleus Projects to the Primary Somatic Sensory Cortex

The ventral posterior lateral nucleus projects to the arm, trunk, and leg areas of the primary somatic sensory cortex (Figure 12.14A, see also Chapter 5). The ventral posterior medial nucleus projects to the *face area* of the primary somatic sensory cortex. This projection, like that from the ventral posterior lateral nucleus, courses in the *posterior limb of the internal capsule*. The face area of the primary somatic sensory cortex is located on the lateral portion of the postcentral gyrus (Figure 12.14). The representation of the body surface takes the form of a map in which body parts extensively used are overrepresented (Chapter 5). In humans, the representations of the fingers, tongue, and perioral region in the primary somatic sensory cortex are larger than the cortical representations of other body parts. In many species of rodents and carnivores, the face representation is more extensive than either that of the fingers or tongue and perioral regions because their large whiskers are their principal tactile

Figure 12.14 A. Lateral view of cerebral hemisphere, with the representations of the limbs, trunk, and face indicated on the postcentral gyrus. *B.* Somatotopic organization of the postcentral gyrus. (*B.* Adapted from Penfield, W. and Rasmussen, T. 1950. The Cerebral Cortex of Man: A Clinical Study of Localization of Function. New York: Macmillan.)

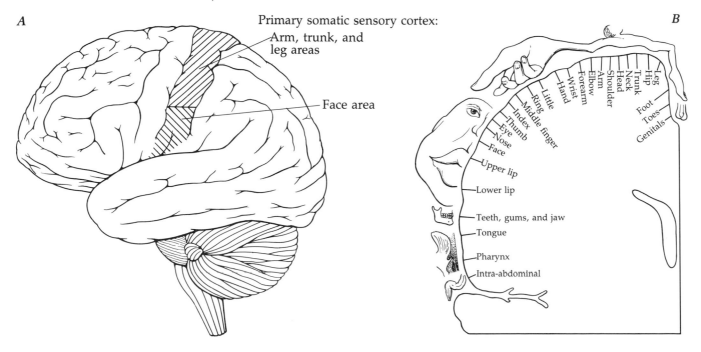

discriminative organs. Three other cortical areas process somatic sensory information from the face: (1) the *secondary somatic sensory cortex*, which is located largely on the parietal operculum, (2) areas in the posterior insular cortex, and (3) cytoarchitectonic area 5, which is sometimes termed the *tertiary somatic sensory cortex* (see Figure 5.18).

Summary

There are 12 cranial nerves (Table 12.1, Figure 12.1). The first two, the *olfactory* nerve and the *optic* nerve, are sensory nerves and enter the telencephalon and diencephalon directly. The third through twelfth cranial nerves enter and exit from the brain stem directly. Two cranial nerves are located in the midbrain, the *oculomotor nerve* (III) and the *trochlear nerve* (IV), both of which are motor nerves. The pons contains the *trigeminal* (V), a mixed nerve; the *abducens* (VI), a motor nerve; the *facial* (VII), a mixed nerve; and the *vestibulocochlear* (VIII), a sensory nerve. The medulla also contains four cranial nerves: *glossopharyngeal* (IX) and *vagus* (X) are mixed nerves, whereas *spinal accessory* (XI) and *hypoglossal* (XII) are motor nerves. There are separate columns of cranial nerve nuclei that course through the brain stem along its rostrocaudal axis (Figures 12.3 and 12.4). Each column subserves a separate sensory (afferent) or motor function, and the nomenclature conforms to that for the cranial nerves: (1) *general somatic motor*, (2) *special visceral motor*, (3) *general visceral motor*, (4) *general and special visceral afferent*, (5) *general somatic afferent*, (6) *special somatic afferent* (Table 12.1). Different columns have a different mediolateral location (Figures 12.3 and 12.4). The *sulcus limitans* separates the sensory from the motor nuclear columns.

Somatic sensation of cranial structures is mediated predominantly by the trigeminal nerve, which has three sensory divisions (Figure 12.7A): *ophthalmic division, maxillary division*, and *mandibular division*. The cell bodies of the primary sensory neurons that innervate the skin and mucous membranes of the head and are located in the *trigeminal ganglion*. Three other cranial nerves also innervate portions of the head. The *intermediate* (a branch of the *facial nerve*) (VII) and *vagus* (X) nerves innervate the skin of the *ear*, and the *glossopharyngeal* (IX) nerve innervates the posterior tongue and portions of the oral cavity, nasal cavity, pharynx, and middle ear (Figure 12.7A). The cell bodies of the primary afferent fibers in the facial nerve are located in the *geniculate ganglion*, and those of the glossopharyngeal and vagus nerves, in the *superior ganglion* of each nerve. Afferent fibers in these four cranial nerves enter the brain stem and ascend and descend in the spinal trigeminal tract (Figures 12.7 and 12.8). The fibers of the trigeminal nerve, whose cell bodies lie in trigeminal ganglion, terminate in two of the three major components of the trigeminal nuclear complex (Figure 12.5): the *main trigeminal sensory nucleus* (Figures 12.5 and 12.9) and the *spinal trigeminal nucleus* (Figures 12.5 and 12.8), which has three subdivisions (Figures 12.5 and 12.9)—the *oral nucleus*, the *interpolar nucleus*, and the *caudal nucleus*. The afferent fibers of the facial, glossopharyngeal, and vagus nerves terminate in the spinal trigeminal nucleus.

Mechanoreceptive afferent fibers of the trigeminal nerve terminate predominantly in the *main trigeminal sensory nucleus*. The majority of the ascending projection neurons of this nucleus (Figure 12.6A) send their axons to the *contralateral ventral posterior medial nucleus* of the thalamus (Figure 12.13). From here, thalamic neurons project, via the posterior limb of the internal capsule, to the face representation of the *primary somatic sensory cortex*, which is located in the lateral portion of the *postcentral gyrus* (Figure 12.14). Other cortical areas are important in processing somatic sensory information from the head, the *secondary somatic sensory cortex*, which is located primarily in the *parietal operculum*, and other higher order sensory areas in the *insular cortex* and posterior parietal lobe.

The pathway for *pain* and *temperature* sensations originates from the *spinal trigeminal nucleus* (Figure 12.6B). The axons of projection neurons of this nucleus either remain on the ipsilateral side or decussate. The ascending fibers course with the anterolateral system in the lateral medulla and pons en route to the rostral brain stem and thalamus. The thalamic nuclei in which the fibers terminate are the *ventral posterior medial* nucleus and in the *intralaminar nuclei*.

Afferent fibers carrying proprioceptive information from the jaw muscles form the *mesencephalic trigeminal tract* (Figures 12.6C, 12.11, and 12.12). Their cell bodies are located in the *mesencephalic trigeminal nucleus* and are unique because they are the only primary sensory neurons with their cell bodies located in the central nervous system (Figure 12.2). ■

References

Arvidsson, J., and Gobel, S. 1981. An HRP study of the central projections of primary trigeminal neurons which innervate tooth pulp in the cat. Brain Res. 210:1–16.

Burton, H., and Craig Jr., A. D. 1979. Distribution of trigeminothalamic projection cells in cat and monkey. Brain Res. 161:515–521.

Cajal, S. Ramon y. 1909, 1911. Histologie du système nerveux de l'homme et des vertèbres. 2 vols. Paris: Maloine.

Craig Jr., A. D., and Burton, H. 1981. Spinal and medullary lamina I projection to nucleus submedius in medial thalamus: A possible pain center. J. Neurophysiol. 45:443–466.

Fukushima, T., and Kerr, F. W. L. 1979. Organization of trigeminothalamic tracts and other thalamic afferent systems of the brainstem in the rat: Presence of gelatinosa neurons with thalamic connections. J. Comp. Neurol. 183:169–184.

Gobel, S., Hockfield, S., and Ruda, M. A. 1981. Anatomical similarities between medullary and spinal dorsal horns. In Kawamura, Y., and Dubner, R. Oral-Facial Sensory and Motor Functions. Tokyo: Quintessence Publishing Co., Inc., pp. 211–223.

Hayashi, H., Sumino, R., and Sessle, B. J. 1984. Functional organization of trigeminal subnucleus interpolaris: Nociceptive and innocuous afferent inputs, projections to thalamus, cerebellum, and spinal cord, and descending modulation from periaqueductal gray. J. Neurophysiol. 51:890–905.

Hu, J. W., and Sessle, B. J. 1984. Comparison of responses of cutaneous nociceptive and nonnociceptive brain stem neurons in trigeminal subnucleus caudalis (medullary dorsal horn) and subnucleus oralis to natural and electrical stimulation of tooth pulp. J. Neurophysiol. 52:39–53.

Kruger, L. Functional subdivision of the brainstem sensory trigeminal nuclear comlex. In Bonica, J. J., Liebeskind, J. C., and Albe-Fessard, D. G. Advances in Pain Research and Therapy, Vol. 3. New York: Raven Press, pp. 197–209.

Nieuwenhuys, R., Voogd, J., and van Huijzen, Chr. 1988. The Human Central Nervous System: A Synopsis and Atlas, Third Edition. Berlin: Springer-Verlag.

Smith, R. L. 1975. Axonal projections and connections of the principal sensory trigeminal nucleus in the monkey. J. Comp. Neurol. 163:347–376.

Selected Readings

Brodal, A. 1957. The Cranial Nerves, Anatomical and Anatomicoclinical Correlations. Oxford: Blackwell Scientific Publications.

Brodal, A. 1981. Neurological Anatomy. New York: Oxford University Press.

Dubner, R., and Bennett, G. J. 1983. Spinal and trigeminal mechanisms of nociception. Ann. Rev. Neurosci. 6:381–418.

Kelly, J. P. 1985. Cranial nerve nuclei, the reticular formation, and biogenic amine-containing neurons. In Kandel, E. R., and Schwartz, J. H. Principles of Neural Science. New York: Elsevier, pp. 539–561.

Kelly, J. P. 1985. Trigeminal system. In Kandel, E. R., and Schwartz, J. H. Principles of Neural Science. New York: Elsevier, pp. 563–570.

The Somatic and Visceral Motor Functions of the Cranial Nerves

13

Motor Functions of Cranial Nerves

In Chapter 12, it was shown that the function and key features of the anatomical organization of the trigeminal system parallel those of the spinal cord ascending pathways. A similar comparison can be made between motor control of cranial structures and that of the limbs and body axis: cranial muscles are innervated by motor neurons that are located in the cranial nerve motor nuclei, whereas limb and axial muscles are innervated by motor neurons in the motor nuclei of the ventral horn. Certain cranial nerves also contain the axons of parasympathetic preganglionic neurons. The autonomic nervous system is considered with the hypothalamus, the principal diencephalic structure that regulates its function, in Chapter 14. However, the autonomic nuclei of the cranial nerves, together with the nuclei subserving skeletal motor control, are examined in this chapter because complete knowledge of the functions of the cranial nerves provides the physician with a remarkably precise probe for localizing the site of injuries.

In this chapter, the organization of the three functional categories of cranial nerve motor nuclei is considered in detail: (1) nuclei in the *general somatic motor* column, which contain motor neurons that innervate striated muscle of somatic origin, (2) nuclei of the *special visceral motor* column, which contain motor neurons innervating striated muscle of visceral (branchiomeric) origin, and (3) nuclei of the *general visceral motor* column, which contain the parasympathetic preganglionic neurons. Then, a series of sections through the brain stem are examined, tracing the locations of the various cranial nerve motor nuclei in relation to the other key brain stem structures. In completing our study of the cranial nerve nuclei, greater knowledge of the regional anatomy of the brain stem will emerge. An in-depth understanding of brain stem regional anatomy is essential for clinical problem solving: *identifying the locus of central nervous system damage using knowledge of the function and location of the cranial nerve nuclei.* This is possible because each of these nuclei has a clearly identifiable sensory or motor function and the integrity of this function can be thoroughly tested by the physician.

As we saw in the preceding chapter, there are 12 cranial nerves and 10 of these enter and exit the brain stem (Figure 13.1A). The 10 brain stem cranial nerves are directly connected to the sensory and motor cranial nerve nuclei. The locations of the cranial nerve nuclei are shown in Figure 13.1B. There are six columns of cranial nerve nuclei that course rostrocaudally in the brain stem (Figure 12.3A). The columns containing nuclei that mediate cranial motor function are located medially whereas the sensory columns are located laterally. On the floor of the fourth ventricle, the *sulcus limitans* is the boundary between the sensory and motor columns.

The General Somatic Motor Cell Column Is Located Close to the Midline

The most medial motor column contains motor neurons that innervate striated muscles that derive from the *occipital somites*. There are four nuclei in this column (Figures 13.1–13.3), and three of these nuclei contain motor neurons that innervate the extraocular muscles: (1) the *oculomotor nucleus* and (2) and the *trochlear nucleus* are located in the rostral and caudal midbrain, respectively, whereas (3) the *abducens nucleus* is located in the pons. The fourth nucleus in this column is the *hypoglossal nucleus*, which innervates tongue muscles. The oculomotor nucleus contributes most of the axons of the *oculomotor (III)* nerve, which exits the rostral midbrain from the medial aspect of the *cerebral peduncle*. The oculomotor nucleus (Figure 13.2) innervates four of the six extraocular muscles: *medial rectus, inferior rectus, lateral rectus,* and *inferior oblique* (Figure 13.2A). This nucleus also innervates bilaterally the *levator palpebrae superioris muscle,* an elevator of the eyelid.[1] Motor neurons that innervate these different muscles are segregated into subregions of the oculomotor nucleus. (It should be recalled that the somatic motor neurons that innervate different body muscles are also segregated into separate motor nuclei in the ventral horn.) Motor neurons in the trochlear nucleus give rise to the fibers in the *trochlear (IV)* nerve. The only cranial nerve that exits from the *dorsal* brain stem surface is the trochlear nerve. It innervates the *superior oblique muscle* (Figure 13.2). This cranial nerve is further distinguished because all of its axons decussate and do so within the central nervous system. The abducens nucleus contains the motor neurons that project their axons to the periphery through the *abducens (VI)* nerve. This nerve exits the brain stem at the *pontomedullary junction.* Abducens motor neurons innervate the *lateral rectus* muscle (Figure 13.2). Whereas the trochlear and abducens nerves contain axons that innervate extraocular muscles only, the oculomotor nerve also contains the axons of autonomic preganglionic neurons (see later).

Unlike other skeletal muscles, the extraocular muscles are not controlled by descending pathways from the primary motor cortex. Rather, two other cortical regions are important in controlling eye movements (Figure 13.2C): the *frontal eye field* (cytoarchitectonic area 8) and the *parieto-occipital eye field* (corresponding roughly to parts of area 17, and areas 18 and 19). The *frontal eye field* is important primarily in controlling the rapid phase of eye movement, termed a *saccade*, which brings the fovea to the image. The frontal eye field is located rostral to the supplementary motor area and the premotor cortex (Chapter 9). The descending axons from the frontal eye field course in the *anterior limb and genu of the internal capsule.* The pathway to the extraocular motor nuclei is complex and involves synaptic relays in the superior colliculus and the reticular formation. The parieto-occipital eye field is thought to play an important role in *smooth pursuit* eye movement, which maintains the position of a moving visual image on the fovea. The descending projection of the parieto-occipital eye field is via the *posterior limb of the internal capsule.* Similar to the frontal eye field, the parieto-occipital eye field also influences extraocular motor neurons indirectly. Two brain stem nuclear regions receive input from the two eye fields of the cerebral cortex and are important sites for controlling eye movements. The (1) *paramedian pontine reticular formation* (PPRF) is believed to participate in controlling horizontal eye movements, and (2) the *rostral interstitial nucleus* of the *medial longitudinal fasciculus,* in vertical eye movements. The medial longitudinal fasciculus (MLF) is the key brain stem tract for coordinating the contraction of extraocular mus-

---

[1] The action of the levator palpebrae superioris muscle is assisted by the tarsal muscle, a smooth muscle under sympathetic nervous system control.

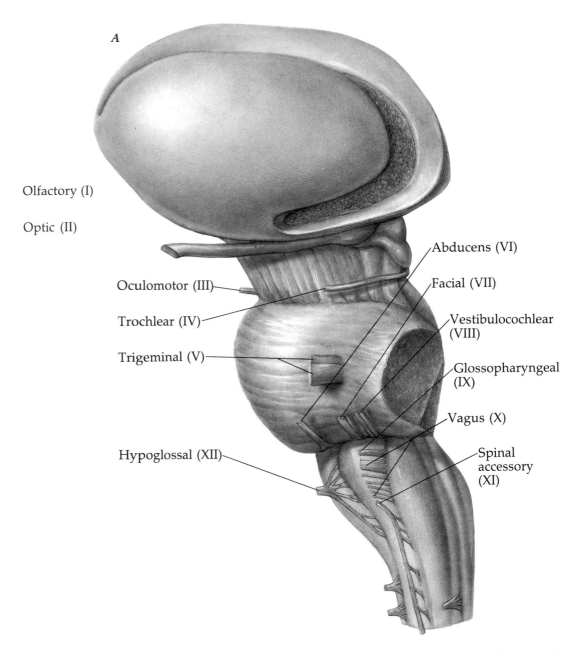

Olfactory (I)

Optic (II)

Oculomotor (III)

Trochlear (IV)

Trigeminal (V)

Hypoglossal (XII)

Abducens (VI)

Facial (VII)

Vestibulocochlear (VIII)

Glossopharyngeal (IX)

Vagus (X)

Spinal accessory (XI)

Figure 13.1 *A.* Locations of the cranial nerves (lateral view of the brain stem). *B.* Locations of the cranial nerve nuclei (dorsal view of the brain stem without cerebellum).

cles. Axons in the MLF originating from the *vestibular nuclei* are especially important in stabilizing eye position when the head is moved. Recall that there is also a descending component of the MLF that originates predominantly from the medial vestibular nucleus (Chapter 9). This descending motor pathway may be important in controlling head position.

B

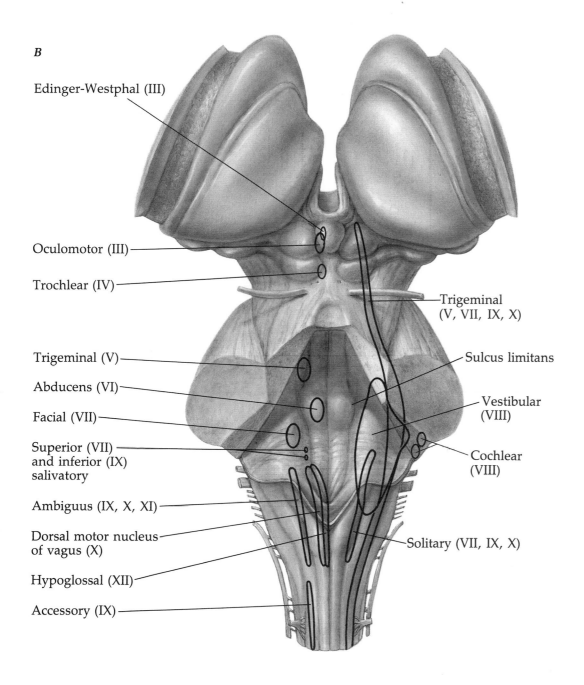

Edinger-Westphal (III)

Oculomotor (III)

Trochlear (IV)

Trigeminal (V, VII, IX, X)

Trigeminal (V)

Abducens (VI)

Facial (VII)

Superior (VII) and inferior (IX) salivatory

Ambiguus (IX, X, XI)

Dorsal motor nucleus of vagus (X)

Hypoglossal (XII)

Accessory (IX)

Sulcus limitans

Vestibular (VIII)

Cochlear (VIII)

Solitary (VII, IX, X)

The *hypoglossal nucleus* is the fourth member of the general somatic motor column (Figure 13.3). The axons of motor neurons in the hypoglossal nucleus course in the hypoglossal nerve (XII) and innervate intrinsic tongue muscles, genioglossus, hypoglossus, and styloglossus muscles. A lesion of the hypoglossal nucleus or nerve produces a classical

A

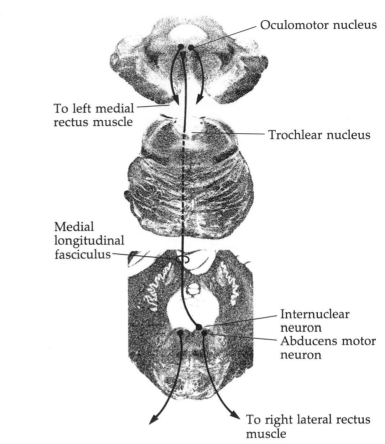

Oculomotor nucleus

To left medial rectus muscle

Trochlear nucleus

Medial longitudinal fasciculus

Internuclear neuron

Abducens motor neuron

To right lateral rectus muscle

B

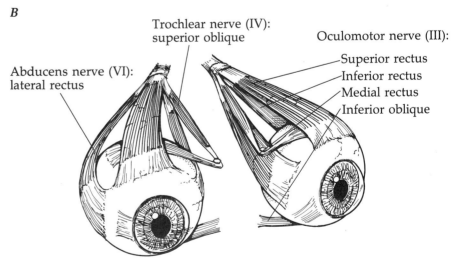

Trochlear nerve (IV): superior oblique

Oculomotor nerve (III):

Abducens nerve (VI): lateral rectus

Superior rectus
Inferior rectus
Medial rectus
Inferior oblique

motor sign: when the patient is asked to protrude the tongue, it deviates to the side of the lesion. Similar to the control of limb muscles (and in contrast to the other three general somatic motor nuclei), the primary motor cortex projects to the hypoglossal nucleus. The axons descend in the *corticobulbar tract*, which courses through the genu of the internal capsule (as well as the rostral part of the posterior limb) and then in the

C

Primary motor cortex

Frontal eye field

Parietal-occipital
eye field

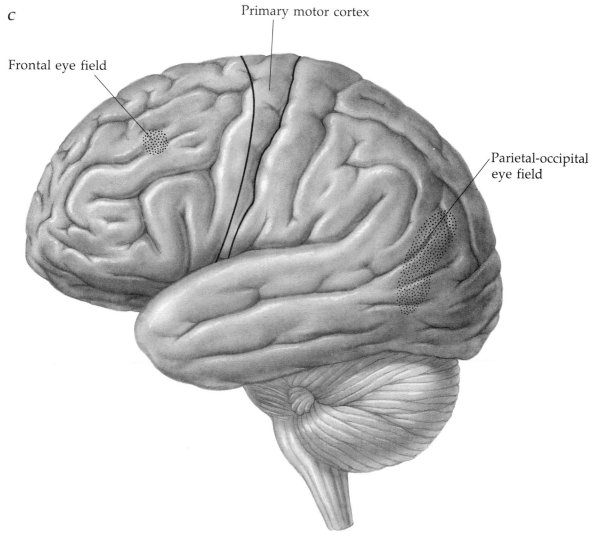

Figure 13.2 ***A.*** Transverse sections through oculomotor, trochlear, and abducens nuclei are shown with key internuclear connections that are important in controlling horizontal eye movements indicated. ***B.*** The two eyes with the various extraocular muscles and their innervation patterns. The levator palpebrae, which is an eyelid elevator (innervated by CN III), is not shown. The extraocular muscles of both eyes operate as three functional pairs. The lateral and medial rectus muscles move the eye horizontally. The superior and inferior rectus muscles elevate and depress the eye, respectively (most importantly when the eye is abducted). Finally, the superior and inferior oblique muscles depress and elevate the eye, but to a greater extent when the eye is adducted. ***C.*** A lateral view of the cerebral cortex shows the approximate locations of the frontal eye field, primary motor cortex, and parieto-occipital eye field.

basis pedunculi, medial to the spinal-projecting axons of the corticospinal tract (Chapter 9). Neurons contributing axons to the corticobulbar tract, as well as all other cortical descending projection neurons, are located in layer V. Cells of origin of the corticobulbar tract are located in the portion of the precentral gyrus close to the *lateral sulcus* (Figure 9.6). This projection is primarily *crossed*.

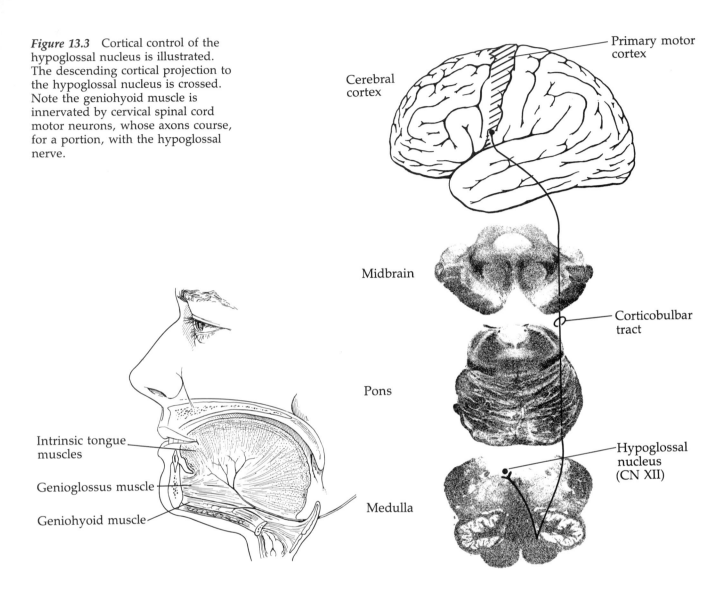

Figure 13.3 Cortical control of the hypoglossal nucleus is illustrated. The descending cortical projection to the hypoglossal nucleus is crossed. Note the geniohyoid muscle is innervated by cervical spinal cord motor neurons, whose axons course, for a portion, with the hypoglossal nerve.

The Special Visceral Motor Cell Column Innervates Skeletal Muscles That Develop from the Branchial Arches

The general and special visceral motor cell columns are located lateral to the general somatic motor column and medial to the sulcus limitans (Figure 13.1). The general visceral motor column, located immediately beneath the floor of the fourth ventricle (Figure 13.1), contains *parasympathetic preganglionic neurons* and will be considered in the next section. Nuclei in the special visceral motor column are located in the *reticular formation* (see Figure 12.3B), and contain motor neurons that innervate the striated muscles derived from the *branchial arches*. Four cranial nerve nuclei constitute this brain stem nuclear column: *trigeminal motor nucleus, facial motor nucleus, nucleus ambiguus,* and *accessory nucleus.* The special visceral motor nuclei in the brain stem each receive a projection from the primary motor cortex via the *corticobulbar tract,* and the accessory nucleus receives a projection from the corticospinal tract because it is located in the cervical spinal cord. These axons of the descending pathways terminate either contralaterally or bilaterally, depending on the particular nucleus (see later). Muscles innervated by motor nuclei that receive a *bilateral* projection from the motor cortex do not become weak after a unilateral lesion of motor cortex (or some portion of its descending pathway). The intact projection is sufficient for normal (or near-normal) control of force. This is not the case, however, for muscles receiving only contralateral motor cortical control. Here, weakness is a characteristic sign of unilateral damage.

The axons of motor neurons of the trigeminal motor nucleus course in the trigeminal (V) nerve and innervate principally the muscles of *mastication:* masseter, temporalis, and external and internal pterygoid muscles. The primary motor cortex projects bilaterally to the trigeminal motor nuclei (Figure 13.4A), and unilateral lesions of the motor cortex or the descending cortical fibers do not produce weakness of the muscles of mastication. Bilateral control by the primary motor cortex may reflect the fact that muscles of mastication on both sides of the mouth are typically activated in tandem (for example, during chewing). This is similar to the bilateral control of axial muscles by the medial descending spinal cord pathways (Chapter 9).

The facial (motor) nucleus contains the motor neurons that innervate the muscles of *facial expression* (Figure 13.4A). These axons course in the *facial (VII) nerve.* There is an interesting organization of descending control by the motor cortex to the facial nucleus (Figure 13.4B). Motor neurons in the facial nucleus that innervate muscles of the *upper face* receive *bilateral control by the motor cortex,* whereas those innervating muscles of the lower face are controlled by the *contralateral* motor cortex. A unilateral lesion of the descending cortical fibers, for example in the genu of the internal capsule, will have differential effects on upper and lower facial muscles. After the lesion, upper facial muscles retain an intact cortical control from the opposite side and, therefore, are unaffected. In contrast, lower facial muscles become weak on the side contralateral to the lesion because their cortical control has been interrupted. This weakness is noted as asymmetry in facial expressions. This is a remarkable example of how knowledge of the specificity of neuroanatomical connections provides important diagnostic insights. This complex pattern of facial motor deficits after lesions of the motor cortex or corticobulbar tract contrasts with deficits occurring on the *ipsilateral face with a facial nerve or nucleus lesion.* In these cases, muscles of both the upper and lower face are affected.

Unlike the cranial nerve nuclei considered up to now, the nucleus ambiguus contains motor neurons whose axons course in three cranial nerves (Figure 13.4C): *glossopharyngeal (IX), vagus (X),* and *spinal accessory (XI).* These axons innervate striated muscles of *palate, pharynx,* and *larynx.* There is a rostrocaudal organization of locations of motor neurons in the nucleus and the cranial nerves through which their axons course (Figure 13.4C). Motor neurons in the rostral portion of the nucleus ambiguus course in the glossopharyngeal nerve and innervate one pharyngeal muscle, the stylopharyngeus. Caudal to these motor neurons, and representing the majority of motor neurons in the nucleus ambiguus, are those that course in the vagus nerve. The axons in the vagus nerve innervate numerous *pharyngeal, palatal,* and *laryngeal* muscles. The caudal portion of the nucleus ambiguus contains motor neurons whose axons course in the spinal accessory nerve (see later) and innervate *laryngeal* muscles. The motor cortex exerts bilateral control of palatal, pharyngeal, and laryngeal muscles (Figure 13.4A).

The *accessory nucleus* (Figure 13.4A) is located in line with the nucleus ambiguus (Figure 13.1) but in the ventral horn of the spinal cord, beginning at the pyramidal decussation and extending numerous segments, as far caudally as the fifth cervical segment (C5). Motor neurons in the accessory nucleus innervate the *sternocleidomastoid* and *trapezius muscles*. The fibers course in the spinal accessory nerve, but in a root separate from that in which fibers of the caudal nucleus ambiguus course: accessory nucleus motor neurons course in the *spinal root* of the spinal accessory nerve, whereas nucleus ambiguus motor neurons course in the *cranial root*. The spinal root leaves the lateral margin of the spinal cord between the dorsal and ventral roots, ascends in the spinal canal, and joins the fibers from the cranial root. After exiting the posterior cranial fossa through the jugular foramen, the cranial and spinal root fibers separate. Fibers of the spinal root go on to innervate the sternocleidomastoid and trapezius muscles and those of the cranial root join the vagus nerve and innervate laryngeal muscles. (The cranial root fibers are considered displaced vagal fibers because their cell bodies are located in the nucleus ambiguus and the fibers join the vagus nerve in the periphery.) The cortical innervation of the accessory nucleus is bilateral (Figure 13.4A), but the crossed component of the projection is proportionally larger compared with that of the other special visceral motor nuclei.

The General Visceral Motor Cell Column Contains Parasympathetic Preganglionic Neurons

The general visceral motor cell column, which is located lateral to the general somatic motor column, contains four nuclei, from rostral to caudal: *Edinger–Westphal, superior salivatory, inferior salivatory,* and *dorsal motor nucleus of the vagus*. (Most parasympathetic preganglionic neurons are located in these nuclei; however, additional ones that course in the vagus nerve are located in and around the nucleus ambiguus.) The general visceral motor column is analogous to the intermediolateral nucleus in the spinal cord, which contains sympathetic preganglionic neurons. The autonomic nervous system is discussed in Chapter 14 with the hypothalamus, which regulates many of its functions.

The Edinger–Westphal nucleus is located in the midbrain dorsal to the oculomotor nucleus and in the pretectal region (Figure 13.5). The proximity of the Edinger-Westphal and oculomotor nuclei makes it easy to remember that the parasympathetic preganglionic neurons in the Edinger–Westphal nucleus send their axons into the *oculomotor* (III) nerve. As with the other parasympathetic nuclei, the Edinger–Westphal nucleus contains *preganglionic neurons* that synapse on *postganglionic neurons* in a peripheral autonomic ganglion. The organization of the efferent projections of parasympathetic preganglionic neurons in this nucleus is schematically illustrated in Figure 13.5A (see also Figure 14.6).[2] The preganglionic neurons in the Edinger–Westphal nucleus synapse on postganglionic neurons in the *ciliary* ganglion, which in turn innervate *constrictor muscles of the iris* and the *ciliary muscle*.

---

[2] Other neurons in and around the Edinger–Westphal nucleus project to the spinal cord.

A

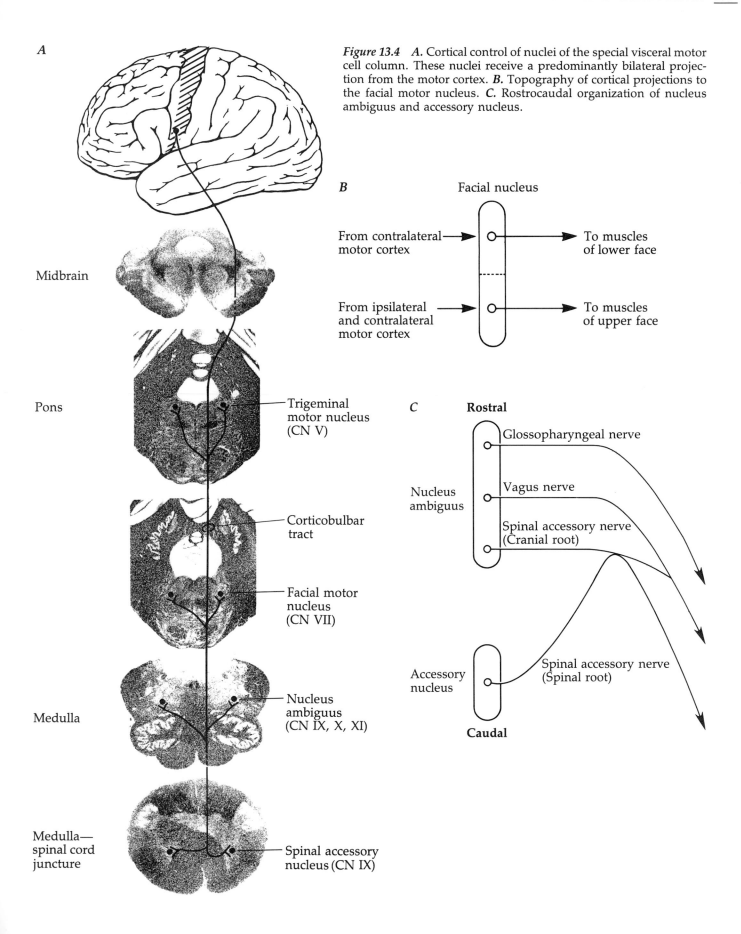

Midbrain

Pons

Medulla

Medulla—
spinal cord
juncture

Trigeminal
motor nucleus
(CN V)

Corticobulbar
tract

Facial motor
nucleus
(CN VII)

Nucleus
ambiguus
(CN IX, X, XI)

Spinal accessory
nucleus (CN IX)

Figure 13.4 **A.** Cortical control of nuclei of the special visceral motor cell column. These nuclei receive a predominantly bilateral projection from the motor cortex. **B.** Topography of cortical projections to the facial motor nucleus. **C.** Rostrocaudal organization of nucleus ambiguus and accessory nucleus.

B   Facial nucleus

From contralateral → To muscles
motor cortex   of lower face

From ipsilateral → To muscles
and contralateral   of upper face
motor cortex

C   **Rostral**

Glossopharyngeal nerve

Nucleus
ambiguus   Vagus nerve

Spinal accessory nerve
(Cranial root)

Accessory
nucleus   Spinal accessory nerve
             (Spinal root)

Caudal

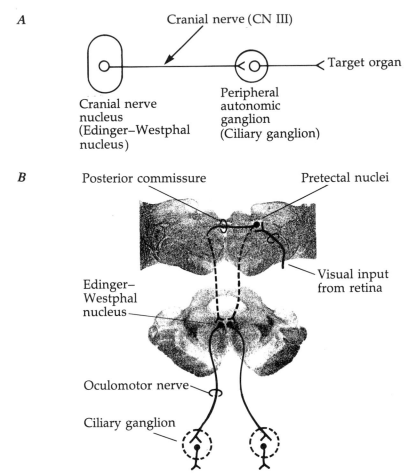

A

Cranial nerve (CN III)

Cranial nerve nucleus (Edinger–Westphal nucleus)

Peripheral autonomic ganglion (Ciliary ganglion)

Target organ

B

Posterior commissure

Pretectal nuclei

Edinger–Westphal nucleus

Visual input from retina

Oculomotor nerve

Ciliary ganglion

Figure 13.5 *A.* The general organization of the cranial parasympathetic nuclei and the projection to the periphery. Edinger–Westphal nucleus and efferent projections to the ciliary ganglion. *B.* The circuit for the pupillary light reflex is shown in relation to sections through the pretectal nuclei (top) and the oculomotor nucleus (bottom).

Parasympathetic preganglionic neurons in the midbrain are the efferent components of two important visual reflexes: the pupillary light reflex and the accommodation reflex. The *pupillary light reflex* is the constriction of the pupil that occurs when the retina is illuminated (Figure 13.5B). Visual input from the retina passes directly to the *pretectal nuclei* via the *brachium of the superior colliculus* (Chapter 6). The pretectal nuclei, in turn, project bilaterally to the parasympathetic preganglionic neurons. The axons cross to the contralateral side in the *posterior commissure*. Parasympathetic preganglionic neurons project to the ciliary ganglion through the *oculomotor nerve*, and from there, postganglionic neurons innervate the constrictor muscles of the iris. The bilateral projection of pretectal neurons to the parasympathetic preganglionic neurons ensures that illumination of one eye causes constriction of the pupil not only on the same side (direct response) but on the other side as well (consensual response). (Pupillary dilation is mediated either by inhibition of the neural circuit for pupillary constriction or by the separate control of the iris by the sympathetic component of the autonomic nervous system.)

Parasympathetic preganglionic neurons of the midbrain participate in a second visual reflex, the *accommodation reflex*, which is the *increase in lens curvature that occurs during near vision*.[3] The accommodation reflex is

---

[3] The majority of postganglionic neurons in the ciliary ganglion actually innervate the ciliary muscle.

normally one part of the *accommodation–convergence reaction*, a complex response that prepares the eyes for near vision by (1) increasing lens curvature, (2) pupillary constriction, and (3) convergence of the eyes. These responses involve the integrated actions of visual areas of the occipital lobe, motor neurons in the oculomotor nucleus that innervate the extraocular muscles, and parasympathetic preganglionic neurons. Central nervous system pathology may distinguish different components of the various visual reflexes. For example, *Argyll Robertson pupils*—a neurologic sign associated with neurosyphilis—are small, fixed, and unreactive to light but get smaller to accommodation.

The other brain stem locations of parasympathetic preganglionic neurons are nuclei of the caudal pons and medulla (Figure 13.1). The *dorsal motor nucleus of the vagus* forms a column of neurons beneath the floor of the *fourth ventricle* in the medulla. Neurons of the *superior salivatory nucleus*, which is located in the pons, and the *inferior salivatory nucleus*, which is located in the medulla, do not form a discrete cell column. The axons of neurons of the superior salivatory nucleus course in the *intermediate nerve* (Figure 13.6). They synapse in two peripheral ganglia: (1) the *pterygopalatine* ganglion, where postganglionic neurons innervate the

Figure 13.6. Organization of the parasympathetic cranial nerve nuclei in the pons and medulla, as well as the peripheral ganglia to which they project.

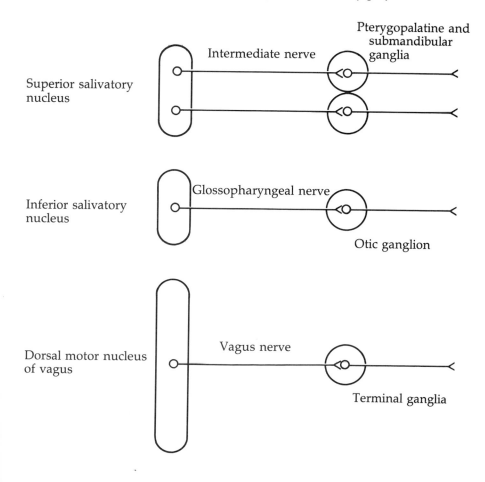

A

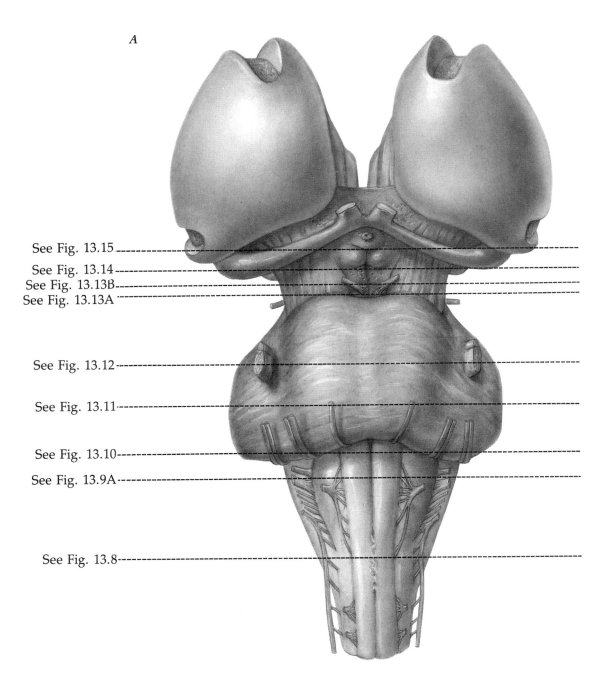

See Fig. 13.15

See Fig. 13.14

See Fig. 13.13B

See Fig. 13.13A

See Fig. 13.12

See Fig. 13.11

See Fig. 13.10

See Fig. 13.9A

See Fig. 13.8

Figure 13.7. Ventral *(A)* and dorsal *(B)* views of the brain stem. Planes of section for Figures 13.8, 13.9, 13.10, 13.11A, 13.12–13.16.

lacrimal glands and glands of the nasal mucosa, and (2) the submandibular ganglion from which postganglionic parasympathetic neurons innervate the submandibular and sublingual salivary glands. The intermediate nerve is sometimes considered to be the "sensory" branch of the *facial nerve* because it contains afferent fibers, which are the axons of pseu-

B

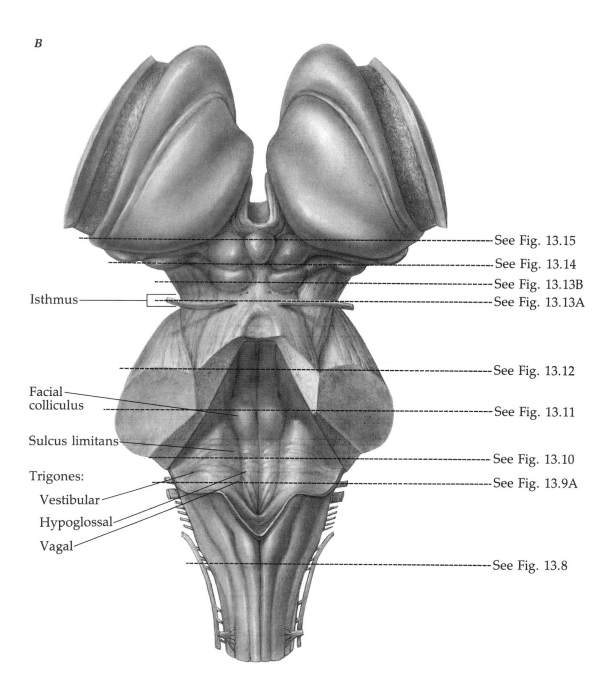

Isthmus

Facial
colliculus

Sulcus limitans

Trigones:

Vestibular

Hypoglossal

Vagal

See Fig. 13.15
See Fig. 13.14
See Fig. 13.13B
See Fig. 13.13A

See Fig. 13.12

See Fig. 13.11

See Fig. 13.10
See Fig. 13.9A

See Fig. 13.8

dounipolar neurons of the *geniculate ganglion* (see Chapters 8 and 12). The inferior salivatory nucleus contains parasympathetic preganglionic neurons whose axons course in the *glossopharyngeal nerve* and synapse on postganglionic neurons in the *otic ganglion* (Figure 13.6). Parasympathetic postganglionic neurons in the otic ganglion, in turn, innervate the parotid gland. The parasympathetic preganglionic neurons in the dorsal motor nucleus of the vagus synapse in extracranial parasympathetic ganglia, termed *terminal ganglia* (Figure 13.6), located in the viscera of the thoracic and abdominal cavities including the gastrointestinal tract proximal to the splenic flexure of the colon. (The colon distal to the flexure is innervated by parasympathetic preganglionic neurons of the sacral spinal cord (see Figure 14.7).)

In the remaining portion of this chapter the regional anatomical organization of the cranial nerve nuclei is considered. The focus is on the spatial relations between nuclei and other important brain stem structures. Serial transverse sections are examined with the goal to obtain a mind's-eye reconstruction, in three dimensions, of the internal structure of the brain stem. To facilitate identification of internal structures of the brain stem, surface landmarks are compared with their internal counterparts. Comparison is also made between the location of cranial nerve nuclei and the sulcus limitans. A sagittal section, close to the midline, is also examined. The level of these slices, in relation to the dorsal and ventral brain stem surfaces, is shown in Figure 13.7.

The Accessory Nucleus Is Located at the Junction of the Spinal Cord and Medulla

The dominant structure in the section through the junction of the spinal cord and medulla (Figure 13.8) is the *pyramidal decussation*, which can also be seen on the ventral brain stem view (Figure 13.7A). The spinal root of the *spinal accessory nerve* contains axons of motor neurons whose cell bodies are located in the accessory nucleus (Figure 13.8). Comparison of this section with the one through the cervical enlargement (see Appendix II.5) reveals the similarity in the locations of the accessory nucleus and other motor nuclei located more caudally in the ventral horn.

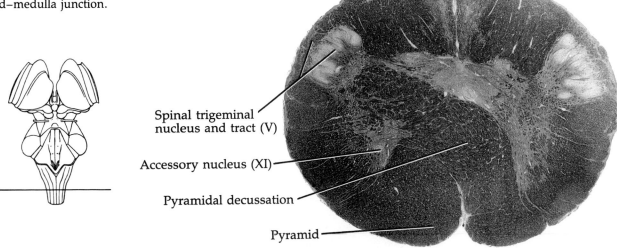

Figure 13.8. Myelin-stained transverse section at the level of the spinal cord–medulla junction.

Spinal trigeminal nucleus and tract (V)

Accessory nucleus (XI)

Pyramidal decussation

Pyramid

A Level through the Midmedulla Reveals the Locations of Six Cranial Nerve Nuclei

The cranial nerve nuclei that are located immediately beneath the floor of the fourth ventricle in the medulla form bulges, termed trigones (or triangles). There are three bulges, from medial to lateral: hypoglossal, vagal, and vestibular (Figure 13.7B). The hypoglossal and vagal trigones overlie nuclei of the same names. The vestibular trigone includes the various vestibular nuclei and, in addition, the solitary nucleus. The boundary between the vagal and vestibular trigones, which is the *sulcus limitans*, is distinct in both gross specimens and in cross section (Figure 13.9). In contrast, the boundary between the hypoglossal and vagal trigones is often not clear and, as a consequence, separate bulges may not be visible on transverse section (Figure 13.9). Compare the locations of

Figure 13.9. *A.* Myelin-stained transverse section through the hypoglossal nucleus in the medulla. *B.* Arterial supply of medulla. Lesion of the posterior inferior cerebellar artery produces a complex set of neurological deficits, termed the lateral medullary syndrome (or Wallenberg's syndrome).

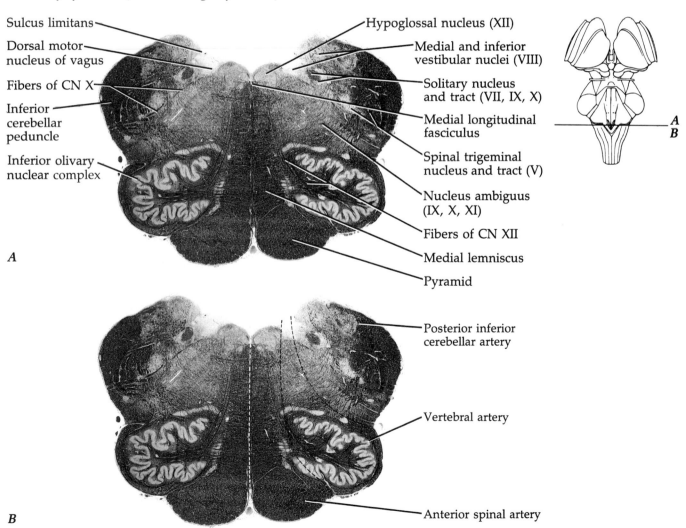

the two landmarks on the ventral medullary surface, the pyramid and the olive, with their counterparts in cross section (Figure 13.9). The hypoglossal nerve exits the brain stem immediately lateral to the pyramid (Figure 13.7A), and in cross section, a segment of hypoglossal nerve axons can be identified (Figure 13.9). Axons from the dorsal motor nucleus of the vagus also can be seen in Figure 13.9. Two cranial nerve nuclei, the spinal trigeminal nucleus and the nucleus ambiguus, are located deeper within the medulla. The actual location of the nucleus ambiguus cannot be determined precisely in myelin-stained sections; its approximate location is indicated in Figure 13.9A. Nucleus ambiguus and accessory nucleus (Figure 13.1B) form an interrupted column of motor neurons that innervate striated muscle.

Infarction in the Territory of Different Arterial Branches Interrupts the Function of Different Cranial Nerve Nuclei

In the medulla, different cranial nerve nuclei receive their arterial supply from different branches of the vertebrobasilar system (Figure 13.9B; see Figure 4.3). The medial portion of the medulla, which contains the *hypoglossal nucleus*, the medial lemniscus, and the pyramid, is supplied by the *anterior spinal artery*. This is a branch of the vertebral artery. When the territory of the anterior spinal artery, or more commonly that of the vertebral artery itself, is infarcted, three deficits result. First, tongue muscles are paralyzed on the side of the lesion because the hypoglossal motor neurons and axons are destroyed. Second, tactile sensation, vibration sense, and limb proprioception sense on the side opposite the lesion are impaired because the medial lemniscus is affected. Third, body musculature on the side opposite the lesion is weak because the *pyramid* is affected.

The dorsolateral portion of the medulla is supplied by the *posterior inferior cerebellar artery* (*PICA*) (Figure 13.9B). When the territory of this artery is infarcted, the functions of the vagal and glossopharyngeal nerves are impaired (the lateral medullary, or Wallenberg's, syndrome), because the *nucleus ambiguus* is affected. This produces difficulty in swallowing, hoarseness, and loss of the ipsilateral gag reflex. Vestibular dysfunction also occurs when the dorsolateral medulla is infarcted. This results in dizziness and nystagmus (involuntary rhythmical oscillation of the eyes). Somatic sensory signs associated with infarction of the territory of the posterior inferior cerebellar artery were considered in earlier chapters. Briefly, there is a loss of pain and temperature sense on the contralateral limbs and trunk and the ipsilateral face.

The Cochlear Nuclei Are Located in the Rostral Medulla

The myelin-stained section through the rostral medulla (Figure 13.10) cuts through the dorsal and ventral cochlear nuclei, which are located at the lateral brain stem margin. The glossopharyngeal (IX) nerve can be seen at the lateral brain stem surface, interposed between the inferior cerebellar peduncle and the spinal trigeminal tract (Figure 13.10). The efferent axons of the glossopharyngeal nerve originate from neurons in two nuclei, the *rostral portion of the nucleus ambiguus* (motor neurons that innervate striated muscle) and the *inferior salivatory nucleus* (para-

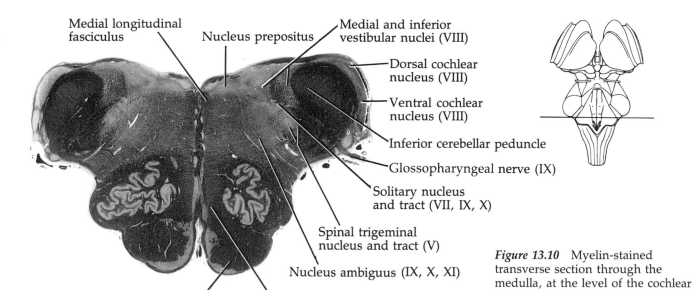

Medial longitudinal fasciculus

Nucleus prepositus

Medial and inferior vestibular nuclei (VIII)

Dorsal cochlear nucleus (VIII)

Ventral cochlear nucleus (VIII)

Inferior cerebellar peduncle

Glossopharyngeal nerve (IX)

Solitary nucleus and tract (VII, IX, X)

Spinal trigeminal nucleus and tract (V)

Nucleus ambiguus (IX, X, XI)

Pyramid   Medial lemniscus

Figure 13.10 Myelin-stained transverse section through the medulla, at the level of the cochlear nuclei.

sympathetic preganglionic neurons). Sensory nuclei are seen in this rostral medullary slice lateral to the sulcus limitans: the spinal trigeminal nucleus, and cochlear and vestibular nuclei. At this level, a large nucleus is located close to the midline beneath the ventricular floor, the *prepositus nucleus* (Figure 13.10). Because of its location, the prepositus nucleus is often incorrectly identified as the hypoglossal nucleus. It is thought to play a role in the regulation of eye movements.

The Fibers of the Facial Nerve Have a Complex Trajectory through the Pons

The pontine section shown in Figure 13.11A cuts through portions of the facial nerve. The axons leave the facial nucleus and follow a path toward the floor of the fourth ventricle (Figure 13.11B). These fibers of the facial nerve are not seen in Figure 13.11A because they do not course in discrete and straight fascicles.[4] As the facial nerve fibers approach the ventricular floor, they first ascend close to the midline. Next, the fibers sweep around the medial and rostral aspects of the abducens nucleus. This component is termed the *genu* of the facial nerve and, with the abducens nucleus, forms a surface landmark on the pontine floor of the fourth ventricle termed the *facial colliculus* (Figure 13.7). The facial nerve fibers then run ventrally and caudally to exit the pons at the *pontomedullary junction*. Fibers of the abducens nerve can be seen exiting the abducens nucleus (Figure 13.11A) and coursing toward the ventral brain stem surface, medial to the central tegmental tract and lateral to the medial lemniscus. They exit the pons medial to the facial nerve (Figures 13.7A and 13.11B).

---

[4] The hook-shaped path of CN VII fibers is not unique among the cranial nerves. Axons of CNs IX, X, and XI that originate in the nucleus ambiguus first course toward the ventricular floor before leaving the medulla. The motor root of CN V is the only component of the special visceral efferent group whose axons exit the brain stem following a direct path to the ventral surface.

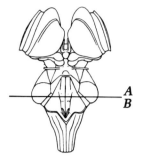

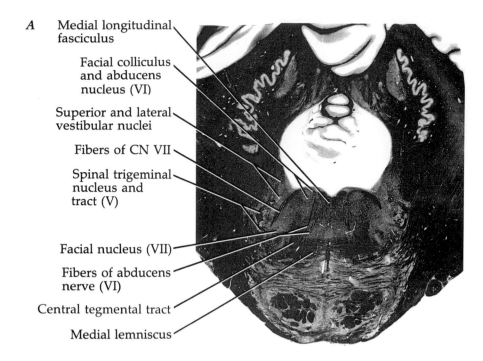

A Medial longitudinal fasciculus

Facial colliculus and abducens nucleus (VI)

Superior and lateral vestibular nuclei

Fibers of CN VII

Spinal trigeminal nucleus and tract (V)

Facial nucleus (VII)

Fibers of abducens nerve (VI)

Central tegmental tract

Medial lemniscus

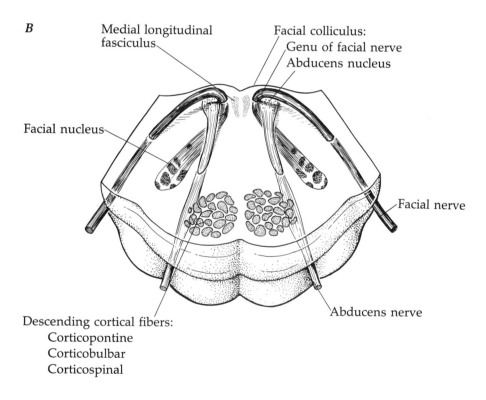

B Medial longitudinal fasciculus

Facial colliculus:
Genu of facial nerve
Abducens nucleus

Facial nucleus

Facial nerve

Abducens nerve

Descending cortical fibers:
Corticopontine
Corticobulbar
Corticospinal

Figure 13.11 *A.* Myelin-stained transverse section through the pons, at the level of the genu of CN VII. *B.* The three-dimensional course of facial nerve in the pons. (*B.* Adapted from Williams, P. L., and Warwick, R. 1975. Functional Neuroanatomy of Man. Philadelphia: W.B. Saunders.)

Eye Movement Deficits after an Abducens Nerve Lesion Differ from Those after an Abducens Nucleus Lesion

A lesion of the abducens nerve produces only *paralysis of the ipsilateral lateral rectus muscle*, thereby preventing ocular abduction on the same side. The unopposed action of the medial rectus muscle causes the affected eye to be adducted. In contrast, an abducens nucleus lesion produces a *lateral gaze palsy* in which the patient cannot direct lateral *gaze* to the side of the lesion. (Lateral gaze requires contraction of the *ipsilateral lateral rectus muscle* and the *contralateral medial rectus muscle*.) The lateral gaze palsy has two components. First, as with the nerve lesion, there is an inability to abduct the ipsilateral eye because of destruction of the lateral rectus motor neurons. Second, the patient cannot contract the contralateral medial rectus muscle when attempting to direct gaze to the side of the lesion. This occurs because the abducens nucleus, in addition to containing motor neurons, contains another class of neurons, termed *internuclear neurons*. The command for lateral gaze is transmitted from the abducens nucleus on one side to the part of the oculomotor nucleus on the contralateral side that contains medial rectus motor neurons by internuclear neurons (Figure 13.2A). The axons of these internuclear neurons decussate in the pons and ascend in the MLF. When the MLF is damaged rostral to the abducens nucleus (for example, at the level shown in Figure 13.12), thereby interrupting this internuclear projection, *anterior internuclear ophthalmoplegia* results. A unilateral lesion of the MLF is characterized, on lateral gaze to the contralateral side, by the inability (or reduced ability) to contract the ipsilateral medial rectus muscle and thereby adduct that eye. In addition, there is nystagmus (more pronounced in the abducting eye) as a result of involvement of the axons of vestibular neurons, which also course in the MLF.

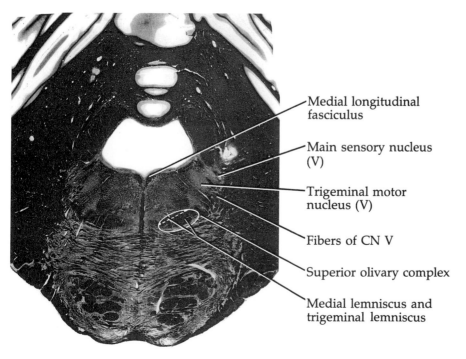

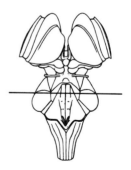

Figure 13.12 Myelin-stained transverse section through the pons, at the level of the main sensory and trigeminal motor nuclei.

Medial longitudinal fasciculus

Main sensory nucleus (V)

Trigeminal motor nucleus (V)

Fibers of CN V

Superior olivary complex

Medial lemniscus and trigeminal lemniscus

The Motor Nucleus of the Trigeminal Nerve Is Located Medial to the Main Sensory Nucleus

The most rostral component of the special visceral motor cell column is the *motor nucleus* of the *trigeminal* nerve (Figure 13.12). At this brain stem level the sulcus limitans is indistinct. However, the mediolateral organization of motor and sensory nuclei is preserved, with the trigeminal motor nucleus located medial to the main trigeminal sensory nucleus. Identification of the *trigeminal root fibers* in Figure 13.12 facilitates localization of the trigeminal sensory and motor nuclei. The trigeminal mesencephalic nucleus and tract, which are also located at this level, extend farther rostrally, where they can be readily identified (see later). The superior olivary complex, which receives input from the ventral cochlear nucleus (Chapter 7), is also illustrated in Figure 13.12.

The Trochlear Nerve Exits the Dorsal Surface of the Pons at the Level of the Isthmus

The junction of the pons and the midbrain is the *isthmus* (Figures 13.7 and 13.13), named for the constriction in the diameter of the brain stem, which is especially noticeable during development (Figure 2.12A). The trochlear nerve exits the brain stem at this level. Two unusual features of the anatomy of the trochlear nerve are apparent in Figure 13.13: its emergence from the *dorsal pontine surface* (see Figure 13.7) and its *decussation*. Trochlear motor neurons are located in the *trochlear nucleus*, which is located in the caudal midbrain at the level of the inferior colliculus (Figure 13.13B). The trochlear nucleus is nested within the MLF. The axons of the trochlear motor neurons course caudally along the lateral margin of the cerebral aqueduct and fourth ventricle, in the *periaqueductal gray matter*. The axons decussate in the isthmus of the pons, dorsal to the cerebral aqueduct, and emerge from the dorsal brain stem surface. Some of the descending, decussating, and emerging fibers of the trochlear nerve can be seen in Figure 13.13A.

The Cranial Nerve Cell Columns Have a Dorsoventral Spatial Organization in the Midbrain

The mediolateral organization of the cranial nerve nuclei that was characteristic of the medulla and caudal pons is not apparent in the midbrain. In fact, the spatial organization of the three cranial nerve nuclear columns in the midbrain is more like that of the spinal cord, because they are oriented dorsal to ventral, than that of the pons and medulla. This can be appreciated by considering the level of the superior colliculus (Figure 13.14). From dorsal to ventral, the three columns are general somatic afferent, general visceral motor, and general somatic motor. The mesencephalic nucleus of CN V is the only member of the general somatic afferent column in the midbrain (Figure 13.14). In Chapter 12 it was noted that the trigeminal mesencephalic nucleus is unique because it is the only central nervous system nucleus that contains the cell bodies of *primary afferent fibers*. The mesencephalic tract of CN V contains the primary afferent fibers and is located lateral to the nucleus. The midbrain nucleus of the general visceral motor column (parasympathetic preganglionic neurons), the *Edinger–Westphal* nucleus, is located at the level of the superior colliculus (Figure 13.14). At the level of the superior colliculus, the nucleus

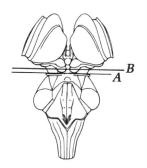

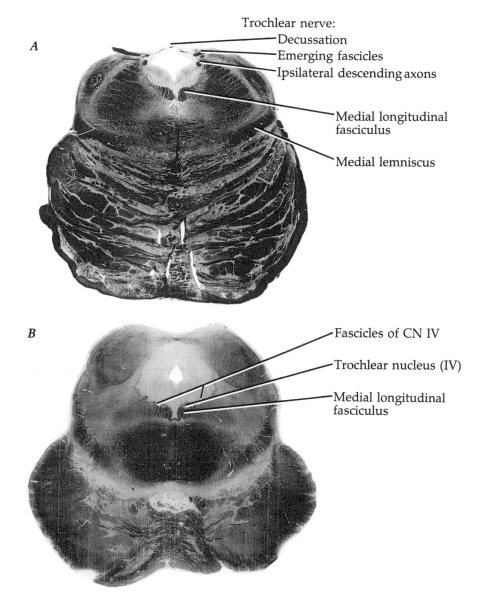

Trochlear nerve:
— Decussation
— Emerging fascicles
— Ipsilateral descending axons

— Medial longitudinal fasciculus

— Medial lemniscus

A

B

— Fascicles of CN IV

— Trochlear nucleus (IV)

— Medial longitudinal fasciculus

Figure 13.13 *A.* Myelin-stained section through the pons, at the level of the isthmus. *B.* Myelin-stained section through the caudal midbrain at the level of the trochlear nucleus.

of the general somatic motor column is the *oculomotor nucleus*. It was shown in the previous section that the trochlear nucleus was located caudally, at the level of the inferior colliculus. Axons from the oculomotor nucleus and the Edinger–Westphal nucleus course through the *red nucleus* en route to the periphery. The oculomotor nerve exits from the medial surface of the cerebral peduncle into the *interpeduncular fossa*. Cerebrospinal fluid collects here, in the *interpeduncular cistern* (see Figure 4.12). The interpeduncular fossa is also the site where numerous perforating arterioles leave the basilar artery and enter the midbrain.[5] Knowledge of regional midbrain anatomy is clinically important because a lesion of this

[5] This region of the floor of the interpeduncular fossa is sometimes termed the posterior perforating substance because of the perforating paramedian branches of the basilar artery. The anterior perforating substance (Chapter 15) is formed by the perforating branches of the anterior cerebral artery.

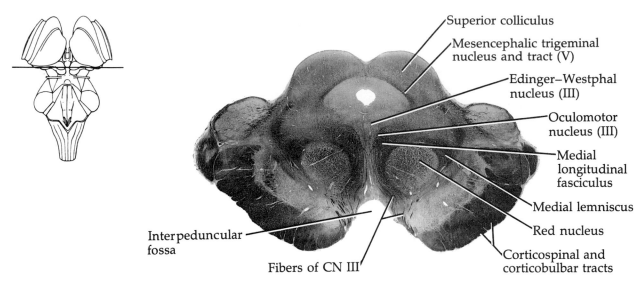

Figure 13.14 Myelin-stained transverse sections through the rostral midbrain at the level of the superior colliculus.

area, such as might be produced by occlusion of the posterior cerebral artery or a perforating basilar artery branch depending on the midbrain level, produces a complex set of neurological deficits that involve control of eye movements, cranial motor function, and limb movements. The control of eye movements and the pupillary and accommodation reflexes is disrupted ipsilaterally because of infarction of the oculomotor and trochlear nuclei and nerves and the Edinger–Westphal nucleus. Cranial and limb motor function is disrupted contralaterally because of involvement of three key motor structures: the red nucleus, the decussation of the superior cerebellar peduncle (or cerebellothalamic fibers more rostrally), and the basis pedunculi, which contains the corticobulbar and corticospinal tracts.

Figure 13.15 Myelin-stained transverse section through the midbrain–diencephalic juncture.

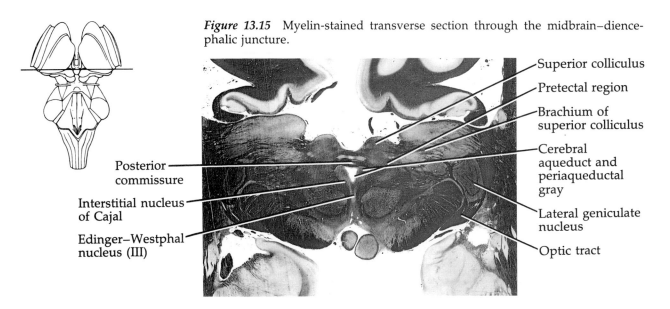

The rostral midbrain merges with the caudal diencephalon (Figure 13.15). This is an important level for the control of eye movements and visual reflexes. Neurons that transmit visual information to parasympathetic preganglionic neurons in Edinger–Westphal nucleus are located in the *pretectal nuclei*. These neurons receive visual input from the ipsilateral optic tract and brachium of the superior colliculus. They send their axons either directly to the Edinger–Westphal nucleus on the same side or, through the *posterior commissure*, to the contralateral side. The interstitial nucleus of Cajal, which is implicated in the coordination of eye and head movements, is located at this level as is the rostral margin of the superior colliculus.

The Medial Longitudinal Fasciculus (MLF) and Components of the General Somatic Motor Column Are Seen on a Midsagittal Section

Three of the four general somatic motor nuclei are seen on the sagittal section, from caudal to rostral: hypoglossal nucleus, trochlear nucleus, and oculomotor nucleus. The rostrocaudal course of the MLF can be identified in a sagittal section located close to the midline (Figure 13.16). In the caudal pons, the MLF is immediately beneath the floor of the fourth ventricle. At progressively more rostral levels, the MLF is displaced ventrally from the ventricular floor as the periaqueductal gray matter becomes larger. (Compare, for example, the location of the MLF in Figure 13.11 and 13.13.) In the midbrain, the MLF is further displaced by the trochlear and oculomotor nuclei. The path of the exiting oculomotor nerve fibers in the midbrain also can be identified. Fascicles of the oculomotor nerve can be seen exiting the ventral midbrain surface.

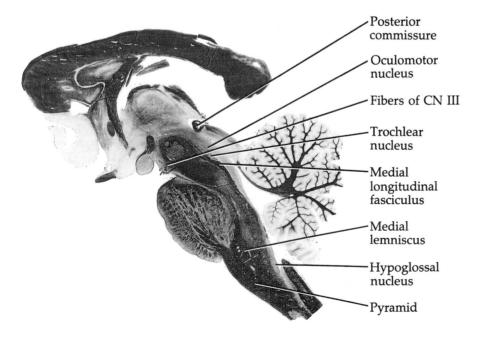

Posterior commissure

Oculomotor nucleus

Fibers of CN III

Trochlear nucleus

Medial longitudinal fasciculus

Medial lemniscus

Hypoglossal nucleus

Pyramid

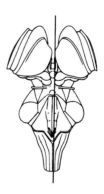

Figure 13.16 Myelin-stained sagittal section through brain stem, close to the midline.

Summary

There are three separate columns of cranial nerve motor nuclei (Figure 13.1), from medial to lateral: *general somatic motor, special visceral motor,* and *general visceral motor.* The most medial motor column, the *general somatic motor* column, consists of four nuclei each of which contains motor neurons that innervate striated muscle derived from the *occipital somites* (Figures 13.4 and 13.5). The *oculomotor nucleus* (1) (Figures 13.2, 13.14, and 13.16) contains motor neurons whose axons course in the *oculomotor nerve* (III) and innervate the following extraocular muscles: *medial rectus, superior rectus, inferior rectus,* and *inferior oblique.* The oculomotor nucleus also innervates the *levator palpebrae superioris* muscle. The *trochlear nucleus* (2) (Figures 13.2, 13.4A, 13.13B, and 13.16), via the *trochlear nerve* (IV), innervates the *contralateral superior oblique* muscle, and the *abducens nucleus* (3) (Figures 13.2 and 13.11), via the *abducens nerve* (VI), innervates the *lateral rectus* muscle. The extraocular motor nuclei receive an indirect projection from two main areas of the cerebral cortex, the *frontal eye field* and the *parieto-occipital eye field* (Figure 13.2C). The *hypoglossal nucleus* (4) gives rise to axons that course in the *hypoglossal nerve* (XII) and innervate tongue muscles (Figures 13.3, 13.9, and 13.15). The hypoglossal nucleus receives a predominantly contralateral projection from the motor cortex.

The *special visceral motor column* is displaced ventrally from the floor of the fourth ventricle (Figures 13.1 and 13.4). It contains four nuclei, each of which innervates striated muscles derived from the branchial arches. The *trigeminal motor nucleus* (1) (Figures 13.4 and 13.12) innervates the muscles of *mastication* via the *trigeminal nerve* (V). This nucleus receives a *bilateral projection from the motor cortex.* The *facial nucleus* (2) (Figures 13.4 and 13.11) innervates the muscles of *facial expression.* The axons of facial motor neurons course in the *facial nerve* (VII). Facial motor neurons that innervate the upper face muscles receive a *bilateral projection* from motor cortex, whereas motor neurons innervating lower face muscles receive a *contralateral projection* (Figure 13.4B). The *nucleus ambiguus* (3) (Figures 13.4 and 13.9) innervates the muscles of the *palate, pharynx,* and *larynx* via the *glossopharyngeal* nerve (IX), the *vagus* nerve (X), and the *cranial root of the spinal accessory nerve* (XI) (see also Figure 13.8). The *accessory nucleus* (4) innervates the sternocleidomastoid and trapezius muscles via the *spinal root of the spinal accessory nerve* (XI).

The *general visceral motor* column contains four nuclei (Figure 13.1). Each nucleus contains *parasympathetic preganglionic neurons.* The *Edinger–Westphal nucleus* (1) is located in the midbrain (Figures 13.5, 13.14, and 13.16). Its axons project via the *oculomotor nerve* to the *ciliary ganglion* where postganglionic neurons innervate the constrictor muscles of the iris and the ciliary muscle. Axons from the *superior salivatory nucleus* (2) (Figure 13.1) course in the *intermediate nerve* (a branch of the *facial nerve*). Via synapses in the pterygopalatine and submandibular ganglia, the nucleus influences the *lacrimal gland* and glands of the *nasal mucosa.* The *inferior salivatory nucleus* (3) (Figure 13.1), via the *glossopharyngeal nerve*, synapses on postganglionic neurons in the *otic ganglion.* From there, postganglionic neurons innervate the *parotid gland.* Axons from the *dorsal motor nucleus of the vagus* (4) (Figures 13.1, 13.6, 13.9, and 13.10) course in the periphery in the *vagus nerve* and innervate *terminal ganglia* in most of the thoracic and abdominal viscera (to the splenic flexure of the colon). ■

References

Akert, K., Glickman, M. A., Lang, W., et al. 1980. The Edinger–Westphal nucleus in the monkey. A retrograde tracer study. Brain Res. 184:491–498.

Carpenter, M. B., and Sutin, J. 1983. Human Neuroanatomy. Baltimore: Williams & Wilkins.

Ferner, H., and Staubestand, J. (eds.) 1983. Sobota Atlas of Human Anatomy. Vol. 1: Head, Neck, Upper Extremities. Baltimore: Urban & Schwarzenberg.

Lowey, A. D., Saper, C. B., and Yamondis, N. D. 1978. Re-evaluation of the efferent projections of the Edinger–Westphal nucleus in the cat. Brain Res. 141:153–159.

Williams, P. L., and Warwick, R. 1975. Functional Neuroanatomy of Man. Philadelphia: W.B. Saunders.

Selected Readings

Brodal, A. 1957. The Cranial Nerves: Anatomical and Anatomicoclinical Correlations. Oxford: Blackwell Scientific Publications.

Brodal, A. 1981. Neurological Anatomy. New York: Oxford University Press.

Kelly, J. P. 1985. Cranial nerve nuclei, the reticular formation, and biogenic amine-containing neurons. In Kandel, E. R., and Schwartz, J. H., Principles of Neural Science. New York: Elsevier, pp. 539–561.

Gouras, P. 1985. Oculomotor System. In Kandel, E. R., and Schwartz, J. H., Principles of Neural Science. New York: Elsevier, pp. 571–583.

Reiner, A., Karten, H. J., Gamlin, P. D. R., et al. 1983. Parasympathetic ocular control: Functional subdivisions and circuitry of the avian nucleus of Edinger–Westphal. Trends in Neurosci. 6:140–145.

Rowland, L. P. 1985. Clinical Syndromes of the Brain Stem. In Kandel, E. R., and Schwartz, J. H., Principles of Neural Science. New York: Elsevier, pp. 597–607.

The Hypothalamus and the Regulation of Endocrine and Visceral Functions

14

The Hypothalamus

The central nervous system plays an important role in maintaining normal organ function, a role played in large measure by the hypothalamus. Through release of pituitary hormones and modulating the actions of the autonomic nervous system, the hypothalamus regulates the function of virtually all organs of the body. The anatomical substrates of central neural control of endocrine and autonomic function are beginning to be unraveled, with the aid of new techniques that allow an assessment of both the projections of hypothalamic neurons and their biochemistry. A second major function of the hypothalamus is in effecting the behavioral changes necessary to achieve such basic needs as feeding, drinking, and mating. Therefore, the functions of the hypothalamus ensure survival not only of the individual but even of the species.

In this chapter the neuroanatomy of the regulation of endocrine and autonomic functions by the hypothalamus is examined. The pituitary gland and neuroendocrine function are considered first. Next, the organization of the autonomic nervous system is surveyed, and then the central neural control of autonomic function by the hypothalamus is examined. The role of the hypothalamus in motivational behavior and reducing drive states will be considered in Chapter 15 along with other brain structures that constitute the limbic system.

The Hypothalamus Is Divided into Three Mediolateral Zones

The hypothalamus is located in the diencephalon, ventral to the thalamus (Figure 14.1). It is bounded dorsally by the hypothalamic sulcus, rostrally by the anterior wall of the third ventricle[1] (the lamina terminalis, Chapter 2), and laterally by the internal capsule. The caudal boundary of the hypothalamus is defined by a line drawn between the caudal edge of the *mammillary body*, a prominent landmark on the ventral hypothalamic surface (see later), and the *posterior commissure* (Figure 14.1). In addition to the mammillary bodies, which mark the location of the mammillary nuclei, the ventral surface of the hypothalamus is characterized by two other prominent landmarks (Figure 14.2). With the pituitary gland removed, we see (1) the *infundibular stalk* caudal to the optic chiasm, and (2) the *tuber cinereum*, surrounding the base of the infundibular stalk. The infundibular stalk connects the pituitary gland with the brain. The tuber cinereum is a swelling under which lie most of the hypothalamic nuclei that regulate the release of anterior pituitary hormones. Two prominent recesses in the rostral floor of the third ventricle can be seen on the medial hypothalamic surface, the *supraoptic recess* and the *infundibular recess* (Figure 14.1). These recesses have characteristic shapes, and provide important radiological information in the localization of space-occupying lesions.

---

[1] A portion of the *preoptic region*, which is part of the forebrain, is located rostral to the lamina terminalis. However, it is typically included as a component of the hypothalamus because it subserves similar functions.

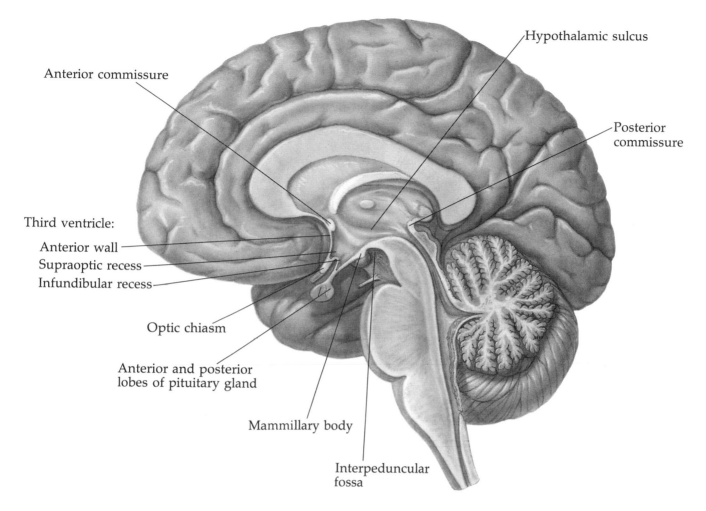

Anterior commissure

Hypothalamic sulcus

Posterior commissure

Third ventricle:

Anterior wall

Supraoptic recess

Infundibular recess

Optic chiasm

Anterior and posterior lobes of pituitary gland

Mammillary body

Interpeduncular fossa

Figure 14.1 A midsagittal view of brain showing key structures in and around the hypothalamus.

A schematic three-dimensional view of the hypothalamic nuclei is shown in Figure 14.3. The major nuclei are organized into three mediolateral zones. Whereas the boundaries between the zones are indistinct, the nuclei and tracts in these zones serve different functions. The *periventricular zone* (1) borders the third ventricle and is important in *neuroendocrine function*. The *medial zone* (2) constitutes a major site of termination of limbic system projections, the components of the central nervous system that participate in emotions and their behavioral expression (Chapter 15). The *lateral zone* (3) functions largely as a relay station, connecting limbic system structures in the telencephalon with other parts of the hypothalamus and the midbrain. This zone is separated from the medial zone by the *fornix*, a C-shaped tract that interconnects limbic system structures. The *medial forebrain bundle* (MFB) is located in the lateral zone. This is a diffuse pathway mediating ascending and descending connections between the brain stem, the hypothalamus, and the cerebral hemisphere. Neurons in the lateral zone are not organized into distinct nuclei, but rather are interspersed along the MFB. The hypothalamus also has an anterior–posterior organization, the boundaries of which are considered later when the regional anatomy of the hypothalamus is examined.

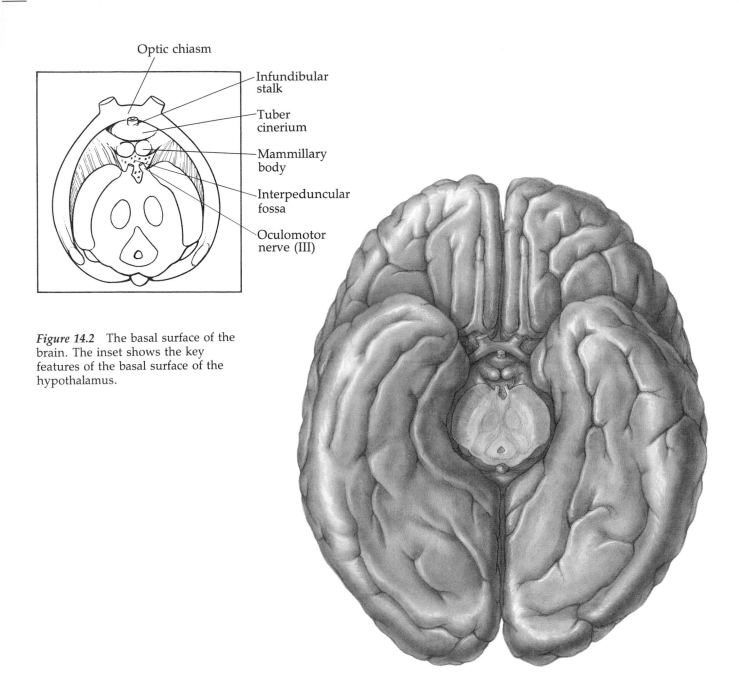

Figure 14.2 The basal surface of the brain. The inset shows the key features of the basal surface of the hypothalamus.

A region related anatomically and functionally to the hypothalamus, the *preoptic region*, is located dorsal to the optic chiasm and extends rostrally. Whereas most of the preoptic region is located caudal to the lamina terminalis, a portion is located rostral, and as a consequence, the preoptic region is traditionally considered as a forebrain region separate from the hypothalamus. It was also thought to develop from the telencephalon, not the diencephalon from which the hypothalamus is derived. Modern work on the embryology of the preoptic region shows a diencephalic origin, and the connections and functions of the preoptic region are similar to those of the hypothalamus proper.

A

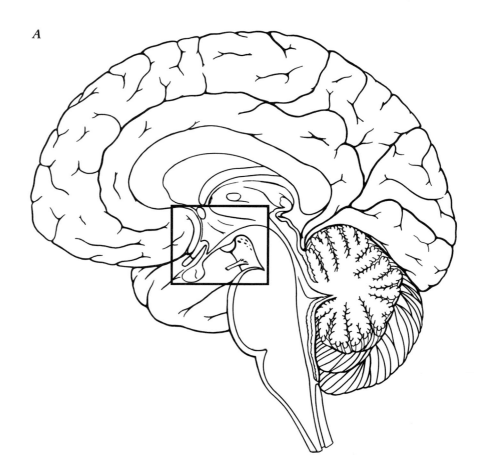

Figure 14.3 The major hypothalamic nuclei are illustrated in the cutaway view shown in *B*. The region illustrated in part B is located within the box shown in *A*. Note that the periventricular nuclei, which are located immediately beneath the walls and floor of the third ventricle, extend dorsally to approximately the level of the hypothalamic sulcus (dorsal margin of cutaway view) but are illustrated as shown to facilitate depiction of the three mediolateral hypothalamic zones: periventricular, middle, and lateral. (Adapted from Nauta, W. J. H., and Haymaker, W. 1969. Hypothalamic Nuclei and Fiber Connections. In Haymaker, W., Anderson, E., and Nauta, W. J. H. The Hypothalamus. Springfield, Ill.: Charles C. Thomas, pp. 136–209.)

B

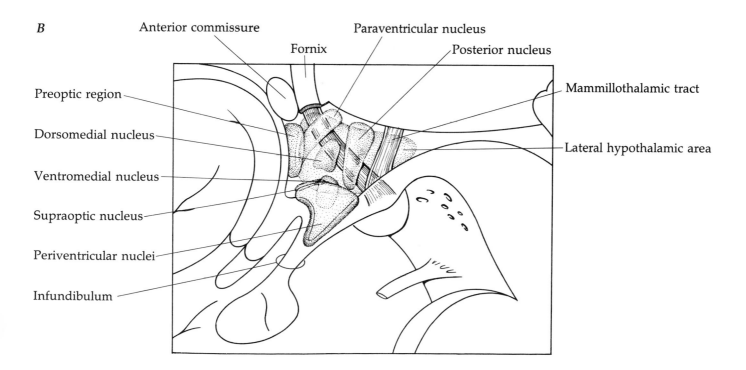

Separate Neurosecretory Systems Regulate Hormone Release from the Anterior and Posterior Lobes of the Pituitary

The pituitary gland (Figure 14.1), or hypophysis, extends from the ventral surface of the hypothalamus. In humans, there are two major anatomical divisions of the pituitary gland which mediate the release of different hormones: the *anterior lobe* (adenohypophysis; Table 14.1), and the *posterior lobe* (neurohypophysis). A third lobe, the intermediate lobe, is prominent in many phylogenetically less advanced mammals, but is vestigial in humans. The lobes of the pituitary gland have different developmental histories. The posterior lobe develops from the *neuroectoderm;* the anterior and intermediate lobes are of *ectodermal* origin, developing from a diverticulum in the roof of the developing oral cavity (Rathke's pouch). Early during development the ectodermal and neuroectodermal portions fuse, thereby forming a single structure.

The release of hormones from the anterior and posterior lobes is regulated by different populations of hypothalamic neurons. The posterior lobe is part of the *magnocellular neurosecretory system* (Figure 14.4A). Here, *large-diameter* hypothalamic neurons in two nuclei project their axons into the posterior lobe, where their terminals release peptide hormones directly onto capillaries of the systemic circulation. The anterior lobe is regulated by the *parvocellular neurosecretory system* (Figure 14.4B) in which *small-diameter* hypothalamic neurons in numerous hypothalamic and extrahypothalamic nuclei regulate anterior lobe hormone release by *neurovasculature* rather than synaptic mechanisms. Specific chemicals (Table 14.1) are secreted into the *portal circulation* (Figure 14.5) of the pituitary gland. The magnocellular system is considered first because its organization is somewhat simpler.

Hypothalamic Neurons Release Vasopressin and Oxytocin from the Posterior Lobe

Vasopressin, a peptide consisting of nine amino acids, has numerous functions, including promotion of water reabsorption from the distal tubules of the kidney to reduce urine volume[2] and elevation of blood pressure through its action on vascular smooth muscle. *Oxytocin*, which has a chemical structure nearly identical to that of vasopressin—differing by amino acids at only two sites—functions primarily to stimulate uterine contractions and to promote ejection of milk from the mammary glands. Despite the fact that oxytocin is best known for its actions on female organs, there do not seem to be differences in oxytocin-containing cells in males and females (see later). It is likely that other major actions of this hormone will be discovered. Both vasopressin and oxytocin are synthesized primarily in two hypothalamic nuclei, the *paraventricular nucleus* and the *supraoptic nucleus*. These nuclei are illustrated in Figure 14.4A which is a midsagittal view of the hypothalamus. It was once thought that vasopressin was synthesized in one nucleus and oxytocin in the other. However, with the use of immunocytochemical techniques (Chapter 11), it has now been established that separate cells in both nuclei produce both hormones. Both vasopressin and oxytocin are synthesized

---

[2] Another name for vasopressin is antidiuretic hormone (ADH).

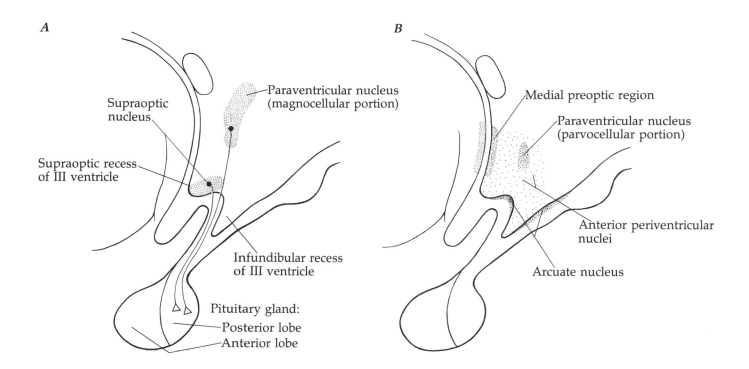

A

Supraoptic
nucleus

Paraventricular nucleus
(magnocellular portion)

Supraoptic recess
of III ventricle

Infundibular recess
of III ventricle

Pituitary gland:
Posterior lobe
Anterior lobe

B

Medial preoptic region

Paraventricular nucleus
(parvocellular portion)

Anterior periventricular
nuclei

Arcuate nucleus

from larger prohormone molecules. These prohormone molecules also contain other proteins, termed *neurophysins*, which are released with vasopressin and oxytocin. A physiological role for neurophysins has not been identified.

The axons of the paraventricular and the supraoptic nuclei course in the *infundibular stalk* (Figure 14.4A) and do not make synaptic contacts with other neurons; rather they terminate on *fenestrated capillaries* in the *posterior lobe* of the pituitary (Figure 14.5). The process by which these hypothalamic neurons release vasopressin or oxytocin from their terminals into the systemic circulation is similar to the release of neurotransmitters at synapses. Immunocytochemical studies have also shown that the magnocellular neurons have a complex biochemistry and contain other peptides that have both central and peripheral actions, peptides that also may be released into the circulation along with oxytocin or vasopressin. An important mystery to be solved is the function of this coordinated peptide release. Vasopressin is an example of a specific brain peptide that has a diversity of coordinated functions. It acts as a circulating hormone that influences the function of specific peripheral target organs (the kidney for example), as a neuroactive peptide involved in control of the autonomic nervous system (see later), and as a releasing hormone to control the anterior pituitary. Peptidergic neurons have a remarkable capacity for plasticity. For example, damage to the infundibular stalk may interrupt the axons of magnocellular neurosecretory cells containing vasopressin as they pass to the posterior pituitary. This results in a condition known as *diabetes insipidus* in which excessive amounts of urine are produced. However, the condition is temporary because the cells form a new, functional "posterior lobe."

An understanding of the projections from other brain regions to the magnocellular hypothalamic neurons provides insight into how the brain

Figure 14.4 A. Locations of neurons constituting the magnocellular system and the trajectory of their axons to the posterior lobe of the pituitary gland are illustrated on this drawing of a midsagittal section. *B.* Locations of neurons of the parvocellular system.

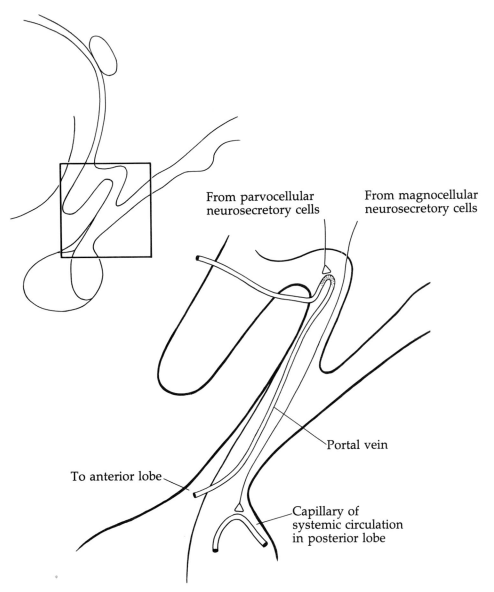

From parvocellular
neurosecretory cells

From magnocellular
neurosecretory cells

Portal vein

To anterior lobe

Capillary of
systemic circulation
in posterior lobe

Figure 14.5 The hypothalamus, pituitary gland, and rostral and ventral portions of the third ventricle are shown in this schematic drawing of the midsagittal brain surface. The region indicated by the box is enlarged below to show the organization of the parvocellular and magnocellular neurosecretory systems in relation to the portal circulation. The primary capillaries of the hypophyseal portal system are indicated by the shaded region. These vessels derive from the superior hypophyseal arteries, which are branches of the *internal carotid* and *posterior communicating arteries*.

controls neurohormone release. Magnocellular neurons that contain vasopressin receive an indirect projection from the *solitary nucleus*. This pathway conveys *baroreceptor* input (Chapter 8) to the hypothalamus, providing important sensory signals for controlling blood pressure and blood volume. Other major inputs are from the *subfornical organ* and the *organum vasculosum of the lamina terminals*. There is no *blood brain barrier* in these telencephalic structures. The blood brain barrier is a specific permeability barrier between capillaries in the central nervous system and the extra-cellular space. This barrier protects the brain from the influence of many chemicals circulating in the blood. The blood brain barrier is believed to be imposed, in part, by specializations in the capillary endothelium and glial processes that end upon the endothelial cells. With no blood brain barrier, these structures can sense plasma osmolality and circulating chemicals and thereby regulate blood pressure and blood volume through their hypothalamic projections. The *preoptic region* is implicated in the central neural mechanisms for regulating the composition and volume of body fluids and, thus, indirectly affects the control of blood pressure. The preoptic region also projects to the magnocellular neurons.

Regulatory Peptides Released by Hypothalamic Neurons into the Portal Circulation Control Secretion of Anterior Lobe Hormones

Anterior pituitary hormones are released from *epithelial secretory cells* into the systemic circulation, in contrast to posterior pituitary hormones which are the neurosecretory products of hypothalamic neurons. The process by which the hypothalamus stimulates anterior lobe secretory cells to release their hormones (or inhibits release) is quite unlike mechanisms of neural action that have been considered so far. Rather than synapse on anterior lobe secretory cells, the hypothalamic parvocellular neurosecretory neurons terminate on capillaries of the *pituitary portal circulation*[3] in the floor of the third ventricle (Figure 14.5). These capillaries are located in a region termed the *median eminence*, which is part of the infundibular stalk.[4] The neurons release chemicals, most of which are peptides, that function either to promote (*releasing hormones*) or to inhibit (*release-inhibiting hormones*) the release of hormones from anterior lobe secretory cells. These chemicals and their principal actions are listed in Table 14.1. The release or release-inhibiting hormones are carried to the *distal part of the anterior lobe* in the portal veins (Figure 14.5), where they act directly on secretory cells. An analogy can be drawn between the capillaries in the *median eminence* and the integrative function of *spinal motor neurons* (Chapter 9). Separate descending pathways and interneuronal systems synapse on the spinal motor neuron. Thus the motor neuron is the "final common path" for the integration of neuronal information controlling skeletal muscle. The "final common path" for control of anterior lobe hormone release is the capillaries of the median eminence. This is because separate hypothalamic neurons secrete releasing or release-inhibiting hormones into the capillaries of the median eminence, and it is at this *vascular site* that summation of neurohormones occurs.

The distribution of neurons that project to the median eminence has been examined extensively in rodents. These neurons are widespread; the major sources are located primarily in four hypothalamic locations, all close to the third ventricle (Figure 14.4B): anterior periventricular zone,

---

[3] Capillary beds in the systemic circulation are interposed between arterial and venous systems. A portal system, such as in the anterior pituitary or the liver, is characterized by the presence of separate portal veins interposed between two sets of capillaries.

[4] The axons from the supraoptic and paraventricular nuclei, en route to the posterior lobe, are segregated (in an internal zone of the median eminence) from the axons and terminals of the parvocellular neurons.

Table 14.1 Anterior Pituitary Hormones and Substances That Control Their Release

Hormone	Releasing Hormone (RH)	Release-Inhibiting Hormone
Growth hormone	Growth hormone RH/ dopamine	Somatostatin
Luteinizing hormone	Gonadotropin RH	
Follicle-stimulating hormone	Gonadotropin RH	
Thyrotropin	Thyrotropin RH	
Prolactin	Prolactin RH	Dopamine
Adrenocorticotropic hormone	Corticotropin RH	
Melanocyte-stimulating hormone[a]	Corticotropin RH	

[a] In humans, the intermediate lobe of the pituitary gland is vestigial. Secretory cells containing melanocyte-stimulating hormone are located in the anterior lobe.

arcuate nucleus, medial preoptic area, and medial "parvocellular" portion of the paraventricular nucleus. The septal nuclei (Chapter 15) are an extrahypothalamic source of gonadotropin-releasing hormone. Interestingly, most of the neurohormones (release and release-inhibiting, Table 14.1) are also found in parts of the hypothalamus that do not project to the median eminence and in other regions of the central nervous system. Moreover, oxytocin and vasopressin also have extrahypothalamic distributions. This widespread distribution of neurosecretory hormones calls attention to the fact that they are *neuroactive compounds* at these other sites and not simply chemicals that regulate anterior pituitary hormone release.

There is an interesting similarity between the biochemistry of the magnocellular and parvocellular neurosecretory systems. As in the magnocellular system, neurons of the parvocellular system synthesize more than one peptide. In certain groups of parvocellular neurons, for example, it is thought that the levels of circulating hormones in blood influence the amount of synthesis by a neuron of one or another peptide. This is one way in which behavior, such as prolonged exposure to stressful situations, may alter the neurohormone composition in the portal circulation and thereby influence anterior pituitary hormone release. In addition, the actions of the neurohormones as neuroactive compounds, such as neurotransmitters and neuromodulators, influence other central nervous system functions.

Descending Projections from the Hypothalamus Regulate Autonomic Function

The other major role of the hypothalamus is in the regulation of the functions of the autonomic nervous system. The autonomic nervous system controls the various organ systems of the body: cardiovascular and respiratory systems, gastrointestinal system, exocrine glands, and urogenital system. There are two divisions of the autonomic nervous system which originate from different parts of the central nervous system, the *parasympathethic* and the *sympathetic nervous systems*. A third division of the autonomic nervous system, the *enteric nervous system*, is located entirely in the periphery. The enteric nervous system is the intrinsic innervation of the gastrointestinal tract and mediates the complex coordinated reflexes for peristalsis. Different autonomic functions rely to a greater or lesser extent on local reflex mechanisms or control by the central nervous system. Thus, visceral functions are organized similar to the control of skeletal musculature, where both reflex and central control mechanisms play important roles. Before regulation of the autonomic nervous system by the hypothalamus is considered, the anatomical organization of the sympathetic and parasympathetic divisions is reviewed briefly.

The Parasympathetic and Sympathetic Divisions of the Autonomic Nervous System Originate from Different Central Nervous System Locations

The innervation of the organs by the sympathetic and parasympathetic divisions of the autonomic nervous system is fundamentally different in organization than innervation of skeletal musculature (Figure 14.6). Innervation by skeletal muscle is mediated directly by motor neurons (Figure 14.6A). For the autonomic innervation, two neurons link the central nervous system with organs in the periphery: the *preganglionic*

Figure 14.6 The circuit for peripheral innervation of skeletal muscle is shown in *A*. The innervation of peripheral autonomic ganglia is shown in *B*. Preganglionic autonomic neurons are located in the intermediate zone of the spinal cord. Their axons exit the spinal cord through the ventral roots and project to ganglia in the sympathetic trunk (paravertebral ganglia) through the spinal nerves and white rami. The axons of postganglionic neurons in the sympathetic ganglia course to the periphery through the gray rami and spinal nerves. The white and gray rami contain, respectively, the myelinated and unmyelinated axons of preganglionic and postganglionic autonomic neurons. A postganglionic neuron in a prevertebral ganglion is also shown with input from a preganglionic neuron. (*B*. Adapted from Appenzeller, O. 1986. Clinical Autonomic Failure. Practical Concepts. Amsterdam: Elsevier.)

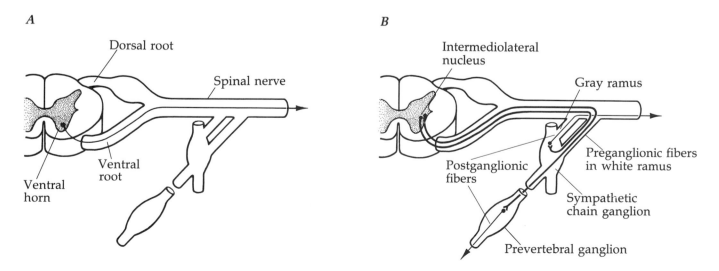

neuron, and the *postganglionic neuron* (Figure 14.6B).[5] The cell body of the preganglionic neuron is located in the central nervous system and its axon follows a tortuous course to the periphery. From the ventral root and through various peripheral neural conduits, the axon of the preganglionic neuron finally synapses on postganglionic neurons in *peripheral ganglia* (Figure 14.6B).

There are two major differences in the neuroanatomical organization of the sympathetic and parasympathetic divisions. The first is the location of the preganglionic neurons in the central nervous system, and the second is the location of the peripheral ganglia. *Preganglionic sympathetic neurons* are located in the intermediate zone of the spinal cord, between the *first thoracic and third lumbar* segments. Most of the neurons are located in the *intermediolateral nucleus* (also termed *intermediolateral cell column* because this nucleus has an extensive rostrocaudal organization). In contrast, parasympathetic preganglionic neurons are located in the *brain stem* and the *first through third sacral* spinal cord segments. The parasympathetic brain stem nuclei were described in Chapter 13 when the cranial nerve nuclei were discussed. They are the Edinger–Westphal nucleus, the superior salivatory nucleus, the inferior salivatory nucleus, and the dorsal motor nucleus of the vagus. The parasympathetic preganglionic neurons in the sacral spinal cord are located laterally in the intermediate zone.

The second major difference in the neuroanatomy of the sympathetic and parasympathetic divisions is the location of the peripheral ganglia in which the postganglionic neurons are located. Parasympathetic ganglia, generally termed *terminal ganglia*, are located on or near the target organ. In contrast, the sympathetic ganglia are located at some distance from the target organs. Postganglionic sympathetic neurons are located in the *paravertebral ganglia*, part of the sympathetic chain, and in the *prevertebral ganglia* (Figure 14.7).

The Hypothalamus Integrates Viscerosensory Information to Control Body Functions

Four hypothalamic nuclear regions contribute axons that synapse on autonomic nuclei in the brain stem and spinal cord (Figure 14.8)[6]: the paraventricular nucleus, the lateral hypothalamic area, the dorsomedial hypothalamic nucleus, and the posterior hypothalamic area. The *paraventricular nucleus* contributes the major projection and the neurotransmitter used by this pathway is thought to be *oxytocin*. Neurons in these four regions project their axons to the brain stem and spinal cord autonomic nuclei, primarily on the ipsilateral side. These axons course through either of two pathways: (1) the dorsal longitudinal fasciculus, or (2) the medial forebrain bundle and its caudal extension in the *dorsolateral tegmentum* of the brain stem (Figure 14.8). In addition to the fibers that

---

[5] A notable exception is the adrenal medulla, which receives direct innervation by preganglionic sympathetic neurons. This is related to the fact that adrenal medullary cells develop from the neural crest (Chapter 2).

[6] Other forebrain regions, in addition to the hypothalamus, participate in the regulation of the autonomic nervous system by projecting to brain stem and spinal cord autonomic nuclei. For example, important regulation of cardiovascular function is mediated by descending autonomic pathways from the pons and medulla; the neurotransmitters are known for many of these pathways.

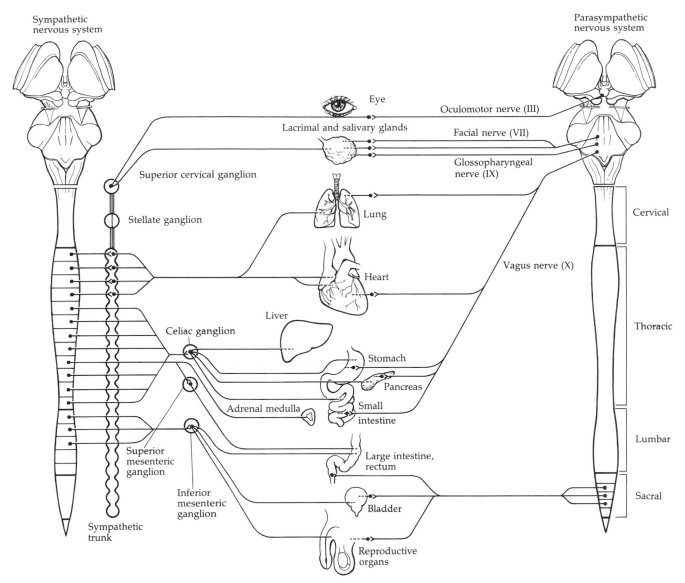

Figure 14.7 Organization of the autonomic nervous system. The sympathetic nervous system is shown on the left and the parasympathetic nervous system is shown on the right. Note that the postganglionic neurons for the sympathetic nervous system are located in sympathetic trunk ganglia and prevertebral ganglia. The postganglionic neurons for the parasympathetic nervous system are located in terminal ganglia which are located close to the target organ. (Adapted from Schmidt, R. F., and Thews, G. (eds.). 1983. Human Physiology. Berlin: Springer.)

synapse on autonomic nuclei, descending and ascending fibers of other functional systems course in these two tracts. The *dorsal longitudinal fasciculus* descends dorsally and medially in the brain stem. Throughout its course, the dorsal longitudinal fasciculus travels in close proximity to the ventricular system. Because the dorsal longitudinal fasciculus descends only as far as the *caudal brain stem*, it is reasoned to regulate principally the functions subserved by the *parasympathetic* division. The *dorsal motor nucleus of the vagus*, which contains parasympathetic preganglionic neu-

Figure 14.8 Regions of origin, course, and termination sites of descending hypothalamic pathways.

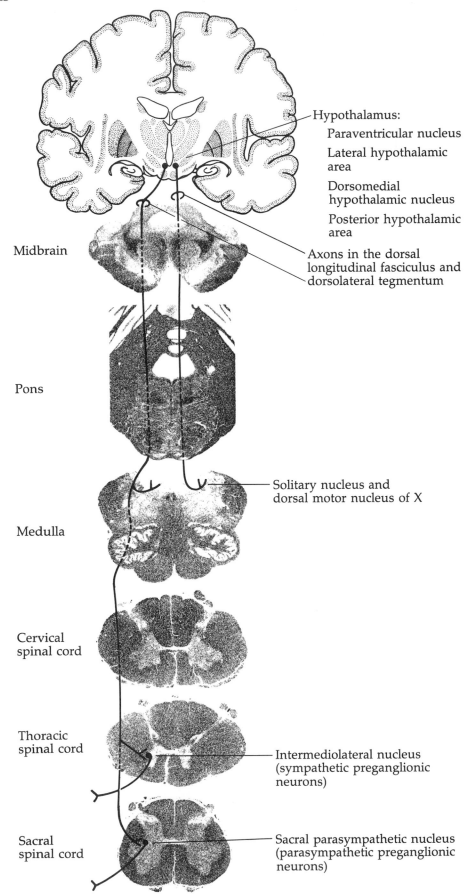

Hypothalamus:
Paraventricular nucleus
Lateral hypothalamic area
Dorsomedial hypothalamic nucleus
Posterior hypothalamic area

Axons in the dorsal longitudinal fasciculus and dorsolateral tegmentum

Midbrain

Pons

Solitary nucleus and dorsal motor nucleus of X

Medulla

Cervical spinal cord

Thoracic spinal cord

Intermediolateral nucleus (sympathetic preganglionic neurons)

Sacral spinal cord

Sacral parasympathetic nucleus (parasympathetic preganglionic neurons)

rons (Chapter 13), and the *solitary nucleus*, which receives visceral sensory input (Chapter 8), receive a projection from the hypothalamus via the dorsal longitudinal fasciculus (Figure 14.8).

The *medial forebrain bundle* is located in the lateral hypothalamus and its descending axons course laterally in the midbrain, pons, and medulla. The medial forebrain bundle is not localized to a discrete tract and it becomes even more scattered caudal in the hypothalamus. (The term *medial forebrain bundle* is more commonly applied to the intrahypothalamic segment.) As we will see later, lateral lesions in the caudal brain stem and spinal cord may interrupt the control of the sympathetic division and produce characteristic autonomic changes. Whereas the dorsal longitudinal fasciculus influences only brain stem parasympathetic function, the hypothalamic axons that descend laterally influence both parasympathetic and sympathetic function. This occurs because they project to the *dorsal motor nucleus of the vagus*, as well as to both the *intermediolateral nucleus* in the spinal cord (which contains sympathetic preganglionic neurons) and the intermediate zone of the sacral spinal cord (which contains parasympathetic preganglionic neurons). The finding that the same hypothalamic areas (and even many of the same neurons) project to regions containing parasympathetic and sympathetic preganglionic neurons is surprising when one considers the opposing functions of these two divisions of the autonomic nervous system.

In addition to projecting to autonomic nuclei in the brain stem and spinal cord, the hypothalamus projects to other sites important in visceral sensory and motor function: solitary nucleus, parabrachial nucleus, and nucleus ambiguus. It should be recalled that the *solitary nucleus* receives viscerosensory information from the glossopharyngeal and vagus nerves and relays this information directly to the hypothalamus, as well as to the thalamus and other forebrain structures (see Chapter 8). The *parabrachial nucleus* is also part of an indirect ascending viscerosensory pathway, and together with the solitary nucleus participates in the complex process of coordinating visceral functions. The *nucleus ambiguus* contains motor neurons that innervate a variety of palatal, laryngeal, and pharyngeal muscles and is important in *food ingestion*.

In the remainder of this chapter, we examine sections through the hypothalamus, as well as sections through the brain stem and spinal cord, that reveal the locations of the descending hypothalamic pathways and autonomic nuclei. The locations of key surface structures are also identified on sections through the hypothalamus to better understand its overall configuration.

The Preoptic Region Influences Release of Reproductive Hormones from the Anterior Pituitary

Figure 14.9 is a section through the *preoptic region*, a region that contains neurons which synthesize gonadotropin-releasing hormone. These neurons are believed to project to the median eminence and regulate pituitary release of reproductive hormones. When the preoptic region is destroyed in experimental animals, reproductive cycles and reproductive behaviors are profoundly altered. The first evidence of *sexual dimorphism* in the brain was obtained for nuclei in the preoptic region of the rat; the morphology of this region differs in males and females. The nuclear organization in the preoptic region is an interesting example of

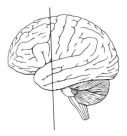

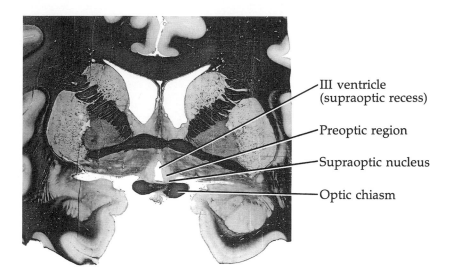

III ventricle
(supraoptic recess)

Preoptic region

Supraoptic nucleus

Optic chiasm

Figure 14.9 Myelin-stained coronal section through the preoptic region.

how sexual differentiation alters brain morphology because perinatal exposure to gonadal steroids influences the size of a sexually dimorphic nucleus in the preoptic region. Sexual dimorphism has also been demonstrated in the human preoptic region. The section shown in Figure 14.9 also cuts through the *supraoptic recess* of the third ventricle (Figure 14.1).

Nuclei of the Magnocellular Neurosecretory System Are Located in the Anterior Hypothalamus

The mediolateral organization of the hypothalamus was briefly considered earlier in the chapter. The three zones—periventricular, middle, and lateral—are located at all anterior–posterior levels of the hypothalamus (see Figures 14.10, 14.12, and 14.14). The hypothalamus also has an anterior-to-posterior organization and knowledge of this organization helps in formulating a framework for the *regional anatomy* of the hypothalamus. The hypothalamus can be divided into three anterior-to-posterior regions. The *anterior region* (1) is located between the lamina terminalis and the posterior edge of the optic chiasm (see inset to Figure 14.10). The *middle region* (2) is between the optic chiasm and the mammillary bodies. The *posterior region* (3) includes the mammillary bodies and the structures dorsal to them. The paraventricular and supraoptic nuclei are located in the anterior region (Figures 14.9 and 14.10). These are the two magnocellular nuclei and release vasopressin and oxytocin in the posterior lobe of the pituitary (Figure 14.4A). The paraventricular nucleus has a remarkable organization. It contains three major functional subdivisions: (1) the parvocellular division, apposed to the third ventricle, projects to the median eminence (Figure 14.4B); (2) the magnocellular division projects to the posterior lobe (Figure 14.4A); and (3) a separate autonomic division projects to brain stem and spinal cord nuclei containing autonomic preganglionic neurons (Figure 14.8). A common feature of the biochemistry of the paraventricular nucleus is that many neurons in each subdivision contain vasopressin or oxytocin. Release of vasopressin or oxytocin at the various target sites of neurons in the paraventricular nucleus may subserve similar sets of functions, for example in regulating blood pressure and blood volume.

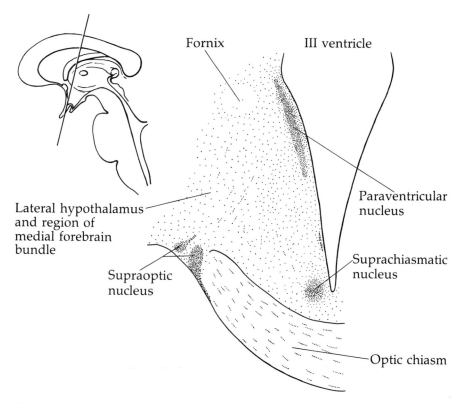

Fornix

III ventricle

Paraventricular nucleus

Lateral hypothalamus and region of medial forebrain bundle

Suprachiasmatic nucleus

Supraoptic nucleus

Optic chiasm

Figure 14.10 Drawing of Nissl-stained section through the anterior hypothalamus (optic chiasm). The inset shows the plane of section. (Adapted from Clarke, W. E. LeGros. 1938. Morphological aspects of the hypothalamus. In Clarke, W. E. LeGros, Beattie, J., Riddoch, G., et al. The Hypothalamus: Morphological, Functional, Clinical and Surgical Aspects. Edinburgh: Oliver & Boyd, pp. 2–68.)

The *suprachiasmatic nucleus*, which is also located at this level (Figure 14.10), functions as the "master clock" for circadian rhythms. It receives a direct projection from the *retina*, thereby allowing visual stimuli to synchronize circadian rhythms. The suprachiasmatic nucleus is believed to control circadian rhythms through local connections with other hypothalamic nuclei more directly involved in behavior, for example, the paraventricular nucleus. The clinical significance of normal circadian rhythms and the function of the suprachiasmatic nucleus are just beginning to be appreciated. For example, defects in circadian rhythms are believed to underlie certain forms of depression and sleeping disorders.

The Middle Hypothalamic Region Contains Parvocellular Neurosecretory Cells That Project to the Median Eminence

The myelin-stained section in Figure 14.11 transects the proximal portion of the infundibular stalk (also termed the infundibulum) (Figure 14.1). This portion contains the *median eminence*, where the primary capillaries of the hypophyseal portal system are located. Because these capillaries are fenestrated, the blood–brain barrier is absent in this region of the central nervous system, and, consequently, the releasing and release-inhibiting hormones secreted by the parvocellular neurosecretory neurons can pass directly into the portal circulation. The *arcuate nucleus* is

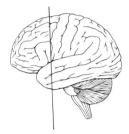

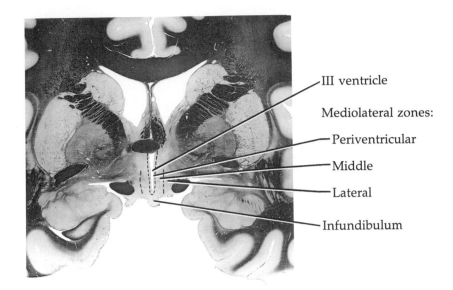

III ventricle

Mediolateral zones:

Periventricular

Middle

Lateral

Infundibulum

Figure 14.11 Myelin-stained coronal section through the infundibular stalk (infundibulum).

located in the middle hypothalamic region (Figure 14.12). Parvocellular neurons in the arcuate nucleus have three readily identifiable functions. First, they may regulate prolactin release from the anterior lobe because they are the major hypothalamic source of dopamine, which inhibits prolactin release. Second, they may regulate the release of growth hormone because they are a major source of growth hormone-releasing hormone. Third, they may play a role in opiate analgesia because they contain β-endorphin, an endogenous opiate that is cleaved from the large peptide *pro-opiomelanocortin* (*POMC*). The neurons that contain β-endorphin project to the periaqueductal gray matter and stimulation of this midbrain

Figure 14.12 Drawings of Nissl-stained section through the middle hypothalamus. The inset shows the plane of section. (Adapted from Clark, W. E. LeGros. 1938. Morphological aspects of the hypothalamus. The Hypothalamus: Morphological, Functional, Clinical and Surgical Aspects. Edinburgh: Oliver & Boyd, pp. 2–68.)

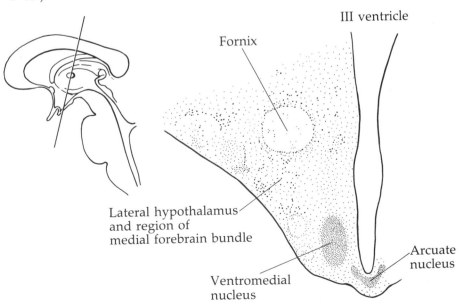

III ventricle

Fornix

Lateral hypothalamus and region of medial forebrain bundle

Ventromedial nucleus

Arcuate nucleus

region produces analgesia (Chapter 5). These neurons and other hypothalamic POMC cells project to various hypothalamic and forebrain sites, and they may participate in endocrine and emotional responses. The *ventromedial hypothalamic nucleus* is located in the middle region of the hypothalamus. This nucleus receives input from a major limbic system structure, the amygdala (Chapter 15), and is important in the regulation of appetite and other consummatory behaviors.

The Posterior Hypothalamus Merges with the Periaqueductal Gray Matter of the Brain Stem

A section through the posterior hypothalamus (Figures 14.13 and 14.14) reveals the mammillary nuclei (or bodies). Each mammillary body contains two nuclei: the prominent medial mammillary nucleus and the smaller *lateral mammillary nucleus*. The mammillary bodies, the principal component of the posterior hypothalamus, establish virtually no intrahypothalamic connections. They receive their major input from the *fornix*

A

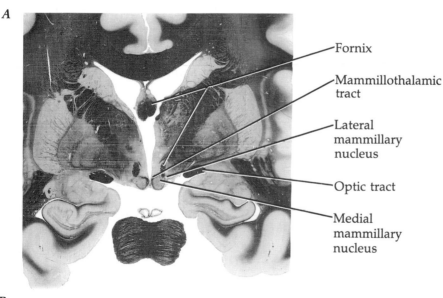

Fornix

Mammillothalamic tract

Lateral mammillary nucleus

Optic tract

Medial mammillary nucleus

B

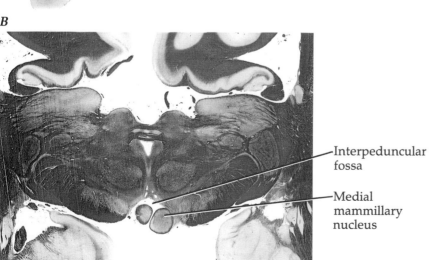

Interpeduncular fossa

Medial mammillary nucleus

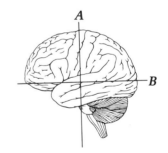

Figure 14.13 Myelin-stained coronal section through the mammillary bodies *(A)* and transverse section through the junction of the midbrain and diencephalon *(B)*. In part B, the mammillary bodies are located in the interpeduncular fossa, separated from the rest of the diencephalon. This is because the mammillary bodies extend from the basal surface of the diencephalon.

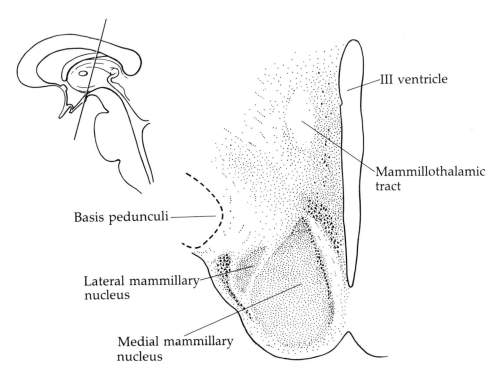

Figure 14.14 Drawings of Nissl-stained section through the posterior hypothalamus (mammillary bodies). The inset shows the plane of section. (Adapted from Clark, W. E. LeGros. 1938. Morphological aspects of the hypothalamus. In Clark, W. E. LeGros, Beattie, J., Riddoch, G., et al. The Hypothalamus: Morphological, Functional, Clinical and Surgical Aspects. Edinburgh: Oliver & Boyd, pp. 2–68.)

(Figure 14.3), a C-shaped tract that originates from the hippocampal formation. The efferent projections of the mammillary bodies are carried primarily in the *mammillothalamic tract*, which projects to the anterior nuclei of the thalamus (see Appendix II.19). The mammillary bodies also have a descending projection to the midbrain. They are considered part of the limbic system and will be discussed further in Chapter 15.

Other nuclei in the posterior hypothalamus, for example, nuclei located in the lateral hypothalamus do not contribute, in a major way, to neuroendocrine function. Rather, this region plays a role in regulating autonomic functions and mediating integrated behavioral responses to environmental stimuli. For example, the posterior hypothalamus is important in conserving body heat, which includes mediation of vasoconstriction and shivering in response to low temperatures.

Descending Autonomic Fibers Course in the Periaqueductal Gray Matter and in the Dorsolateral Tegmentum

Hypothalamic regulation of the autonomic nervous system is mediated, at least in part, by direct projections to brain stem parasympathetic nuclei, the intermediolateral nucleus in thoracic and lumbar spinal segments, and the lateral intermediate zone of the sacral spinal cord. The

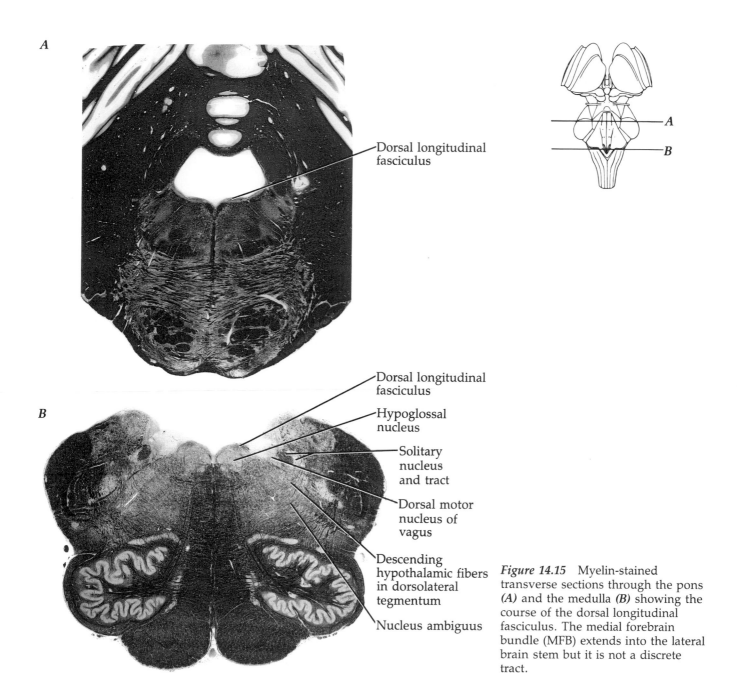

A

Dorsal longitudinal
fasciculus

B

Dorsal longitudinal
fasciculus

Hypoglossal
nucleus

Solitary
nucleus
and tract

Dorsal motor
nucleus of
vagus

Descending
hypothalamic fibers
in dorsolateral
tegmentum

Nucleus ambiguus

Figure 14.15   Myelin-stained
transverse sections through the pons
(A) and the medulla *(B)* showing the
course of the dorsal longitudinal
fasciculus. The medial forebrain
bundle (MFB) extends into the lateral
brain stem but it is not a discrete
tract.

dorsal longitudinal fasciculus, through which fibers that terminate in brain
stem parasympathetic nuclei descend, courses within the gray matter of
the caudal portion of the third ventricle, the midbrain periaqueductal gray
matter, and the gray matter in the floor of the fourth ventricle. Although
diffuse in the diencephalon and midbrain, fibers constituting this path
can be identified in the pons, at the level of the motor nucleus of the
trigeminal nerve (Figure 14.15A), and in the medulla in the dorsal portion
of the hypoglossal nucleus (Figure 14.15B).

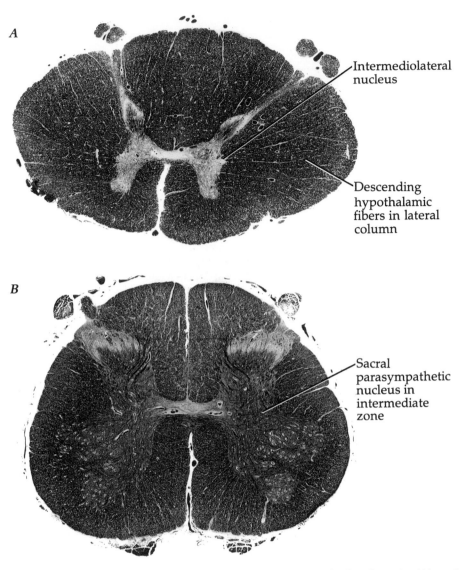

Figure 14.16 Myelin-stained transverse sections through the thoracic *(A)* and sacral *(B)* spinal cord.

Dorsolateral Brain Stem Lesions Interrupt Descending Sympathetic Fibers

Damage to the dorsolateral pons or medulla typically produces *Horner's syndrome*, a disturbance in which the normal balance between sympathetic and parasympathetic function is profoundly disrupted. Such damage may occur as a consequence of occlusion of the posterior inferior cerebellar artery (see Figure 4.3) The three most common signs of Horner's syndrome are: (1) *ipsilateral miosis* resulting from the unopposed action of the pupillary constrictor innervation of the oculomotor nerve (Chapter 13), (2) *dropping of the eyelid* caused by removal of the sympathetic control of the smooth muscle assisting the action of the levator palpebrae, and (3) *decreased sweating* and *increased warmth and redness of the ipsilateral face* resulting from reduced sympathetic control of facial blood flow. Horner's syndrome can also occur after damage to the white matter of the cervical spinal cord, where the hypothalamic projection descends, or pathology in the periphery, where axons of the sympathetic postganglionic neurons course to reach the head.

Preganglionic Neurons Are Located in the Lateral Intermediate Zone of the Spinal Cord

The descending sympathetic fibers from the hypothalamus course in the lateral column of the spinal cord (Figure 14.16) and terminate in the intermediolateral nucleus (or cell column). This is the nucleus in which most sympathetic preganglionic neurons are located. Additional preganglionic neurons are scattered medially in the intermediate zone. At certain levels, the intermediolateral nucleus extends into the lateral column (Figure 14.16A), which explains why this region is sometimes called the *intermediate horn* of the spinal cord gray matter. The spinal cord parasympathetic preganglionic neurons are located in the lateral intermediate zone of the first through third sacral segments (Figure 14.16B). This region is not distinguished by protruding into the lateral column. The sacral parasympathetic preganglionic neurons also receive a projection from the hypothalamus.

Summary

The hypothalamus regulates the functions of the neuroendocrine system and the autonomic nervous system. It is a portion of the diencephalon, bounded by the *lamina terminalis* rostrally, the *hypothalamic sulcus* dorsally, and the *internal capsule* laterally (Figure 14.1). The posterior boundary of the hypothalamus is formed by a line drawn between the *mammillary bodies* and the *posterior commissure* (Figure 14.1). The hypothalamus has a mediolateral functional organization, with separate periventricular, medial, and lateral zones (Figure 14.3). It also has an anterior–posterior regional organization, with the anterior, middle, and posterior regions bounded by key landmarks on the ventral brain surface (Figures 14.2, 14.10, 14.12, and 14.14). The *preoptic region* is also part of the hypothalamus.

Neuroendocrine control by the hypothalamus is mediated by separate *magnocellular* and *parvocellular neurosecretory systems*, which control hormone release from the posterior and anterior pituitary, respectively (Figure 14.4). Two nuclei form the magnocellular system: the magnocellular division of the *paraventricular nucleus* and the *supraoptic nucleus* (Figures 14.3 and 14.10). Magnocellular neurons in these nuclei projects their axons into the *infundibular stalk*, which connects the pituitary with the brain (Figure 14.4). Their termination site is the posterior lobe, where they release *vasopressin* and *oxytocin* directly into the systemic circulation. Separate neurons in the paraventricular and supraoptic nuclei synthesize either vasopressin or oxytocin. *Parvocellular* neurosecretory neurons (Figure 14.4B) regulate anterior lobe hormone release by secreting *releasing* or *release inhibiting hormones* (Table 14.1) into the *portal circulation* in the *median eminence* (Figure 14.5). Four hypothalamic regions contribute to the parvocellular system: anterior periventricular zone, arcuate nucleus, medial paraventricular nucleus, and medial preoptic region. Additional hypothalamic and extrahypothalamic sites project to the median eminence and release gonadotropin-releasing hormones. Both magno- and parvocellular neurons co-localize neuroactive peptides.

The other major function of the hypothalamus is control of the autonomic nervous system. There are three anatomical components of the autonomic nervous system: *sympathetic division, parasympathetic division*, and *enteric nervous system*, which is the intrinsic innervation of the gut. For both the sympathetic and the parasympathetic divisions, two neurons link the central nervous system with their target organs (Figure 14.6B): a *preganglionic neuron*, located in the central nervous system, and a *postganglionic neuron*, located in peripheral ganglia (Figure 14.7). The sympathetic division originates from the spinal cord, between the *first thoracic and third lumbar* segments (Figure 14.7). Preganglionic neurons of this division are located in the *intermediolateral nucleus* (Figure 14.16B). The parasympathetic division originates from the *brain stem* and the *sacral spinal cord*. There are four parasympathetic nuclei in the brain stem containing preganglionic neurons (Chapter 13): Edinger–Westphal nucleus, superior salivatory nucleus, inferior salivatory nucleus, and dorsal motor nucleus of the vagus. The lateral intermediate zone of the *first through third sacral* segments contains parasympathetic preganglionic neurons.

Hypothalamic control of the autonomic nervous system (Figure 14.8) originates from four regions: paraventricular nucleus, lateral hypothalamic area, dorsomedial hypothalamic nucleus, and posterior hypothalamus. The major projection is from the *paraventricular nucleus*. Two pathways transmit information from the hypothalamus to autonomic centers in the brain stem and spinal cord. The first, the *dorsal longitudinal fasciculus*, is located close to or within the gray matter of the floor of the ventricular system. This path descends only as far as the caudal brain stem and thus influences the cranial components of the parasympathetic system. The axons terminate on neurons in the *dorsal motor nucleus of the vagus* where parasympathetic preganglionic neurons are located) and the *solitary nucleus* (which is important in visceral sensory mechanisms) (Figure 14.15). The second descending hypothalamic pathway courses through the *medial forebrain bundle* (Figure 14.12), located laterally in the hypothalamus, and its caudal extension in the lateral tegmentum of the brain stem and the lateral column of the spinal cord. Disruption of this pathway produces *Horner's syndrome*. The hypothalamus also projects to other sites important in visceral sensory and motor function: parabrachial nucleus, solitary nucleus, and nucleus ambiguus.

References

Clarke, W. E. LeGros. 1938. Morphological Aspects of the Hypothalamus. In Clark, W. E. LeGros, Beattie, J., Riddoch, G., et al. The Hypothalamus: Morphological, Functional, Clinical and Surgical Aspects. Edinburgh: Oliver & Boyd, pp. 2–68.

Lowey, A. D., Saper, C. B., and Yamondis, N. D. 1978. Re-evaluation of the efferent projections of the Edinger–Westphal nucleus in the cat. Brain Res. 141:153–159.

Saper, C. B., Loewy, A. D., Swanson, L. W., et al. 1976. Direct hypothalamo-autonomic connections. Brain Res. 117:305–312.

Schmidt, R. F., and Thews, G. (eds.) 1983. Human Physiology. Berlin: Springer.

Swanson, L. W., and Kuypers, H. G. J. M. 1980. The paraventricular nucleus of the hypothalamus: Cytoarchitectonic subdivisions and organization of projections to the pituitary, dorsal vagal complex, and spinal cord as demonstrated by retrograde fluorescence double-labeling methods. J. Comp. Neurol. 1984:555–570.

Watson Jr., R. E., Hoffmann, G. E., and Wiegand, S. J. 1986. Sexually dimorphic opioid distribution in the preoptic area: Manipulation by gonadal steroids. Brain Res. 398:157–163.

Selected Readings

Appenzeller, O. 1986. Clinical Autonomic Failure: Practical Concepts. Amsterdam: Elsevier.

Gershon, M. 1981. The Enteric Nervous System. Ann. Rev. Neurosci. 4:227–272.

Kupferman, I. 1985. Hypothalamus and Limbic System I: Peptidergic Neurons, Homeostasis, and Emotional Behavior. In Kandel, E. R., and Schwartz, J. H., Principles of Neural Science. New York: Elsevier, pp. 611–625.

Kupferman, I. 1985. Hypothalamus and Limbic System II: Motivation. In Kandel, E. R., and Schwartz, J. H., Principles of Neural Science. New York: Elsevier, pp. 626–635.

Nauta, W. J. H., and Haymaker, W. 1969. Hypothalamic Nuclei and Fiber Connections. In Haymaker, W., Anderson, E., and Nauta, W. J. H., The Hypothalamus. Springfield, Ill.: Charles C. Thomas, pp. 136–209.

Silverman, A. J., Zimmerman, E. A. 1983. Magnocellular neurosecretory system. Ann. Rev. Neurosci. 6:357–380.

Swanson, L. W. 1986. Organization of mammalian neuroendocrine system. In Bloom, F. E. (ed), Intrinsic Regulatory Systems of the Brain. Bethesda, Md.: American Physiological Society, pp. 317–363.

Swanson, L. W., and Mogenson, G. J. 1981. Neural mechanisms for the functional coupling of autonomic, endocrine and somatomotor responses in adaptive behavior. Brain. Res. Rev. 3:1–34.

Swanson, L. W., and Sawchenko, P. E. 1983. Hypothalamic integration: Organization of the paraventricular and supraoptic nuclei. Ann. Rev. Neurosci. 6:269–324.

The Limbic System

15

The Limbic System

From a historical perspective, knowledge of the regional anatomy of the cerebral hemisphere has played an important role in the understanding of the anatomical substrates of emotion. In the nineteenth century, the French neurologist Pierre Paul Broca first called attention to the importance of the C-shaped structures on the medial brain surface in emotions. These structures, encircling the diencephalon, were at the border of the cerebral cortex. Hence, he termed the region *le grande lobe limbique* (*limbus* is Latin for "border"). It was not until 1937 that James Papez, a neuroanatomist at Cornell University, suggested that a complex set of interconnections among these midline structures formed an anatomical circuit for emotion, much like neural circuits for sensory or motor function. As the cortical structures were thought to be important in emotion, subcortical limbic system structures were thought to mediate their behavioral expression. A key participant in emotional reactions is the hypothalamus (Chapter 14).

In addition to its role in emotion, the limbic system has long been known to play an important role in olfaction. This is because parts of the limbic system receive a direct projection from the olfactory bulb (Chapter 8). In fact, various components of the limbic system are often referred to as the *rhinencephalon* (nose brain). Projections from the olfactory bulb are a major input to the limbic system of many mammals, for example, rodents and carnivores. In these creatures much of what is termed emotional behavior, for example, fear or sexual behavior, is under important control by olfactory cues. In higher primates, the input to limbic system structures appears to be dominated not by olfactory input but rather by connections from association areas of the cerebral cortex.

In this chapter, the various components of the limbic system are surveyed, including their three-dimensional configurations, connections, and functional organization. Later in the chapter, sections through the cerebral hemisphere are examined and the locations of the various components of the limbic system identified.

Components of the Limbic System Are Located Close to the Midline and Have a Complex Three-Dimensional Configuration

The limbic system includes regions of the cerebral hemisphere, diencephalon, and midbrain (Table 15.1) that collectively mediate emotion and the behavioral expression of emotion. This is accomplished by influencing the function of the three efferent systems: the autonomic nervous system, the somatic motor system, and pituitary hormone release. Limbic system structures also play a critical role in *learning* and *memory*. Many components of the limbic system have a complex C-shaped configuration as do components of the basal ganglia (Chapter 11). C-shaped configurations are a consequence of the extensive development of the cerebral cortex (Chapter 2). There are *three C-shaped telencephalic components of the limbic system:* (1) the limbic association cortex (Figures 15.1 and 15.2) and the corticocortical association pathway the cingulum, and (2) the hippocampal formation and its efferent pathway, the fornix (Figure 15.3). Whereas the amygdaloid complex (3) itself does not have a C-shape, one of its pathways, the stria terminalis, does (Figure 15.5).

Table 15.1   Components of the Limbic System

Major Brain Division	Structure	Component Part
Cerebral hemisphere (telencephalon)	Limbic association cortex	Orbito-frontal
		Cingulate
		Entorhinal
		Temporal pole
	Hippocampal formation	Hippocampus (Ammon's horn)
		Subiculum
		Dentate gyrus
	Amygdaloid complex	Corticomedial
		Basolateral
		Central nucleus
	Basal ganglia	Ventral striatum and ventral pallidum
	Septal nuclei	Medial and lateral septal nuclei
	Bed nucleus of the stria terminalis	
Diencephalon	Thalamus	Anterior nuclei
		Dorsomedial nucleus
	Hypothalamus	Mammillary nuclei
		Ventromedial nucleus
		Lateral hypothalamic area
	Epithalamus[a]	Habenula
Midbrain	Portions of the periaqueductal gray matter and reticular formation	

[a] In addition to the two major divisions of the diencephalon, there is a third division that includes the pineal gland, located along the midline, and the bilaterally paired habenula nuclei.

Limbic Association Cortex Is Located on the Medial Surface of the Frontal, Parietal, and Temporal Lobes

The *limbic association cortex* consists of morphologically and functionally diverse regions on four sets of gyri on the medial and orbital surfaces of the cerebral hemisphere (Figures 15.1 and 15.2): the cingulate gyrus, the parahippocampal gyrus, the medial orbital gyri, and the gyri of the temporal pole. Lesions of the limbic association cortex produce deficits in *memory* and characteristic *emotional changes*. With the exception of olfactory input, these regions of cortex receive sensory input indirectly from higher order sensory areas in the insula and temporal lobe. Limbic association areas, in turn, convey this sensory information, as well as input from association areas on the lateral surface of the parietal, temporal, and frontal lobes, to the hippocampal formation and the amygdala. Together, the *cingulate and parahippocampal gyri* form an incomplete ring

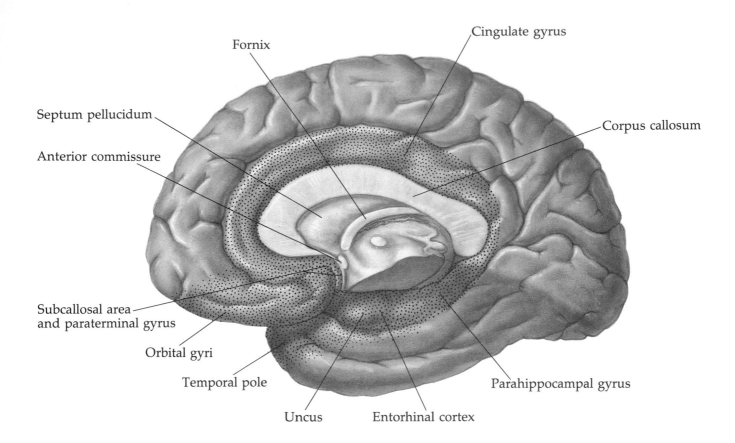

Fornix

Cingulate gyrus

Septum pellucidum

Anterior commissure

Corpus callosum

Subcallosal area
and parateminal gyrus

Orbital gyri

Temporal pole

Parahippocampal gyrus

Uncus   Entorhinal cortex

Figure 15.1 Midsagittal view of the right cerebral hemisphere, with brain stem removed. The limbic association cortex is indicated by the dotted regions.

of cortex that encircles the corpus callosum, diencephalon, and midbrain (Figures 15.1 and 15.2). Rostral to this cortical ring are the *medial orbital gyri of the frontal lobe* and the cortex of the *temporal pole*. The *cingulum* (or *cingulum bundle*) is a collection of axons that courses in the white matter deep within the cingulate and parahippocampal gyri. Cortical association fibers course in the cingulum and terminate in the parahippocampal gyrus. On the ventral brain surface (Figure 15.2), the lateral boundary of the limbic association cortex is marked by the *collateral sulcus* and its rostral extension, the *rhinal sulcus* (or fissure). These sulci also separate cortical regions of different morphologies. The cortex located lateral to the rhinal and collateral sulci is *neocortex*, with a characteristic six-layered configuration, whereas the cortex medial to these sulci is *paleocortex* and consists of fewer than six layers (Chapter 8).

The Hippocampal Formation Plays a Role in Memory Consolidation

The second C-shaped component of the limbic system is the *hippocampal formation* and its efferent pathway the *fornix* (Figure 15.3). These two structures appear to form a concentric ring, nested within the cortical limbic areas (Figures 15.1 and 15.3). The hippocampal formation is located deep to the medial surface of the temporal lobe. The first important insights into the function of the hippocampal formation were obtained by studying the behavior of patients that have had the medial temporal lobe ablated to ameliorate the symptoms of temporal lobe epilepsy. In

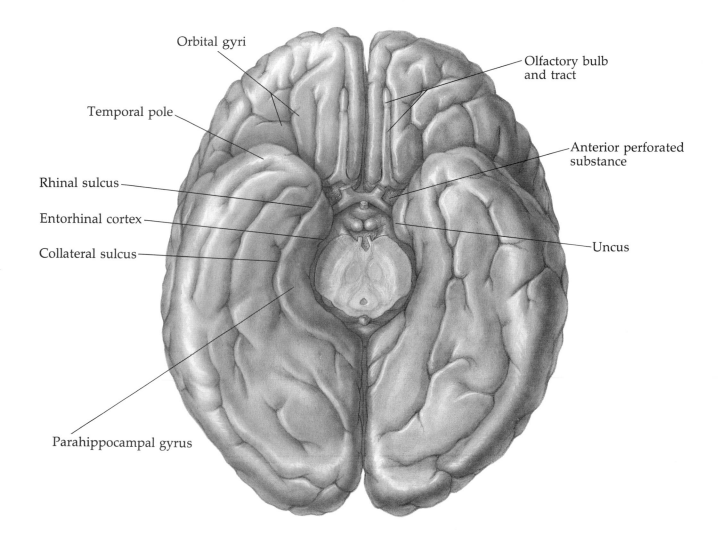

Orbital gyri

Olfactory bulb
and tract

Temporal pole

Anterior perforated
substance

Rhinal sulcus

Entorhinal cortex

Collateral sulcus

Uncus

Parahippocampal gyrus

Figure 15.2 Ventral surface of cerebral hemisphere showing key components of the limbic system as well as other basal forebrain structures.

one of the most extensively examined cases, a patient named "H.M." had the medial portion of the temporal lobes removed bilaterally. After surgery, H.M. lost the capacity for consolidating *short-term memory* into long-term memory but retained the remembrance of things before the lesion.

There are three components of the *hippocampal formation* (Figures 15.4 and 15.12A; Table 15.1): the *subiculum*, the *hippocampus* proper or Ammon's horn, and the *dentate gyrus*.[1] These three components are roughly organized as a linear sequence of strips running the rostrocaudal length of the hippocampal formation (Figure 15.4). During development (Figure 15.11; see later) these strips fold upon one another in a complex manner to assume a "jelly role" configuration. Each component of the hippocampal formation has a *laminar organization* and is termed the *archicortex* (see Figure 15.12). It should be recalled that the other types of cortex are paleocortex (for example, piriform cortex) and neocortex (for example, primary somatic sensory cortex). Parts of the hippocampal formation have

---

[1] The term *hippocampus* is sometimes used to include both Ammon's horn and the dentate gyrus.

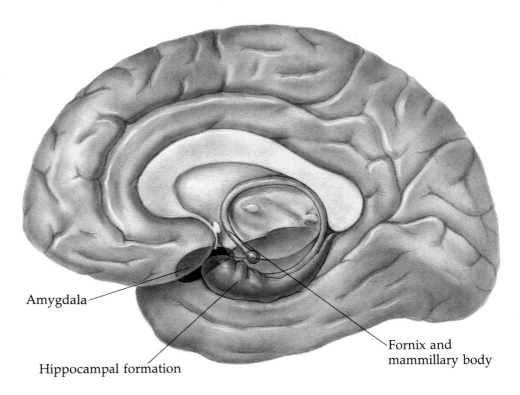

Amygdala

Hippocampal formation

Fornix and
mammillary body

Figure 15.3 Three-dimensional view of the amygdala and the hippocampal formation. The fornix, which is the output pathway of the hippocampal formation, is also illustrated as well as a target to which it projects, the mammillary body.

a layering pattern that rivals the cerebellum in its geometric regularity. Like the cerebellum, knowledge of hippocampal cytoarchitecture has facilitated an understanding of its synaptic organization as well as the intrinsic and extrinsic connectivity (see later).

The hippocampal formation receives a dense projection from the *limbic association cortex* (Figure 15.4), especially from the cingulate gyrus via the cingulum. A restricted portion of the parahippocampal gyrus, termed the *entorhinal cortex*, plays a key role in transmitting most of this information to the *hippocampal formation*. The flow of information through the hippocampal formation is largely *unidirectional*, and it forms a closed anatomical loop (see Figure 15.12B). In the simplest "through-put" circuit, input from the entorhinal cortex is directed to the dentate gyrus, which projects to the hippocampus. Intrinsic connections within the hippocampus end on cells that, in turn, project to the subiculum. The subiculum projects back to the entorhinal cortex (Figure 15.4). The hippocampus and the subiculum also have extrinsic connections (see later). Other hippocampal afferents include a cholinergic input from the *septal nuclei*, which are in the basal and medial telencephalon (Table 15.1, and see later text).

Pyramidal cells are the projection neurons of the hippocampal formation, and they are located in both the hippocampus and the subiculum; pyramidal cells of the *neocortex* are also projection neurons. (The dentate gyrus, which does not contain pyramidal cells, only projects to the hippocampus.) The pyramidal cell axons that form extrinsic connections collect on the surface of the hippocampal formation and eventually form a compact fiber bundle, the *fornix* (Figures 15.1, 15.3, and 15.4). Axons in the fornix synapse on structures in the rostral telencephalon and diencephalon. It was once thought that the hippocampus gave rise to most

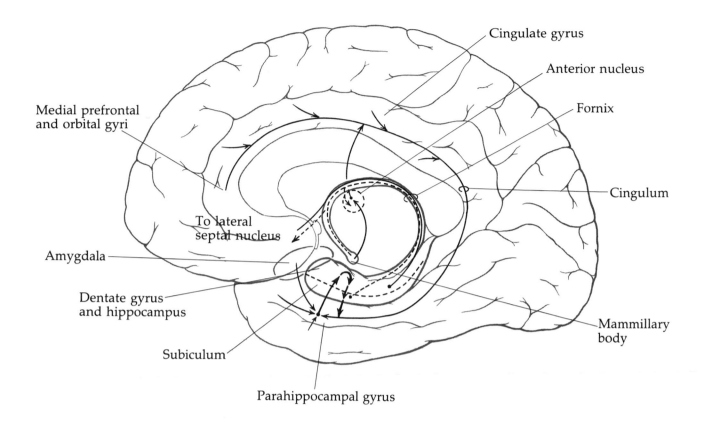

Medial prefrontal
and orbital gyri

Cingulate gyrus

Anterior nucleus

Fornix

Cingulum

To lateral
septal nucleus

Amygdala

Dentate gyrus
and hippocampus

Subiculum

Mammillary
body

Parahippocampal gyrus

of the axons in the fornix that terminate in the rostral forebrain. It has been demonstrated, however, that the *subiculum*, not the hippocampus, is the principal source of these axons (Figure 15.4). About one half of the fibers in the fornix terminate in the *mammillary* body (Figure 15.3), and these fibers originate in the subiculum. The projection from the subiculum to the mammillary body completes an anatomical loop. This is because the mammillary body projects to the *anterior nuclei of the thalamus* via the *mammillothalamic tract;* the anterior thalamic nuclei, in turn, project to the *cingulate gyrus* (Figure 15.4). It should be recalled that the hippocampal formation receives input from the cingulate gyrus. The pathway from the hippocampal formation through the hypothalamus and back to the cingulate gyrus is the circuit postulated by Papez to play an important role in emotion. It is now known that the Papez circuit is part of a complex network of bidirectional limbic system connections and many components of this network play a more important role in memory than emotions. For example, profound memory loss is a key sign of *Korsakoff's syndrome*. In this condition, which is believed to result from thiamine deficiency accompanying alcoholism, the mammillary bodies as well as portions of the medial thalamus are destroyed. The subiculum also projects, via the fornix, to other telencephalic and diencephalic structures, in particular (1) the septal nuclei, (2) directly to the anterior thalamic nuclei, (3) the *bed nucleus of the stria terminalis*, which is a point of convergence for limbic system projections to the hippocampus, and (4) the *nucleus accumbens*, a component of the ventral striatum and part of the limbic loop of the basal ganglia (Chapter 11).

Figure 15.4 Principal afferent and efferent connections of the hippocampal formation. Inputs from cingulate gyrus and other association areas of the cerebral cortex are transmitted to the hippocampal formation from the entorhinal cortex. Efferent projections from the subiculum and hippocampus to the rostral diencephalon and telencephalon are located in the fornix.

The target of the extrinsic projections from the *hippocampus* is the *septal nuclei*. Some neurons in the septal nuclei project back to the hippocampus and subiculum, forming another anatomical loop. These axons course in parallel with, but in opposite directions to, pyramidal cell axons in the *fornix*. The projection from the hippocampus, as well as that from the subiculum, to the septal nuclei is part of a pathway between limbic cortical regions, the lateral portion of the hypothalamus, and nuclei in the midbrain reticular formation. The *limbic midbrain area* is the caudal part of a complex system of connections believed to be important in the behavioral expression of emotions, such as the body's response to stress, reaction to pain, pleasure, and satiety. Septal neurons project to the midbrain reticular formation via neurons of the *lateral hypothalamus*. Neurons of the lateral hypothalamus are interspersed throughout the *medial forebrain bundle* (Chapter 14). From these midbrain regions, the actions of neurons in wide areas of the reticular formation can be modified by the limbic system.

The Amygdaloid Complex Contains Three Functional Divisions

The *amygdaloid complex* (or simply termed *amygdala*) is a collection of nuclei within the rostral temporal lobe (rostral to the hippocampal formation) and portions of the overlying cerebral cortex (Figure 15.3). Because of its developmental heritage (Chapter 2), the amygdaloid complex was once considered to be a component of the basal ganglia. However, it is clearly associated with the function of the limbic system. Although the amygdaloid complex is almond-shaped (*amygdala* is Greek for "almond"), together with one of its pathways, the *stria terminalis*, it constitutes the third C-shaped component of the limbic system (Figure 15.5). The components of the amygdaloid complex are morphologically and histochemically heterogeneous. The functions and connections of the amygdaloid complex with other brain regions are also heterogeneous. When the amygdaloid complex is destroyed, emotional reactions are profoundly altered. A characteristic feature of primate behavior after amygdaloid complex damage is that ongoing experiences lose their significance; for example, threatening objects no longer elicit fear or food is no longer distinguished from nonfood items. Electrical stimulation of the amygdaloid complex, depending on the particular site, evokes such diverse responses as visceral and defense reactions in carnivores, and in humans undergoing testing during neurosurgery, memory-like phenomena, such as *déjà vu*.

The numerous components of the amygdaloid complex can be grouped into three principal divisions. Each division has different afferent and efferent connections and therefore appears to be part of a different functional system (Figure 15.5). Collectively, these divisions link sensory systems with the motivational and autonomic regulatory systems of the hypothalamus. The *corticomedial* division (1) is reciprocally connected with olfactory structures. As a consequence it may play a role in olfactory perception (Chapter 8). The corticomedial division also projects to the *ventromedial nucleus* of the hypothalamus, predominantly via the *stria terminalis* and to a lesser extent the other efferent path of the amygdaloid complex, the *ventral amygdalofugal* pathway. The ventromedial nucleus mediates diverse functions associated with appetitive behaviors, such as

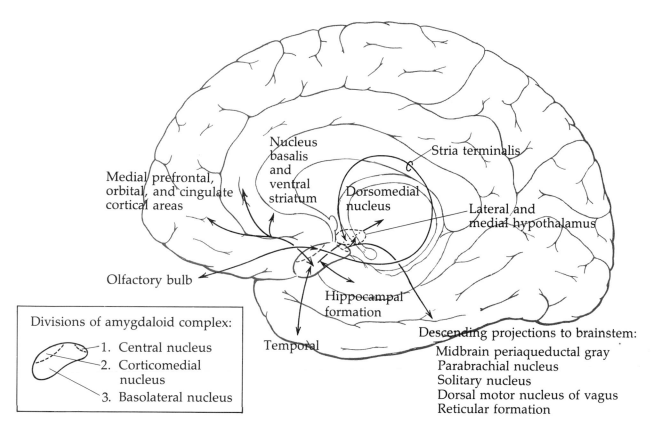

Figure 15.5 Principal connections of the amygdaloid complex. Inset shows the three divisions of the amygdaloid complex. The corticomedial nuclei have reciprocal connections with the olfactory bulb and efferent projections to the ventromedial nucleus of the hypothalamus. The basolateral nuclei are reciprocally connected with the cortex of the temporal lobe, including higher-order sensory areas and association cortex. The basolateral amygdala also projects to the dorsomedial nucleus of the thalamus and the nucleus accumbens. The central nucleus receives input from the brain stem, especially viscerosensory relay nuclei (solitary nucleus and parabrachial nucleus) and projects to the hypothalamus as well as descending projections to autonomic nuclei in the brain stem.

the consumatory phase of food intake. The corticomedial division may transmit important olfactory information to portions of the hypothalamus directly involved in food intake. The *basolateral division* (2) is reciprocally connected with the cerebral cortex, receiving input from association cortical areas and higher order sensory areas. Whereas the basolateral division also projects to the hypothalamus, the largest number of efferent connections are made with the neocortex and the thalamic relay nucleus for association areas in the frontal lobe, the *dorsal medial nucleus*. The basolateral division of the amygdaloid complex may play a key role in attaching the emotional significance to a stimulus. The *central nucleus* (3) is interconnected with the brain stem and autonomic control centers in the hypothalamus. This component of the amygdala receives viscerosensory input from the brain stem, in particular the solitary nucleus and the parabrachial nucleus (Chapter 8). It exerts important control of visceral and cardiovascular function through projections to the hypothalamus and brain stem. The various divisions of the amygdaloid complex also project to the nucleus basalis and nucleus accumbens. The nucleus accumbens is part of the ventral striatum, a component of the basal ganglia limbic loop (Chapter 11).

There Are Connections between Components of the Limbic System and the Efferent Systems

The ultimate "targets" for the limbic system include the *three effector systems for the behavioral expression of emotion*: somatic motor system, endocrine system, and autonomic nervous system. The *somatic motor system* mediates most of the overt behavioral signs of emotion. The limbic system may influence the planning of movement, rather than movement execution, through projections to the ventral striatum. The ventral striatum, in turn, influences prefrontal association cortex and perhaps the supplementary motor area.

The visceral consequences of emotion are mediated by the *endocrine system* and the *autonomic nervous system*, especially the sympathetic division (Chapter 14). Paths by which the limbic system may influence anterior and posterior lobe hormone secretion involve both direct and indirect connections with the hypothalamus. One such path, for example, involves the projection from the corticomedial division of the amygdala to the ventromedial nucleus. This nucleus, in turn, projects to a key component of the parvocellular neurosecretory system, the *arcuate nucleus* (Chapter 14). The central amygdaloid nucleus projects directly to brain stem autonomic centers (Figure 15.5), including direct projections to the *dorsal motor nucleus of the vagus nerve*. The amygdala also projects to the paraventricular nucleus of the hypothalamus, from which descending projections to parasympathetic and sympathetic nuclei originate.

In the following sections the anatomy of the limbic system is explored by examining coronal and sagittal slices through the cerebral hemisphere. The objectives are to identify the locations of the structures considered in the first part of the chapter and, using three-dimensional form, to follow the changes in the locations of these structures through progressive serial sections.

Basal Forebrain Cholinergic Systems Have Diffuse Limbic and Neocortical Projections

The nucleus accumbens and olfactory tubercle (in the region of the anterior perforated substance) can be seen in Figure 15.6. These two regions, together with the ventromedial caudate nucleus and putamen (Figure 15.6), form the ventral striatum, the input nuclei of the basal ganglia limbic loop (Chapter 11). The *septal nuclei*, consisting of separate medial and lateral subdivisions, are located in the rostral forebrain (Figures 15.6 and 15.7). They are adjacent to the *septum pellucidum*, a connective tissue structure that separates the anterior horns of the lateral ventricles of the two cerebral hemispheres. [A small portion of the septal nuclei actually

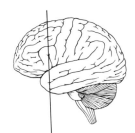

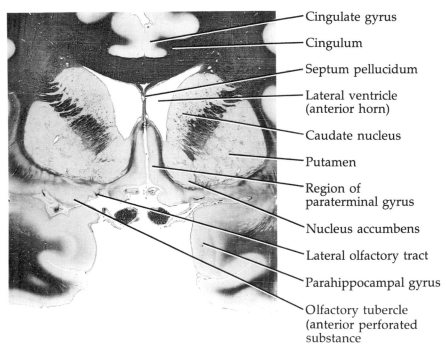

Cingulate gyrus

Cingulum

Septum pellucidum

Lateral ventricle
(anterior horn)

Caudate nucleus

Putamen

Region of
paraterminal gyrus

Nucleus accumbens

Lateral olfactory tract

Parahippocampal gyrus

Olfactory tubercle
(anterior perforated
substance

Figure 15.6   Myelin-stained coronal section through the rostral forebrain.

climb up the septum pellucidum (Figure 15.7).] The septal nuclei are continuous with the gray matter on the medial surface of the cerebral hemisphere, just rostral to the lamina terminalis (Chapter 2). This region is
termed the paraterminal gyrus. The paraterminal gyrus merges with the

Figure 15.7   Myelin-stained coronal section through the septal nuclei, nucleus
basalis, and amygdaloid complex.

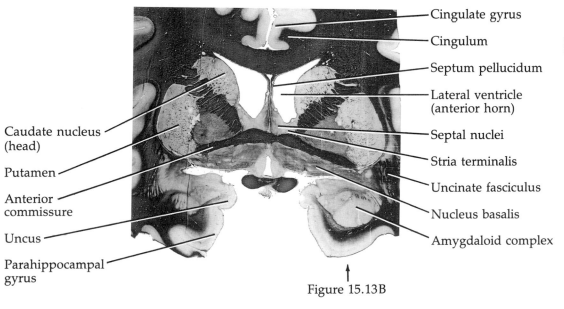

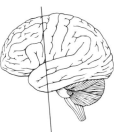

Cingulate gyrus

Cingulum

Septum pellucidum

Lateral ventricle
(anterior horn)

Septal nuclei

Stria terminalis

Uncinate fasciculus

Nucleus basalis

Amygdaloid complex

Caudate nucleus
(head)

Putamen

Anterior
commissure

Uncus

Parahippocampal
gyrus

Figure 15.13B

diagonal band of Broca (see Appendix II, Figure II.24), inferiorly, and a vestigial portion of the hippocampal formation, superiorly.[2]

Little is known of the function of this telencephalic region in humans. In a fascinating series of experiments in the early 1950s, it was discovered that laboratory rats, when given the choice of receiving either electrical stimulation of the septal nuclei or food and water, preferred the electrical stimulation! Investigators studying this behavorial phenomenon reasoned that this region is a "pleasure center," and likely to play an important role in consummatory behaviors, such as reproductive behaviors or feeding. Three different pathways carry the efferent axons from the septal nuclei: a return path to the hippocampus via the *fornix*, brain stem projections via the *medial forebrain bundle*, and a path to the *habenula* via a tract in the wall of the third ventricle, the *stria medullaris* (see Figure 15.10). The habenula, a component of the diencephalon, is located lateral and ventral to the pineal gland (see Appendix I, Figure I.7). It is part of a limbic system neural circuit to the midbrain medial dopaminergic system, the ventral tegmental area (Chapter 11), and the serotonergic system, the raphe nuclei (see Figure 11.14).

Many projection neurons of the medial septal nucleus use *acetylcholine* as their neurotransmitter and project back to the hippocampus, via the fornix. Another group of cholinergic neurons are located ventral to the septal nuclei in the *nucleus basalis*[3] (Figure 15.7). Whereas septal neurons project to the hippocampal formation, nucleus basalis neurons project to the *neocortex*. The actions of acetylcholine on *muscarinic receptors* on cortical neurons is excitatory and may facilitate cortical responses to other inputs. The medial septal nucleus and nucleus basalis, through widespread projections to archicortical and neocortical structures, respectively, may also serve to modulate cortical excitability levels.

C-Shaped Limbic System Structures Are Revealed Multiple Times in Coronal Sections through the Cerebral Hemisphere

It is important to recognize that knowledge of the three-dimensional configuration of individual limbic system structures is essential for understanding their locations in two-dimensional slices. As noted earlier in this chapter, three components of the limbic system have a C-shape: (1) the limbic association cortex, especially the cingulate and parahippocampal gyri (Figure 15.1), (2) the hippocampal formation and its output pathway, the fornix (Figure 15.3), and (3) the amygdala and one of its pathways, the stria terminalis (Figures 15.3 and 15.5). As a consequence of their C-shapes, a coronal section through the cerebral hemisphere may transect these structures twice: first *dorsally* and then *ventrally*.

---

[2] It should be recalled that early in the development of the brain, the hippocampal formation is located dorsal to the corpus callosum. Later in development, it is "dragged" into the temporal lobe. The portions of the hippocampal formations located dorsal to the corpus callosum in the mature brain are miniscule. This portion is termed the indusium gresium. The portion of the hippocampus that is located ventral to the rostrum of the corpus callosum is larger than the indusium gresium.

[3] Nucleus basalis (of Meynert) is located within the region termed the substantia innominata, which lies on the basal surface of the cerebral hemisphere.

The Cingulum Courses beneath the Cingulate and Parahippocampal Gyri

Two cortical limbic areas, the cingulate gyrus and the parahippocampal gyrus, are seen in the series of coronal sections (Figures 15.6–15.10): the cingulate gyrus is located dorsally and the parahippocampal gyrus, ventrally. The *cingulum* is located beneath the cingulate gyrus. This pathway connects regions of the orbitofrontal gyri and the cingulate gyrus with the parahippocampal gyrus. The pathway from the cingulate gyrus to the *entorhinal cortex* courses in the cingulum. Unlike the cingulum, another limbic system cortical association pathway, the *uncinate fasciculus* (Figures 15.7 and 15.8), has a more direct (i.e., not C-shaped) trajectory for interconnecting anterior portions of the temporal lobe with medial orbital gyri of the frontal lobe.

The Amygdaloid Complex Is Located in the Temporal Pole

The amygdaloid complex is located in the rostral temporal lobe deep to the parahippocampal gyrus (Figures 15.2, 15.7, and 15.8). Figures 15.7 and 15.8 transect a bulging surface landmark, the *uncus*. The uncus, which is formed by the underlying rostral hippocampal formation and the amygdaloid complex, also can be seen on Figures 15.1 and 15.2. Expanding space-occupying lesions above the cerebellar tentorium (Chapter 10), especially those of the temporal lobe, may cause the uncus to become displaced medially and ventrally. This is termed *uncal herniation*, and structures in the midbrain and the oculomotor nerves, which exit from the ventral midbrain surface, are compressed. This results in third nerve dysfunction (palsy) and even death.

As can be seen in Figures 15.7 and 15.8, the amygdala merges with the overlying cortex. This is the *corticomedial* division of the amygdala,

Figure 15.8 Myelin-stained coronal section through the column of fornix.

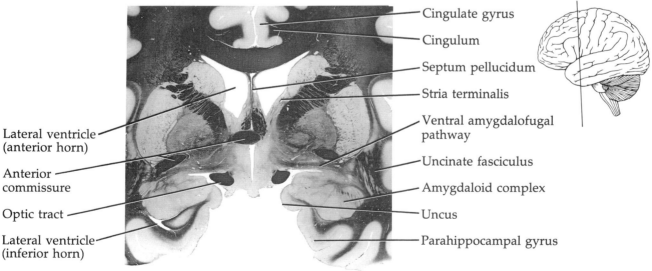

Cingulate gyrus
Cingulum
Septum pellucidum
Stria terminalis
Ventral amygdalofugal pathway
Uncinate fasciculus
Amygdaloid complex
Uncus
Parahippocampal gyrus

Lateral ventricle (anterior horn)
Anterior commissure
Optic tract
Lateral ventricle (inferior horn)

and it is this division that receives input directly from the *olfactory bulb*. Other divisions of the amygdala also receive olfactory input, however, not directly from the olfactory bulb but rather from the olfactory cortex. The parasagittal section in Figure 15.13B reveals the location of the amygdala in the temporal pole, rostral and slightly dorsal to the hippocampal formation. (Compare this with the drawing in Figure 15.3.) The laterally placed arrow in Figure 15.7 shows the approximate plane of section in Figure 15.13B.

The C-chaped efferent path from the amygdala, the *stria terminalis*, parallels the course of the lateral ventricle and the caudate nucleus. The stria terminalis is consistently located medial to the caudate nucleus in the roof of the inferior horn of the lateral ventricle and the floor of the body and anterior horn of the lateral ventricle. The stria terminalis courses in a shallow groove formed at the junction of the thalamus and the caudate nucleus, termed the *terminal sulcus*. The terminal vein runs with the stria terminalis. The terminal vein is also termed the *thalamostriate vein* because it drains portions of the thalamus and caudate nucleus. The location of the caudate nucleus and the stria terminalis in the floor of the anterior horn and body of the lateral ventricle can be followed in Figures 15.8, 15.9, and 15.10. The stria terminalis is not darkly stained because its axons are not heavily myelinated. The *bed nucleus of the stria terminalis* runs along with the tract for much of its length and is larger rostrally (for example, compare Figures 15.8 and 15.9). The other efferent path of the amygdala, the *ventral amygdalofugal pathway* (Figure 15.8) is located ventral to the anterior commissure and globus pallidus (Chapter 11). The efferent projections of more rostral portions of the amygdala tend to course in the ventral amygdalofugal pathway and more caudal regions course in the stria terminalis. The dorsomedial nucleus (Figures 15.10 and 15.13B) is one important site of termination of these efferent axons from the amygdala.

Figure 15.9 Myelin-stained coronal section through the mammillary bodies.

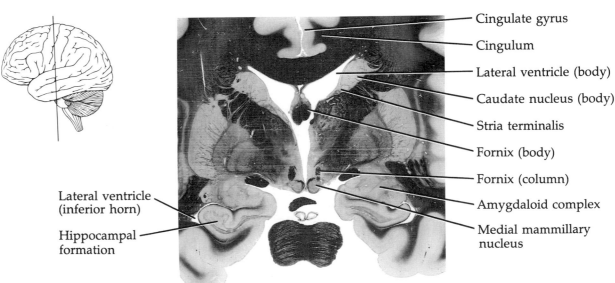

Cingulate gyrus

Cingulum

Lateral ventricle (body)

Caudate nucleus (body)

Stria terminalis

Fornix (body)

Fornix (column)

Amygdaloid complex

Medial mammillary nucleus

Lateral ventricle (inferior horn)

Hippocampal formation

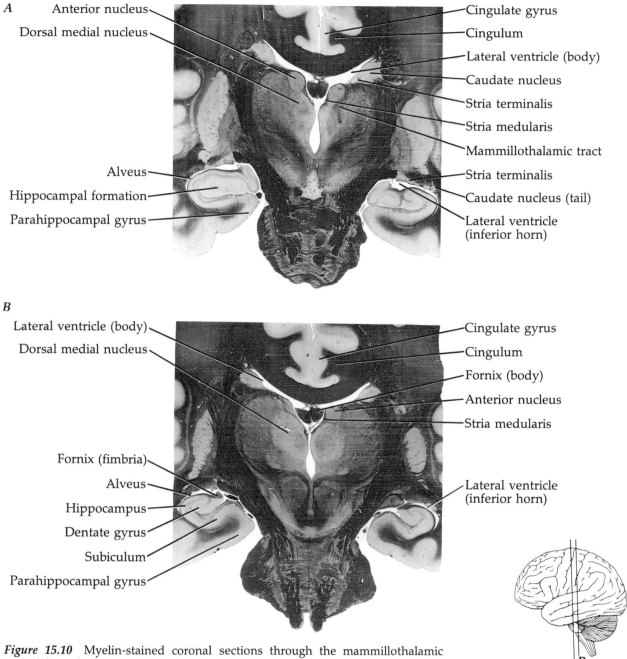

A

Anterior nucleus
Dorsal medial nucleus

Cingulate gyrus
Cingulum
Lateral ventricle (body)
Caudate nucleus
Stria terminalis
Stria medularis
Mammillothalamic tract

Alveus
Hippocampal formation
Parahippocampal gyrus

Stria terminalis
Caudate nucleus (tail)
Lateral ventricle (inferior horn)

B

Lateral ventricle (body)
Dorsal medial nucleus

Cingulate gyrus
Cingulum
Fornix (body)
Anterior nucleus
Stria medularis

Fornix (fimbria)
Alveus
Hippocampus
Dentate gyrus
Subiculum
Parahippocampal gyrus

Lateral ventricle (inferior horn)

B
A

Figure 15.10 Myelin-stained coronal sections through the mammillothalamic tract *(A)*, and through the caudal diencephalon *(B)*. In part A, the mammillo-thalamic tract is seen on right side only because the section is asymmetric.

The Hippocampal Formation Is Archicortex and Is Located beneath the Cortical Surface

Figures 15.9 and 15.10 transect the hippocampal formation; this structure is not located on the medial surface of the temporal lobe, but rather deep within the lobe. In fact, the hippocampal formation forms part of the *floor of the inferior horn of the lateral ventricle*. As noted in Chapter 2, during development, the hippocampal formation (as well as its efferent

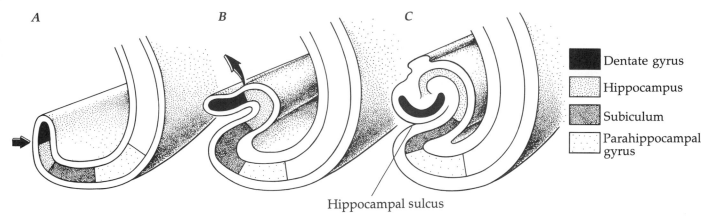

Hippocampal sulcus

Figure 15.11 Schematic of the developmental of the hippocampal formation. (Adapted from Williams, P. L., and Warwick, R. 1975. Functional Neuroanatomy of Man. Philadelphia: W.B. Saunders.)

pathway, the fornix) becomes C-chaped as a result of proliferation of the neocortex. In addition, the hippocampal formation undergoes an *infolding into the temporal lobe*, and this developmental process is illustrated in Figure 15.11. The simple sequence of the component parts of the temporal lobe, from the parahippocampal gyrus on the lateral surface to the dentate nucleus on the medial surface, becomes more complex later in development. Formation of the *hippocampal sulcus* results in apposition of the dentate gyrus and the subiculum, and there is actually fusion of the pial surfaces of these two structures.

Figure 15.12A is a Nissl-stained section through the hippocampal formation, entorhinal cortex, and ventromedial temporal lobe. A schematic diagram indicating the various divisions of the hippocampal formation and the principal circuitry is shown in Figure 15.12B. The three divisions of the hippocampal formation—the *dentate gyrus*, *hippocampus*, and *subiculum*—are illustrated. Each of the three divisions of the hippocampal formation have three principal cell layers. The three layers of the dentate gyrus are indicated in Figure 15.12A: *molecular layer* (abbreviated ML on photograph), *granule cell layer* (GL), and *polymorphic layer* (PL). The layers of the hippocampus and subiculum are similar to those of the dentate gyrus. They are marked on the schematic drawing *molecular layer*, *pyramidal cell layer* (which replaces the granule cell layer of the dentate gyrus), and *polymorphic layer*. The molecular layer in the hippocampus and subiculum contains the apical dendrites of the pyramidal cells, and, in the dentate gyrus, the apical dendrites of granule cells. Axons from various sources are also located in the molecular layer. The pyramidal cell layer contains the cell bodies of the hippocampal projection neurons, the *pyramidal cells*. The polymorphic layer contains various interneurons, including the *basket cells*, inhibitory interneurons that make powerful inhibitory synaptic contacts on pyramidal cell bodies. (A similar inhibitory interneuron is located in the cerebellar cortex. It makes powerful inhibitory synapses on Purkinje cells—see Chapter 10.) The molecular layer of the hippocampal formation is analogous to layer I of the neocortex and the pyramidal cell and polymorphic layers are analogous to the cellular layers of the neocortex (II–VI).

A

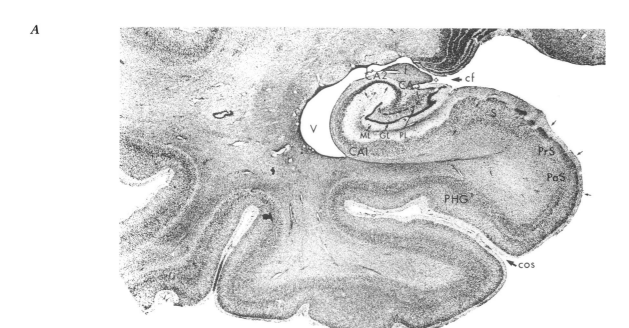

B

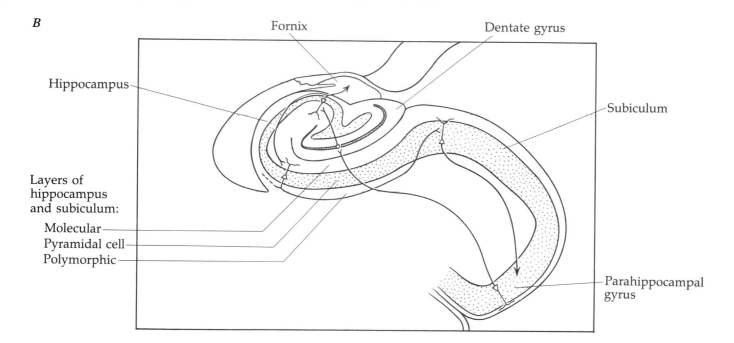

Figure 15.12 *A.* Nissl-stained transverse section of human hippocampal formation, parahippocampal gyrus, and ventral temporal lobe. *B.* Schematic diagram
of the layers of the hippocampus and subiculum and the circuitry of the hippocampal formation. (*A.* Courtesy of Dr. David Amaral, Salk Institute; *B.* Adapted
from Zola-Morgan, S., Squire, L. R., and Amaral, D. G. 1986. Human amnesia
and medial temporal lobe region: Enduring memory impairment following a bilateral lesion limited to field CA1 of the hippocampus. J. Neurosci. 6:2950–2967.)

With this background information about hippocampal formation cytoarchitecture, we are in a better position to consider hippocampal circuitry. As we have seen earlier, the entorhinal cortex (Figure 15.4) provides the major input to the hippocampal formation. Two projection pathways are distinguished: the perforant path and the alvear path. The *perforant path* is illustrated in the schematic diagram (Figure 15.12B). Axons of the perforant path course through the region of fusion previously described and synapse on the dendrites of granule cells of the dentate gyrus and hippocampal pyramidal cells (Figure 15.12B).[4] The *alvear path* courses along the ventricular surface in the *alveus* (Figure 15.10B). The ventricular surface of the hippocampal formation contains myelinated axons of the hippocampal efferents (see later) as well as afferents.

The cytoarchitectonic divisions of the hippocampus—abbreviated CA for cornus ammonis, or Ammon's horn—are also indicated in Figure 15.12. The CA1, CA2, and CA3 regions of the hippocampus are separate processing stages in a sequence of intrinsic connections. As described earlier, the flow of information through the hippocampal formation is largely unidirectional. This circuit is indicated on the schematic diagram in Figure 15.12B. Pyramidal cells of the entorhinal cortex send their axons to the dentate gyrus to synapse on granule cells. Granule cell axons, termed *mossy fibers*, **synapse** on pyramidal cells of the CA3 region of the hippocampal formation, which in turn send their axons (termed the *Schaefer collaterals*) to pyramidal cells of the CA1 region. (These axon collaterals spare the CA2 region.) The subiculum receives the next projection in the sequence, from the CA1 region, and it projects back to the entorhinal cortex. This forms a closed anatomical loop. The pyramidal cells of the hippocampal formation also send their axons to a variety of forebrain structures. The major extrinsic projections arise from the subiculum. The axons course in the fornix and terminate in the mammillary body, lateral septal nucleus, anterior thalamic nuclei, and the nucleus accumbens. The subiculum also projects to the amygdala. The hippocampus also projects to the lateral septal nucleus. An important goal is to understand the nature of the processing carried out by these circuits.

A Sagittal Cut through the Mammillary Bodies Reveals the Fornix and Mammillothalamic Tract

Structures that have a C-shape are oriented approximately in the sagittal plane. The sagittal section in Figure 15.13A is located close to the midline and it transects the fornix, although not through its entire length. The sagittal section in Figure 15.13B cuts through the long axis of the hippocampal formation. The fornix contains four anatomical divisions (Figure 15.3); following the C-shape of the fornix from caudal to rostral, they are the *fimbria*, the *crus*, the *body*, and the *column*. Axons of the alveus (Figure 15.13B) collect on the medial side of the hippocampal formation to form the fimbria. The body of the fornix and the columns can be seen in Figure 15.13A. The column of the fornix can be identified descending *caudal to the anterior commissure* to terminate in the *mammillary body*; this

---

[4] Portions of the diencephalon and telencephalon fuse and the descending cortical axons in the internal capsule pierce through this line of fusion (Chapter 2).

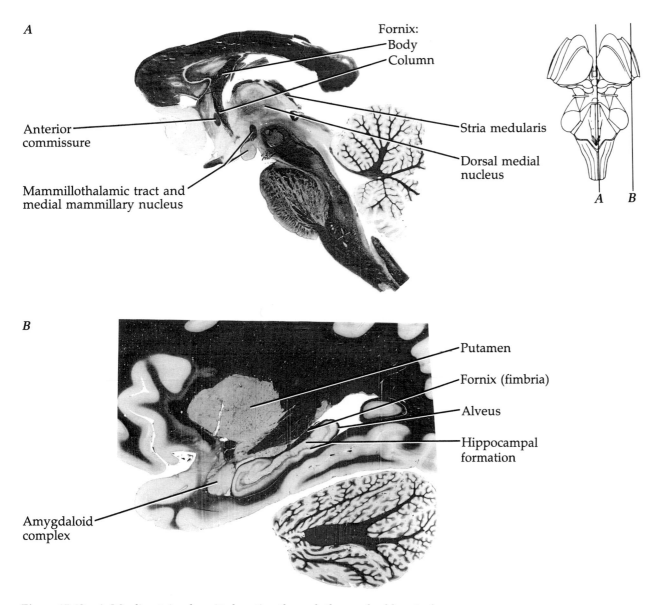

Figure 15.13 *A.* Myelin-stained sagittal section through the cerebral hemisphere, diencephalon, and brain stem close to midline. *B.* A parasagittal section through the amygdaloid complex and hippocampal formation.

is the *postcommissural fornix*. Axons of the *mammillothalamic tract* can be seen leaving the mammillary body.[5] These axons are coursing toward the *anterior thalamic nuclei*, which can be seen in Figure 15.10A along with a portion of the mammillothalamic tract.

Fibers of the fornix also terminate in locations other than the mammillary bodies. Other fibers of the postcommissural fornix terminate directly in the anterior thalamic nuclei. There is also a component of the

---

[5] Fasciculus mammillaris princeps is the name given to the axons as they emerge from the mammillary body. In addition to axons of the mammillothalamic tract, there are also axons that descend to the midbrain and rostral pontine reticular formation.

fornix rostral to the anterior commissure, the *precommissural fornix*, which is smaller than the postcommissural portion and courses away from the midline. It cannot be seen in this section. The precommissural fornix, which contains the axons from both the subiculum and hippocampus, terminates in the lateral septal nucleus. A portion of the *stria medullaris*, which has a rostrocaudal course, is also revealed in this section (Figure 15.13A).

Summary

The limbic system encompasses a set of structures located predominantly on the *medial surface* of the cerebral hemisphere (Figures 15.1 and 15.2).The diverse functions of the limbic system include important roles in *memory, emotion, control of visceral functions*, and *olfaction*. Many of the structures have a *C-shaped configuration*. There are three C-shaped components to the limbic system (Figures 15.1–15.4): (1) *limbic cortical association areas* and the *cingulum*, (2) *hippocampal* formation and the *fornix*, and (3) *amygdaloid complex* and the *stria terminalis*. The limbic cortical areas include (Figures 15.1 and 15.2): the *medial orbital gyri* of the frontal lobe, the *cingulate gyrus* in the frontal and parietal lobes, the *parahippocampal gyrus* in the temporal lobe, and the cortex of the *temporal pole*. The limbic cortical areas receive sensory input from higher order sensory areas in the temporal lobe and other input from the *prefrontal association cortex* and the *association area on the lateral surface of the parietal lobe*. The two principal pathways carrying cortical association axons to and from other limbic system structures are the *cingulum* (beneath the cingulate gyrus, Figure 15.1), which is also C-shaped, and the *uncinate fasciculus* (Figure 15.8). Limbic association cortex has a different cytoarchitecture compared with other cortical regions. The cortex on the external surface of the parahippocampal gyrus, medial to the *collateral* and *rhinal sulci* (Figure 15.2), has fewer than six cell layers and is termed *paleocortex* (Figure 15.12). Lateral to these sulci, the cortex has at least six layers (*neocortex*).

The *hippocampal formation* (Figure 15.3) includes three cytoarchitectonically distinct subdivisions (Figures 15.4 and 15.12): the *dentate gyrus*, the *hippocampus*, and the *subiculum*. Collectively these regions constitute the *archicortex*, primitive three-layered cortex. *Memory disorders* are a characteristic feature of hippocampal formation lesions. The limbic association cortex provides the major input to the hippocampal formation. The *entorhinal cortex*, a specific portion of the rostral parahippocampal gyrus, projects directly to the hippocampal formation (Figure 15.4) via the *perforant path* and the *alvear path*. Other portions of the limbic association cortex influence the hippocampal formation *indirectly*, via the entorhinal cortex. Hippocampal efferents originate predominantly from the subiculum and to a lesser extent from the hippocampus proper; the dentate gyrus projects to the hippocampus only. The major hippocampal output path is the fornix, which has four component parts, from caudal and inferior to rostral (Figures 15.4 and 15.13): *fimbria, crus, body*, and *column*. Most of the axons in the fornix are the axons of *pyramidal cells* of the *subiculum*, and they synapse in the *mammillary body* (Figures 15.3, 15.9, and 15.13A). These axons course in the *postcommissural fornix* (Figure 15.13A). The projection to the mammillary body is part of an anatomical loop (*Papez's circuit*): the mammillary bodies project, via the *mammillothalamic tract* (Figures 15.9 and 15.13A), to the *anterior thalamic nuclei* (Figure 15.10A), which in turn project to the *cingulate gyrus* (Figures 15.1, 15.6–15.10). The hippocampus projects, via the *precommissural* fornix, to the *lateral septal nucleus*. The subiculum also projects to the anterior thalamic nuclei and parahippocampal gyrus directly.

There are three major nuclear divisions of the amygdaloid complex (Figure 15.3) which collectively are involved in *emotion*, control of *visceral function*, and *olfaction* (Figure 15.5). The *corticomedial division* (1) receives direct olfactory input. This division may play a role in appetitive behaviors through its projection to the *ventromedial nucleus* of the hypothalamus. The *basolateral division* (2) is reciprocally connected with the *cerebral cortex*. Projections of the basolateral division to the prefrontal association cortex and the ventral striatum may participate in the planning of movements. The *central nucleus* (3) is reciprocally connected with *visceral sensory* and *visceral motor nuclei* of the brain stem. The amygdaloid complex has two output pathways: (1) the *stria terminalis* (Figures 15.5 and 15.10), which is C-shaped, carries the efferent projection from the corticomedial division, and (2) the *ventral amygdalofugal pathway* (Figure 15.7) carries the efferents from the *central nucleus*, which descend to the *brain stem*, and those from the *basolateral nucleus* to the *hypothalamus* and *thalamus*, especially those to the *dorsal medial nucleus* (Figure 15.10). ■

References

Andy, O. J., and Stephan, H. 1968. The septum of the human brain. J. Comp. Neurol. 133:383–410.

Carlsen, J., and Heimer, L. 1988. The basolateral amygdaloid complex as a cortical-like structure. Brain Res. 441:377–380.

Carpenter, M. B., and Sutin, J. 1983. Human Neuroanatomy. Baltimore: Williams & Wilkins.

Hedren, J. C., Strumble, R. G., Whitehouse, P. J., et al. 1984. Topography of the magnocellular basal forebrain system in the human brain. J. Neuropath. Expt. Neurol. 43:1–21.

Levitt, P. 1984. A monoclonal antibody to limbic system neurons. Science 223:299–301.

Millhouse, O. E., and DeOlmos, J. 1983. Neuronal configurations in lateral and basolateral amygdala. Neurosci. 10:1269–1300.

Nauta, W. J. H., and Haymaker, W. 1969. Hypothalamic nuclei and fiber connections. In Haymaker, W., Anderson, E., and Nauta, W. J. H., The Hypothalamus. Springfield, Ill.: Charles C. Thomas, pp. 136–209.

Nieuwenhuys, R., Voogd, J., and van Huijzen, Chr. 1988. The Human Central Nervous System: A Synopsis and Atlas, Third Edition. Berlin: Springer-Verlag.

Papez, J. W. 1937. A proposed mechanism of emotion. Arch. Neurol. Psych. 38:725–743.

Price, J. L., and Amaral, D. G. 1981. An autoradiographic study of the projections of the central nucleus of the monkey amygdala. J. Neurosci. 1:1242–1259.

Williams, P. L., and Warwick, R. 1975. Functional Neuroanatomy of Man. Philadelphia: W.B. Saunders.

Zola-Morgan, S., Squire, L. R., and Amaral, D. G. 1986. Human amnesia and the medial temporal lobe region: Enduring memory impairment following a bilateral lesion limited to field CA1 of the hippocampus. J. Neurosci. 6:2950–2967.

Selected Readings

Amaral, D. G. 1987. Memory: Anatomical organization of candidate brain regions. In Plum, F. (ed.), Handbook of Physiology. Section 1: The Nervous System. Vol. V. Higher Functions of the Brain. Bethesda, Md.: American Physiological Society, pp. 211–294.

Kupferman, I. 1985. Hypothalamus and Limbic System I: Peptidergic Neurons, Homeostasis, and Emotional Behavior. In Kandel, E. R., and Schwartz, J. H., Principles of Neural Science. New York: Elsevier, pp. 611–625.

Kupferman, I. 1985. Hypothalamus and Limbic System II: Motivation. In Kandel, E. R., and Schwartz, J. H., Principles of Neural Science. New York: Elsevier, pp. 626–635.

Swanson, L. W., and Mogenson, G. J. 1981. Neural mechanisms for the functional coupling of autonomic, endocrine and somatomotor responses in adaptive behavior. Brain. Res. Rev. 3:1–34.

Price, J. L., Russchen, F. T., and Amaral, D. G. 1987. The Limbic Region. II: The amygdaloid complex. In Björklund, A., Hökfelt, T., and Swanson, L. W. (eds.), Handbook of Chemical Neuroanatomy, Vol. 5. Integrated Systems of the CNS, Part I. New York: Elsevier, pp. 279–388.

Atlas of Surface Topography of the Central Nervous System

APPENDIX I

The surface topography atlas is a collection of drawings of the brain and rostral spinal cord. The various views are based on specimens and brain models. Key features are labeled on an accompanying line drawing of each view.

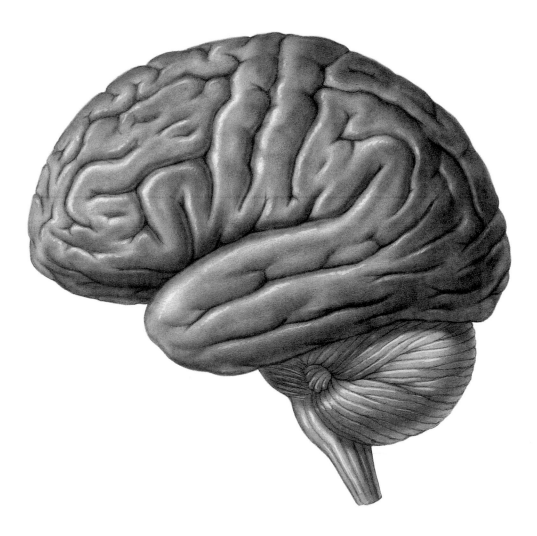

Figure I.1 Lateral surface of the cerebral hemisphere, brain stem, cerebellum, and rostral spinal cord.

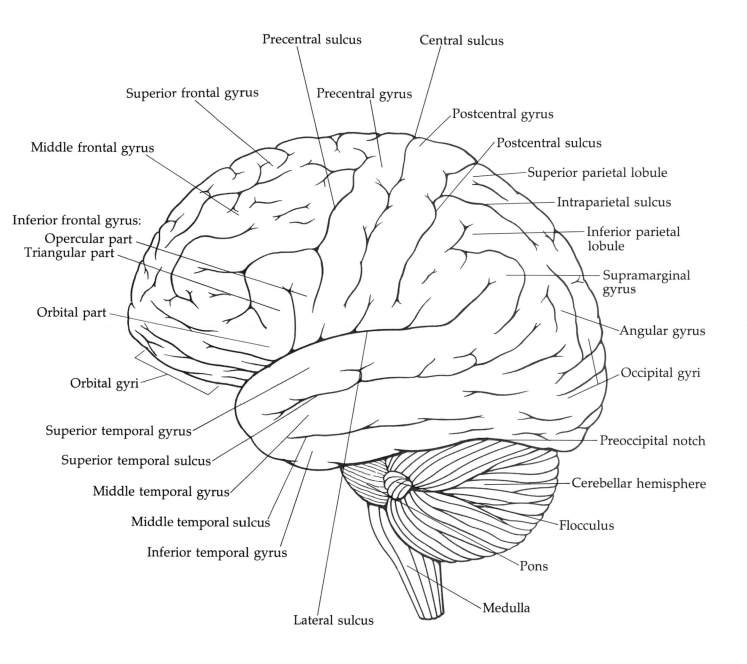

Precentral sulcus

Central sulcus

Superior frontal gyrus

Precentral gyrus

Postcentral gyrus

Middle frontal gyrus

Postcentral sulcus

Superior parietal lobule

Intraparietal sulcus

Inferior frontal gyrus:

Inferior parietal lobule

Opercular part

Triangular part

Supramarginal gyrus

Orbital part

Angular gyrus

Orbital gyri

Occipital gyri

Superior temporal gyrus

Preoccipital notch

Superior temporal sulcus

Cerebellar hemisphere

Middle temporal gyrus

Flocculus

Middle temporal sulcus

Inferior temporal gyrus

Pons

Medulla

Lateral sulcus

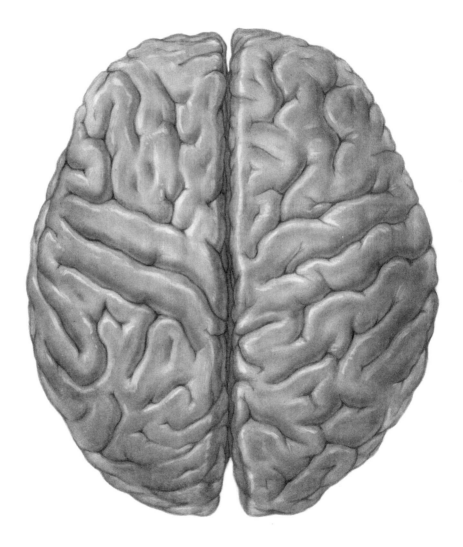

Figure I.2 Superior surface of the cerebral hemisphere.

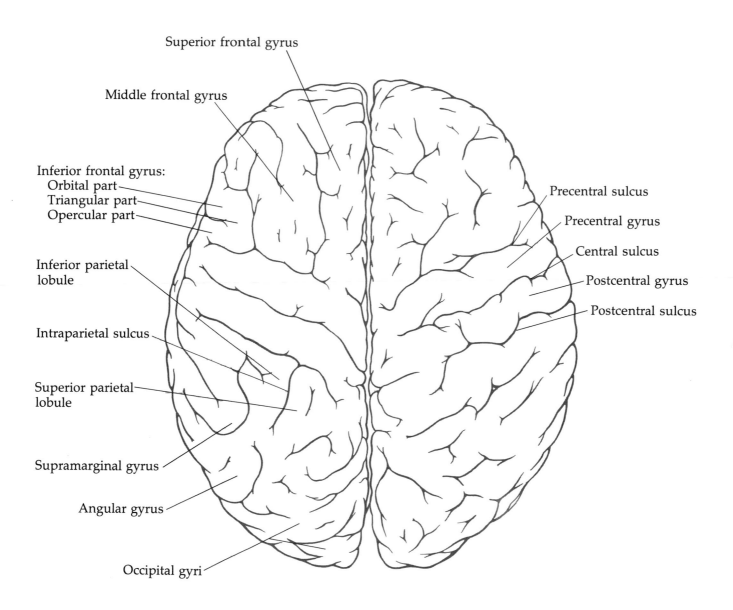

Superior frontal gyrus

Middle frontal gyrus

Inferior frontal gyrus:
Orbital part
Triangular part
Opercular part

Inferior parietal
lobule

Intraparietal sulcus

Superior parietal
lobule

Supramarginal gyrus

Angular gyrus

Occipital gyri

Precentral sulcus

Precentral gyrus

Central sulcus

Postcentral gyrus

Postcentral sulcus

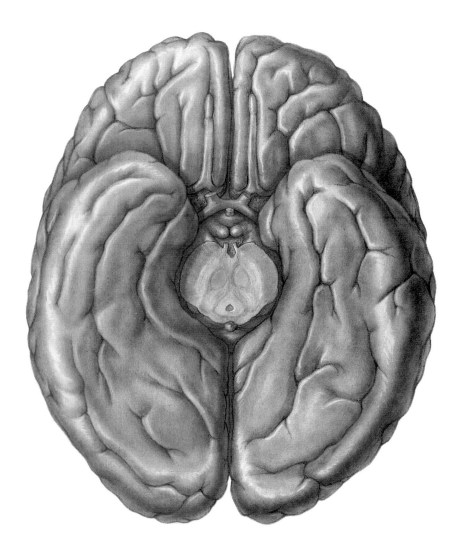

Figure I.3 Inferior surface of the cerebral hemisphere and diencephalon. The brain stem is transected at the rostral midbrain.

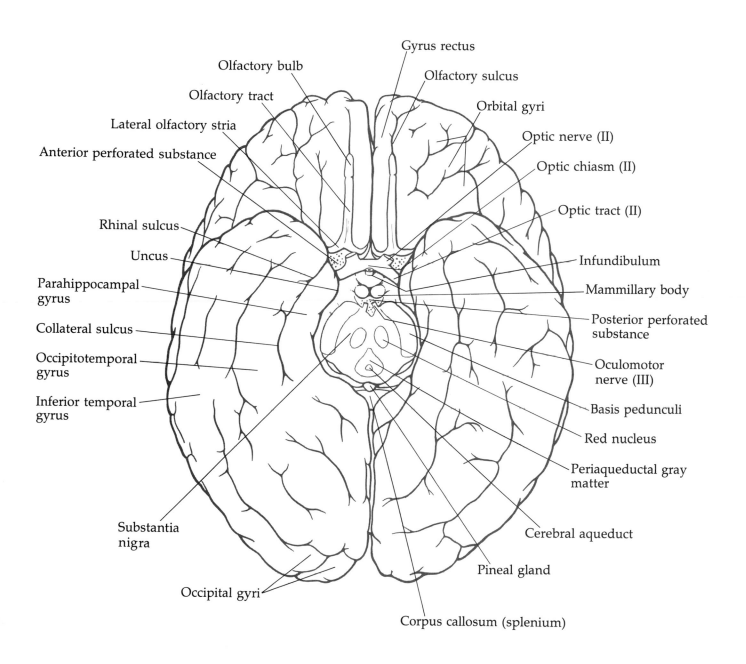

Gyrus rectus

Olfactory bulb

Olfactory sulcus

Olfactory tract

Orbital gyri

Lateral olfactory stria

Optic nerve (II)

Anterior perforated substance

Optic chiasm (II)

Optic tract (II)

Rhinal sulcus

Infundibulum

Uncus

Mammillary body

Parahippocampal gyrus

Posterior perforated substance

Collateral sulcus

Oculomotor nerve (III)

Occipitotemporal gyrus

Basis pedunculi

Inferior temporal gyrus

Red nucleus

Periaqueductal gray matter

Substantia nigra

Cerebral aqueduct

Occipital gyri

Pineal gland

Corpus callosum (splenium)

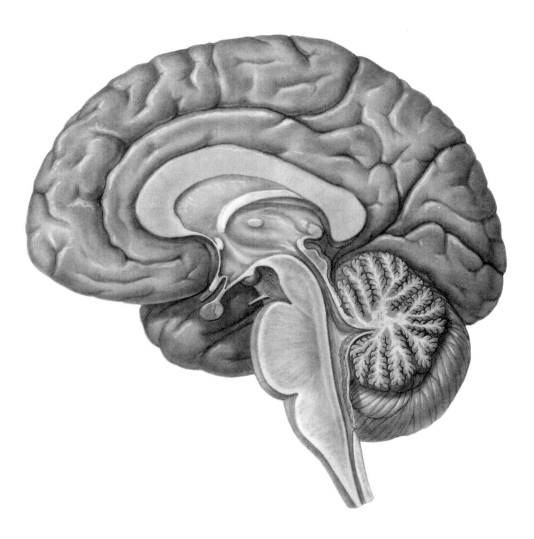

Figure I.4 Medial surface of the cerebral hemisphere and midsagittal section through the diencephalon, brain stem, cerebellum, and rostral spinal cord.

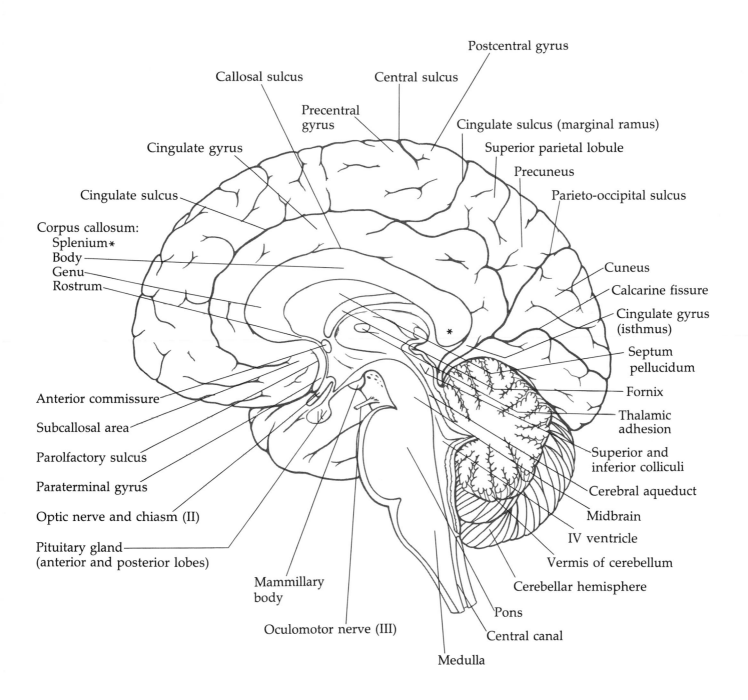

Postcentral gyrus

Callosal sulcus Central sulcus

Precentral gyrus

Cingulate sulcus (marginal ramus)

Cingulate gyrus

Superior parietal lobule

Precuneus

Cingulate sulcus

Parieto-occipital sulcus

Corpus callosum:
Splenium*
Body
Genu
Rostrum

Cuneus

Calcarine fissure

Cingulate gyrus
(isthmus)

Septum
pellucidum

Fornix

Anterior commissure

Thalamic
adhesion

Subcallosal area

Parolfactory sulcus

Superior and
inferior colliculi

Paraterminal gyrus

Cerebral aqueduct

Optic nerve and chiasm (II)

Midbrain

IV ventricle

Pituitary gland
(anterior and posterior lobes)

Vermis of cerebellum

Cerebellar hemisphere

Mammillary
body

Pons

Oculomotor nerve (III)

Central canal

Medulla

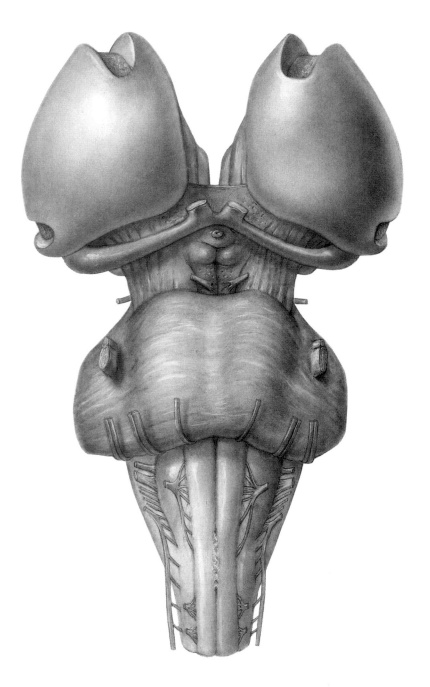

Figure I.5 Ventral surface of the brain stem and rostral spinal cord. The striatum and diencephalon are also shown.

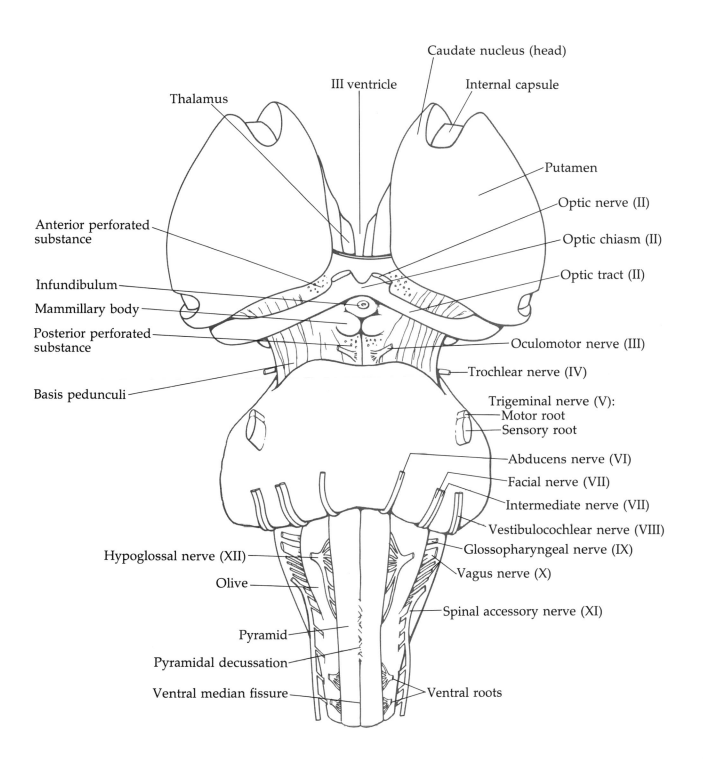

Caudate nucleus (head)

III ventricle

Internal capsule

Thalamus

Putamen

Optic nerve (II)

Anterior perforated substance

Optic chiasm (II)

Optic tract (II)

Infundibulum

Mammillary body

Oculomotor nerve (III)

Posterior perforated substance

Trochlear nerve (IV)

Trigeminal nerve (V):
Motor root
Sensory root

Basis pedunculi

Abducens nerve (VI)

Facial nerve (VII)

Intermediate nerve (VII)

Vestibulocochlear nerve (VIII)

Glossopharyngeal nerve (IX)

Hypoglossal nerve (XII)

Vagus nerve (X)

Olive

Spinal accessory nerve (XI)

Pyramid

Pyramidal decussation

Ventral median fissure

Ventral roots

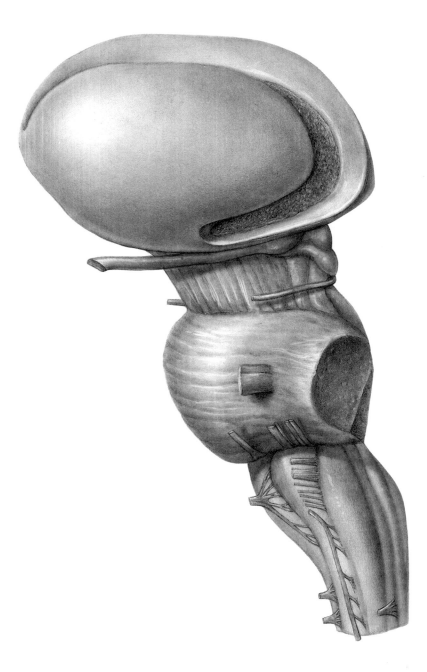

Figure I.6   Lateral surface of the brain stem and rostral spinal cord. The striatum and diencephalon are also shown.

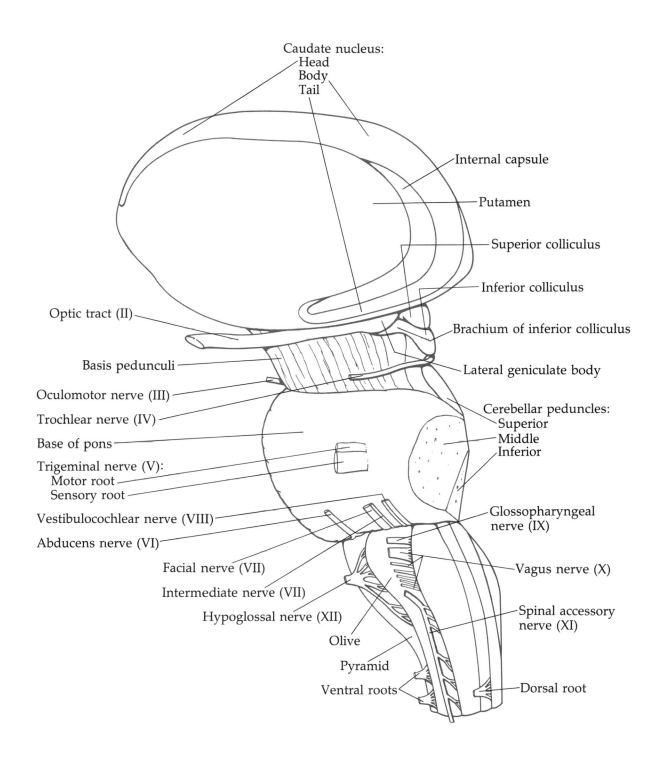

Caudate nucleus:
Head
Body
Tail

Internal capsule

Putamen

Superior colliculus

Inferior colliculus

Optic tract (II)

Brachium of inferior colliculus

Basis pedunculi

Lateral geniculate body

Oculomotor nerve (III)

Cerebellar peduncles:
Superior
Middle
Inferior

Trochlear nerve (IV)

Base of pons

Trigeminal nerve (V):
Motor root
Sensory root

Vestibulocochlear nerve (VIII)

Glossopharyngeal
nerve (IX)

Abducens nerve (VI)

Vagus nerve (X)

Facial nerve (VII)

Intermediate nerve (VII)

Spinal accessory
nerve (XI)

Hypoglossal nerve (XII)

Olive

Pyramid

Ventral roots

Dorsal root

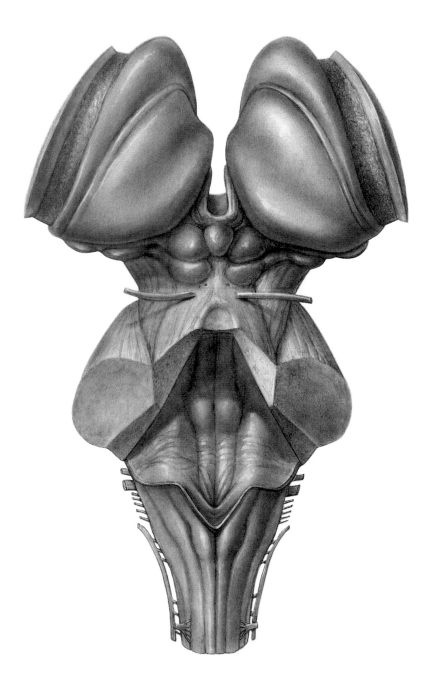

Figure I.7 Dorsal surface of the brain stem and rostral spinal cord. The striatum and diencephalon are also shown. The cerebellum was removed to reveal the structure of the floor of the fourth ventricle.

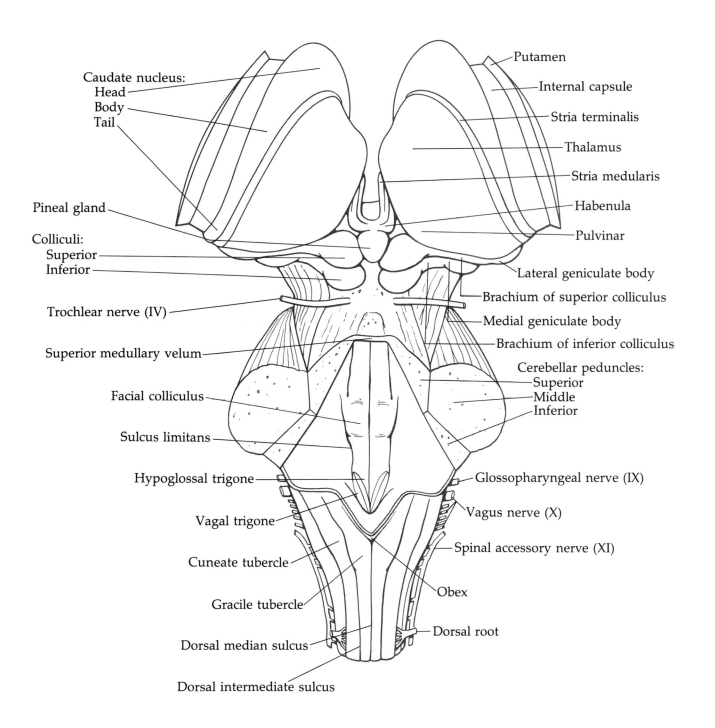

Caudate nucleus:
Head
Body
Tail

Putamen

Internal capsule

Stria terminalis

Thalamus

Stria medularis

Pineal gland

Habenula

Colliculi:
Superior
Inferior

Pulvinar

Lateral geniculate body

Brachium of superior colliculus

Trochlear nerve (IV)

Medial geniculate body

Superior medullary velum

Brachium of inferior colliculus

Cerebellar peduncles:
Superior
Middle
Inferior

Facial colliculus

Sulcus limitans

Hypoglossal trigone

Glossopharyngeal nerve (IX)

Vagus nerve (X)

Vagal trigone

Spinal accessory nerve (XI)

Cuneate tubercle

Gracile tubercle

Obex

Dorsal root

Dorsal median sulcus

Dorsal intermediate sulcus

References

Carpenter, M. B., and Sutin, J. 1983. Human Neuroanatomy. Baltimore: Williams & Wilkins.

Crosby, E. C., Humphrey, T., and Lauer, E. W. 1962. Correlative Anatomy of the Nervous System. New York: Macmillan.

Ferner, H., and Staubesand, J. 1983. Sobotta Atlas of Human Anatomy. Baltimore: Urban & Schwartzenberg.

Nieuwenhuys, R., Voogd, J., and van Huijzen, Chr. 1981. The Human Central Nervous System. Berlin: Springer-Verlag.

Williams, P. L., and Warwick, R. 1975. Functional Neuroanatomy of Man. Philadelphia: Saunders.

Atlas of Myelin-Stained Sections through the Central Nervous System

APPENDIX II

The atlas of myelin-stained sections through the central nervous system is in three planes: *transverse, horizontal,* and *sagittal.* (See Figure 1.13 for schematic views of these planes of section.) Transverse sections through the cerebral hemispheres and diencephalon are termed *coronal* sections because they are approximately parallel to the coronal suture. These sections also cut the brain stem, but *parallel to its long axis.* In addition, there are three sections cut in planes oblique to the transverse and horizontal sections.

In this atlas, each level through the central nervous system is printed without labeled structures as well as with labels on an accompanying photograph (printed at reduced contrast to preserve the essence of the structure). Typically, the border of a structure is indicated either when the structure's location is extremely important for understanding the functional consequences of brain trauma, or the structure is clearly depicted on the section and it is didactically important to emphasize the border. Axons of cranial nerves and primary afferent fibers are indicated by bold lines to distinguish them from the other fibers.

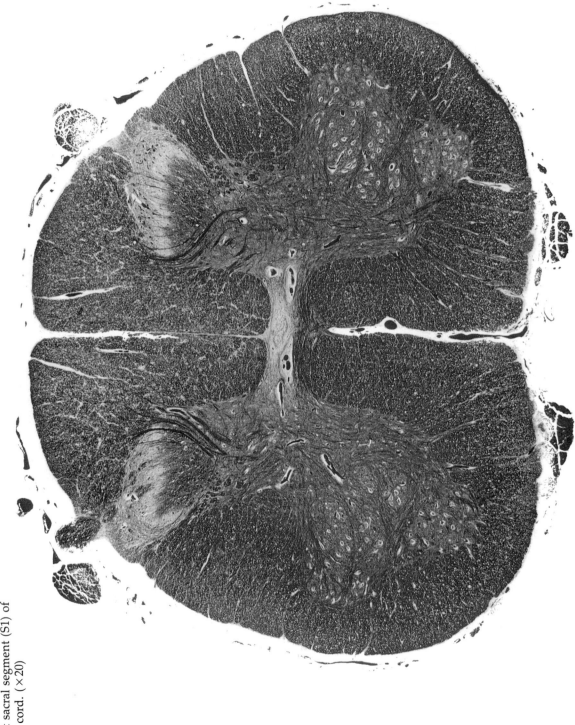

Figure II.1 Transverse section of the first sacral segment (S1) of the spinal cord. (×20)

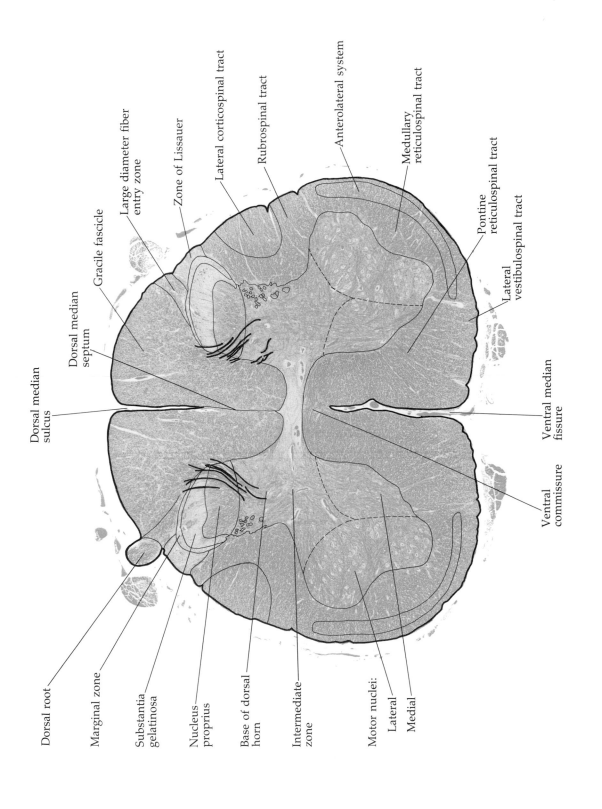

Dorsal median sulcus

Dorsal median septum

Gracile fascicle

Large diameter fiber entry zone

Zone of Lissauer

Lateral corticospinal tract

Rubrospinal tract

Anterolateral system

Medullary reticulospinal tract

Pontine reticulospinal tract

Lateral vestibulospinal tract

Ventral median fissure

Ventral commissure

Dorsal root

Marginal zone

Substantia gelatinosa

Nucleus proprius

Base of dorsal horn

Intermediate zone

Motor nuclei:

Lateral

Medial

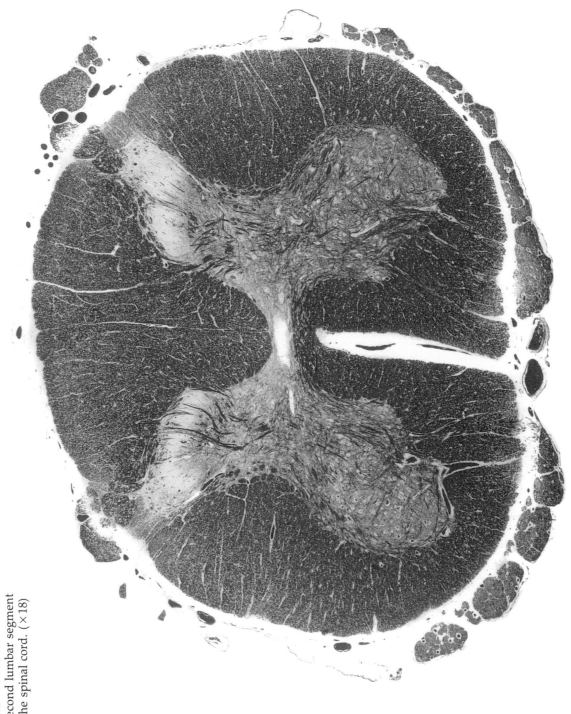

Figure II.2 Transverse section
of the second lumbar segment
(L2) of the spinal cord. (×18)

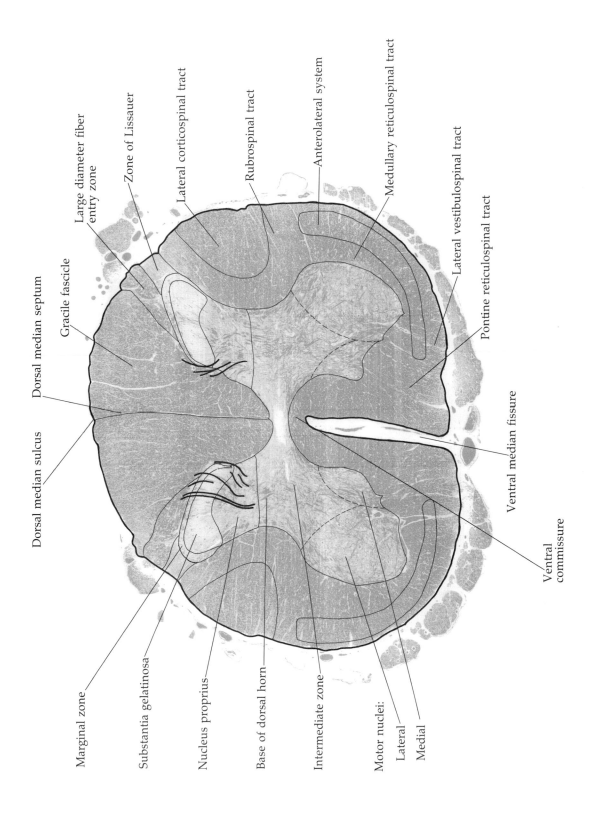

Dorsal median sulcus

Dorsal median septum

Gracile fascicle

Large diameter fiber entry zone

Zone of Lissauer

Lateral corticospinal tract

Rubrospinal tract

Anterolateral system

Medullary reticulospinal tract

Lateral vestibulospinal tract

Pontine reticulospinal tract

Ventral median fissure

Ventral commissure

Marginal zone

Substantia gelatinosa

Nucleus proprius

Base of dorsal horn

Intermediate zone

Motor nuclei:

Lateral

Medial

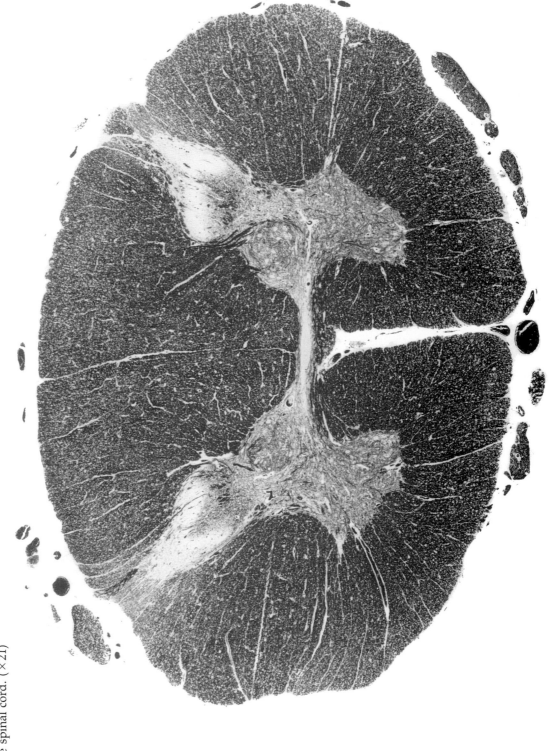

Figure II.3 Transverse section of the first lumbar segment (L1) of the spinal cord. (×21)

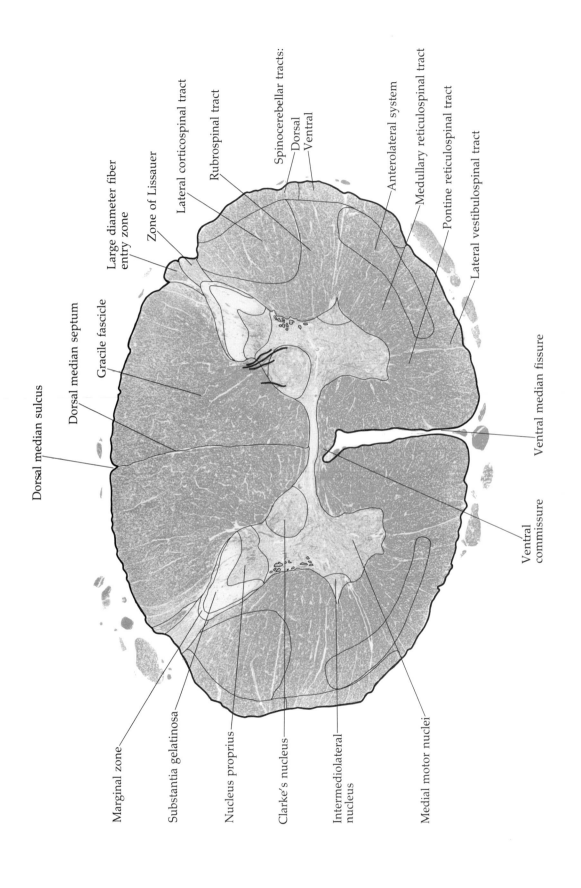

Dorsal median sulcus

Dorsal median septum

Gracile fascicle

Large diameter fiber entry zone

Zone of Lissauer

Lateral corticospinal tract

Rubrospinal tract

Spinocerebellar tracts:
Dorsal
Ventral

Anterolateral system

Medullary reticulospinal tract

Pontine reticulospinal tract

Lateral vestibulospinal tract

Ventral median fissure

Ventral commissure

Medial motor nuclei

Intermediolateral nucleus

Clarke's nucleus

Nucleus proprius

Substantia gelatinosa

Marginal zone

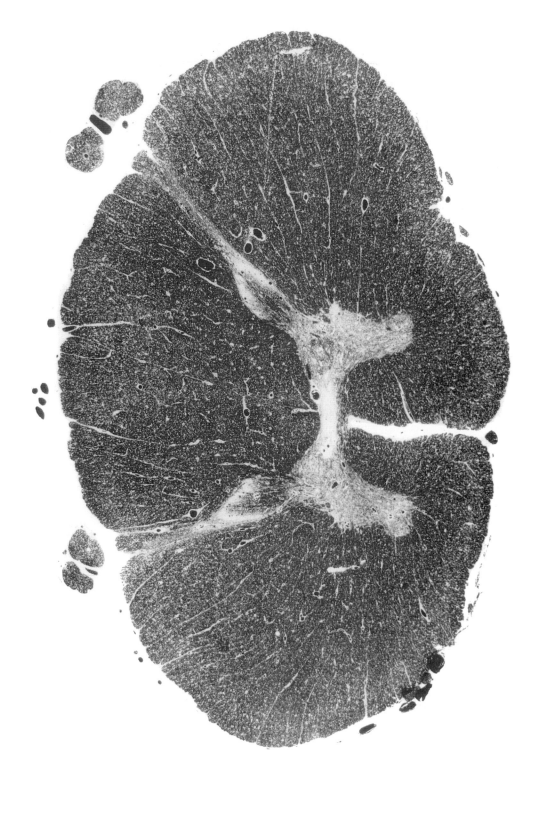

Figure II.4 Transverse section of the third thoracic segment (T3) of the spinal cord. (×23)

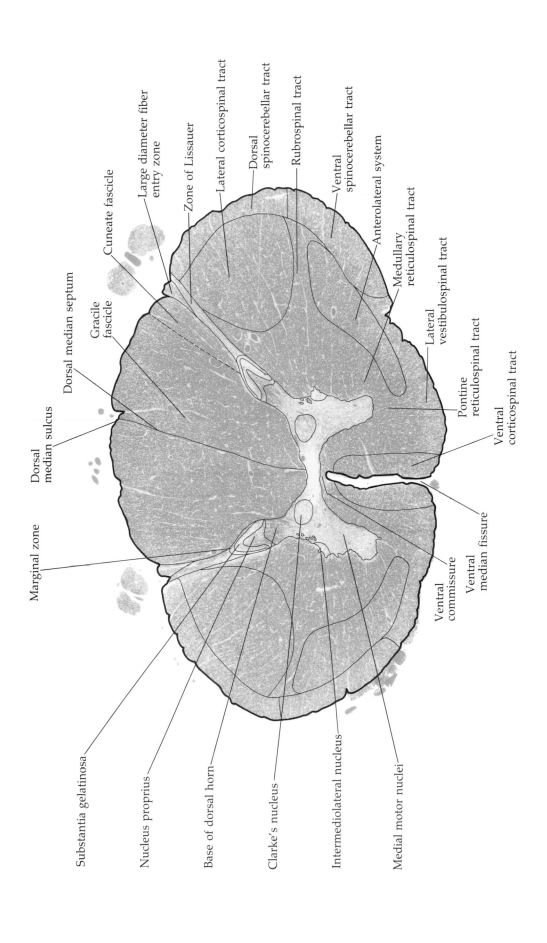

Dorsal median septum

Gracile fascicle

Cuneate fascicle

Large diameter fiber entry zone

Zone of Lissauer

Lateral corticospinal tract

Dorsal spinocerebellar tract

Rubrospinal tract

Ventral spinocerebellar tract

Anterolateral system

Medullary reticulospinal tract

Lateral vestibulospinal tract

Pontine reticulospinal tract

Ventral corticospinal tract

Dorsal median sulcus

Marginal zone

Substantia gelatinosa

Nucleus proprius

Base of dorsal horn

Clarke's nucleus

Intermediolateral nucleus

Medial motor nuclei

Ventral commissure

Ventral median fissure

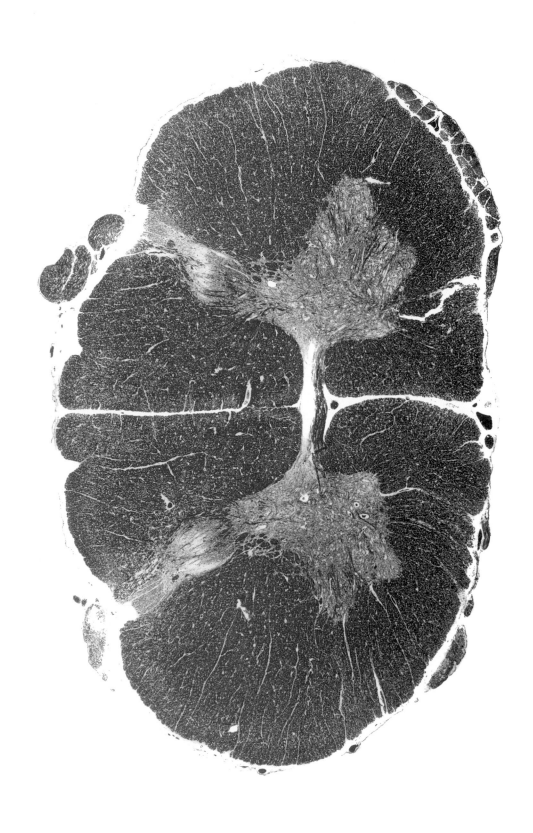

Figure II.5 Transverse section of the seventh cervical segment (C7) of the spinal cord. (×16)

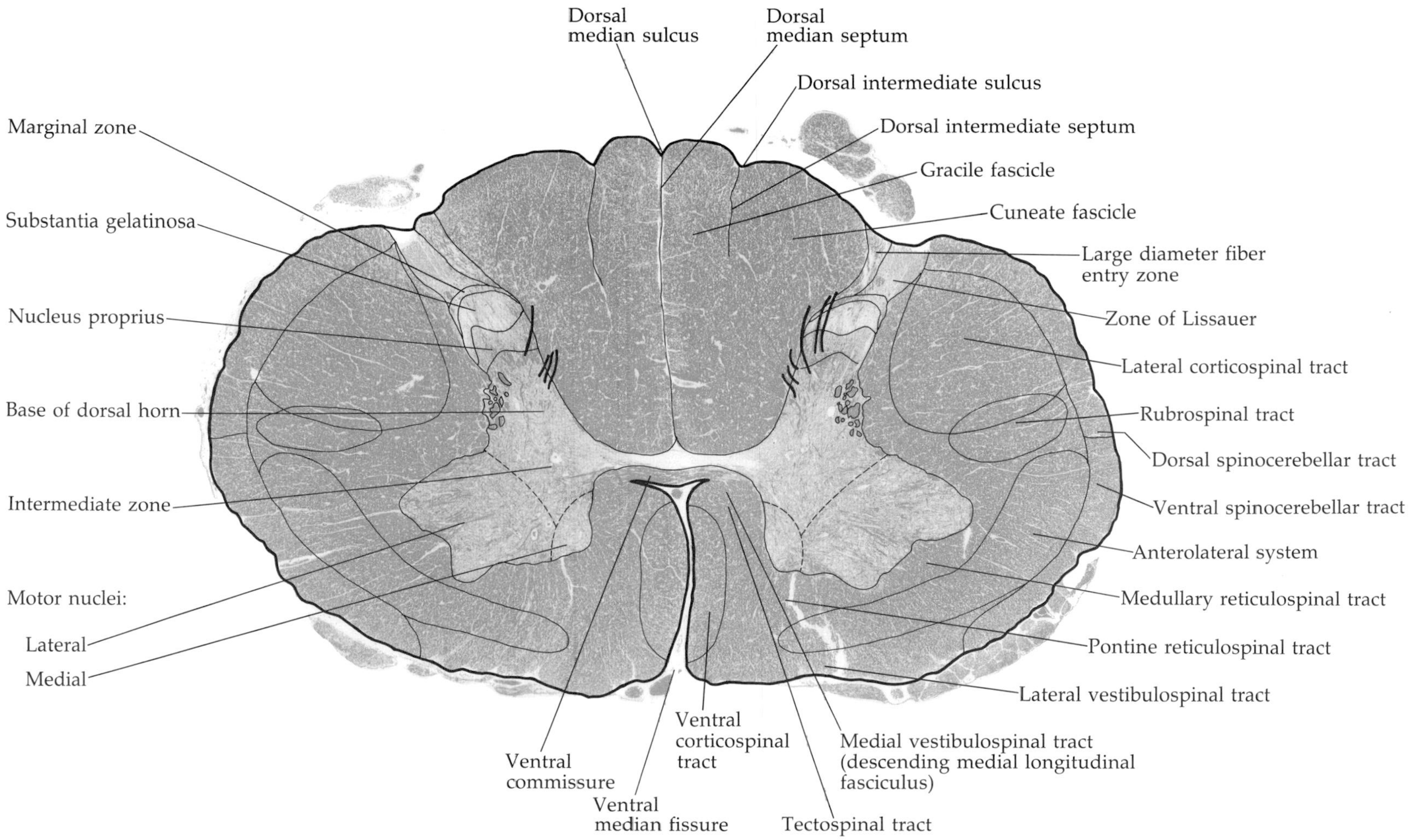

Dorsal median sulcus

Dorsal median septum

Dorsal intermediate sulcus

Dorsal intermediate septum

Gracile fascicle

Cuneate fascicle

Large diameter fiber entry zone

Zone of Lissauer

Lateral corticospinal tract

Rubrospinal tract

Dorsal spinocerebellar tract

Ventral spinocerebellar tract

Anterolateral system

Medullary reticulospinal tract

Pontine reticulospinal tract

Lateral vestibulospinal tract

Medial vestibulospinal tract (descending medial longitudinal fasciculus)

Tectospinal tract

Ventral corticospinal tract

Ventral median fissure

Ventral commissure

Motor nuclei:

Lateral

Medial

Intermediate zone

Base of dorsal horn

Nucleus proprius

Substantia gelatinosa

Marginal zone

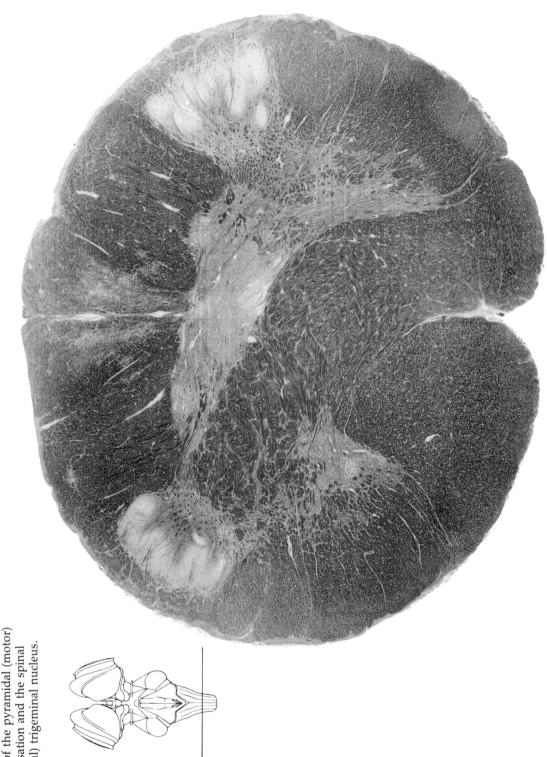

Figure II.6 Transverse section of the caudal medulla at the level of the pyramidal (motor) decussation and the spinal (caudal) trigeminal nucleus. (×17)

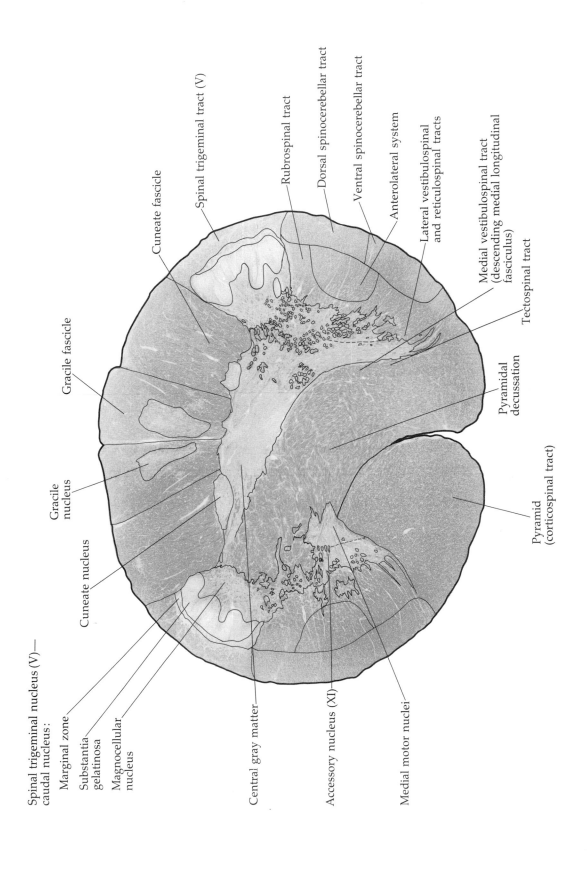

Spinal trigeminal nucleus (V)—
caudal nucleus:

Marginal zone

Substantia
gelatinosa

Magnocellular
nucleus

Gracile fascicle

Gracile
nucleus

Cuneate nucleus

Central gray matter

Accessory nucleus (XI)

Medial motor nuclei

Cuneate fascicle

Spinal trigeminal tract (V)

Rubrospinal tract

Dorsal spinocerebellar tract

Ventral spinocerebellar tract

Anterolateral system

Lateral vestibulospinal
and reticulospinal tracts

Medial vestibulospinal tract
(descending medial longitudinal
fasciculus)

Tectospinal tract

Pyramidal
decussation

Pyramid
(corticospinal tract)

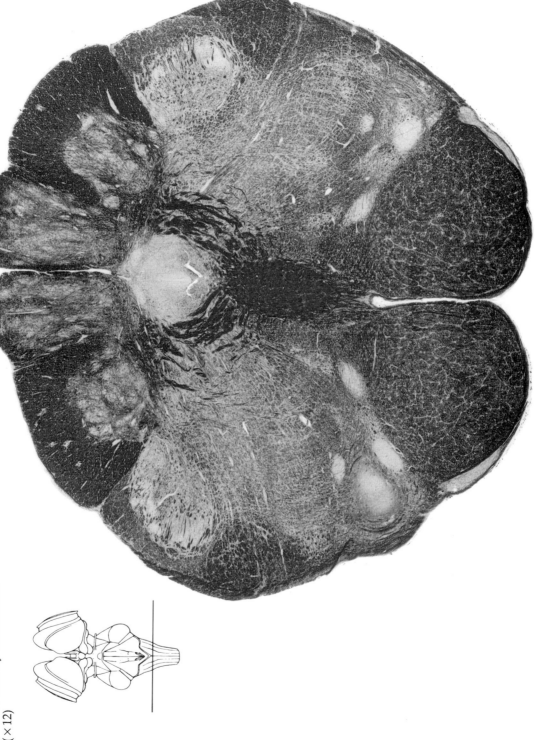

Figure II.7 Transverse section of the medulla at the level of the dorsal column nuclei and the somatic sensory decussation. (×12)

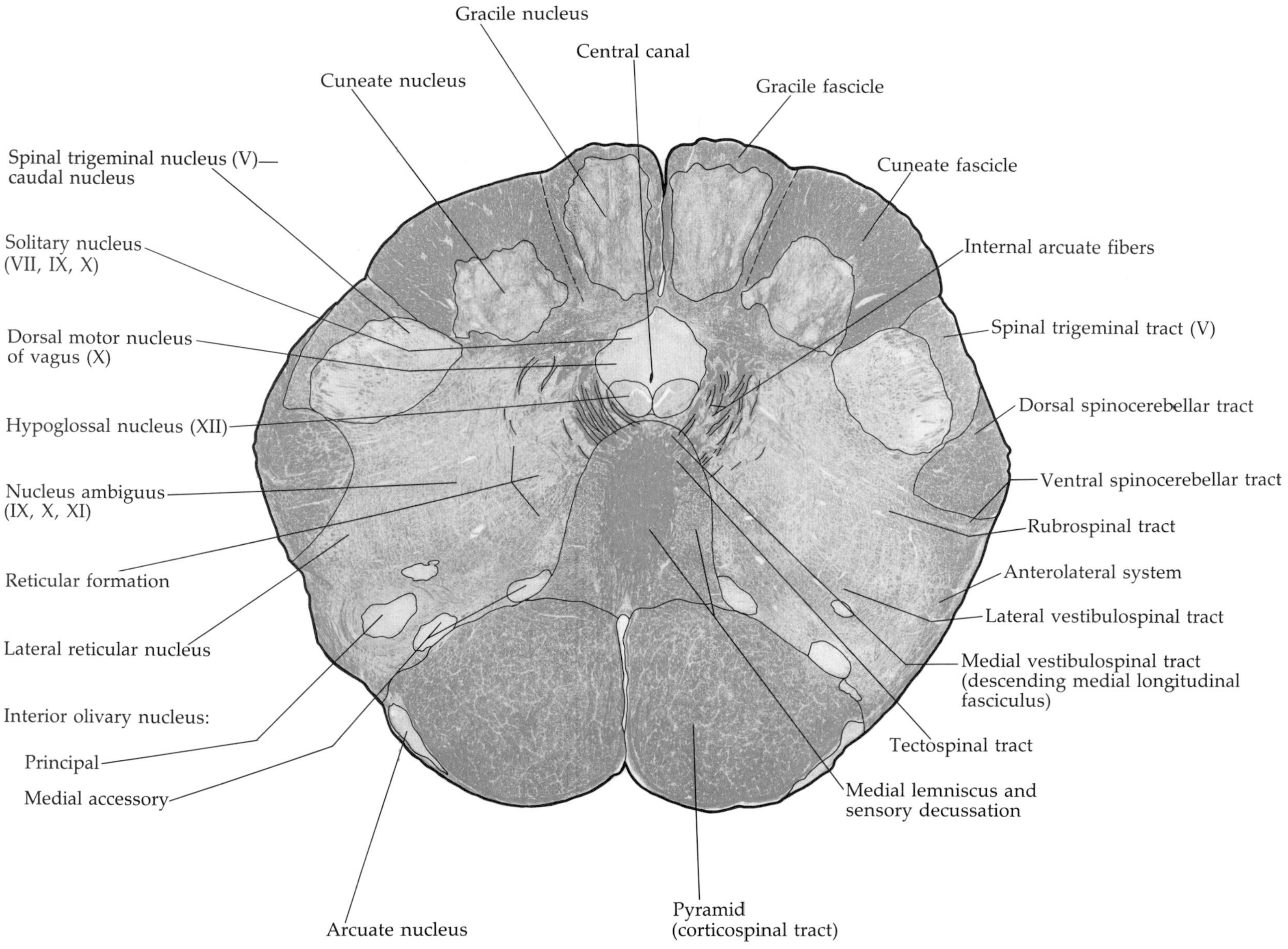

Gracile fascicle

Cuneate fascicle

Internal arcuate fibers

Spinal trigeminal tract (V)

Dorsal spinocerebellar tract

Ventral spinocerebellar tract

Rubrospinal tract

Anterolateral system

Lateral vestibulospinal tract

Medial vestibulospinal tract
(descending medial longitudinal
fasciculus)

Tectospinal tract

Medial lemniscus and
sensory decussation

Gracile nucleus

Central canal

Cuneate nucleus

Spinal trigeminal nucleus (V)—
caudal nucleus

Solitary nucleus
(VII, IX, X)

Dorsal motor nucleus
of vagus (X)

Hypoglossal nucleus (XII)

Nucleus ambiguus
(IX, X, XI)

Reticular formation

Lateral reticular nucleus

Interior olivary nucleus:

Principal

Medial accessory

Arcuate nucleus

Pyramid
(corticospinal tract)

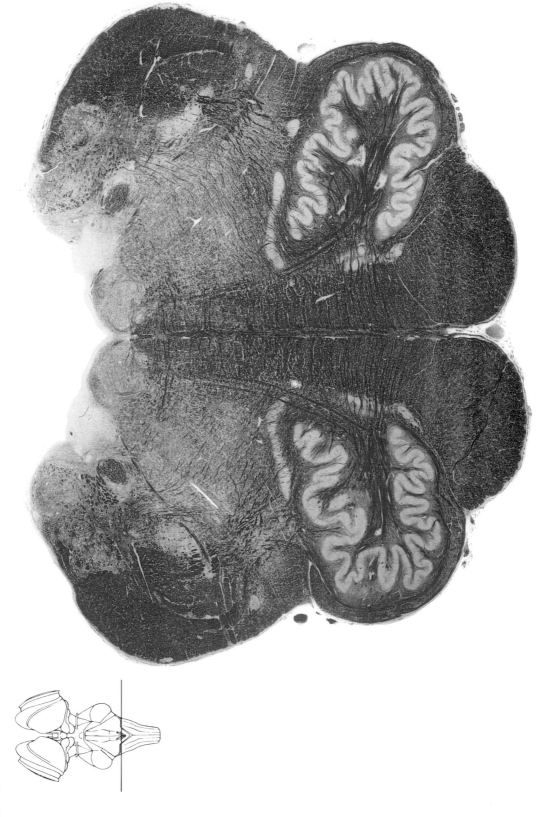

Figure II.8 Transverse section of the medulla through the hypoglossal nucleus. (×9)

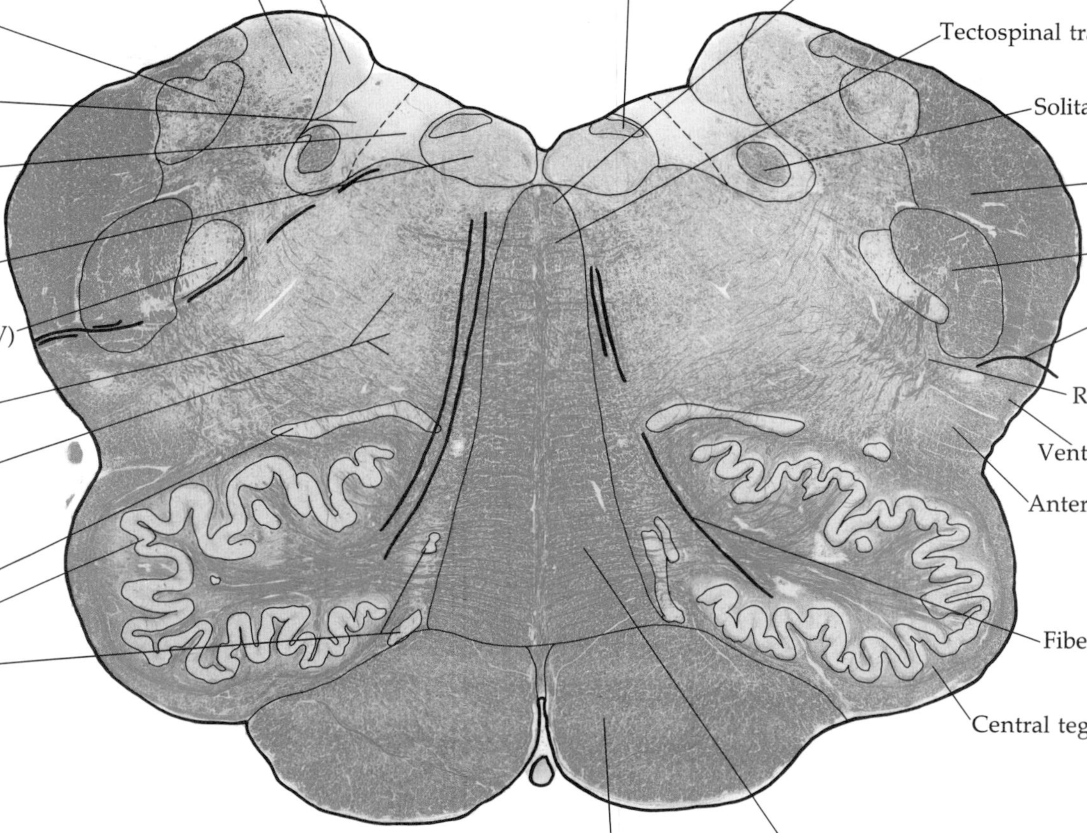

Dorsal longitudinal
fasciculus

Vestibular nuclei (VIII):
Medial
Inferior

Accessory cuneate nucleus

Solitary nucleus
(VII, IX, X)

Dorsal motor nucleus
of vagus (X)

Hypoglossal nucleus (XII)

Spinal trigeminal nucleus (V)
—interpolar nucleus

Nucleus ambiguus
(IX, X, XI)

Reticular formation

Inferior olivary nucleus:
Dorsal accessory
Principal
Medial accessory

Medial longitudinal fasciculus

Tectospinal tract

Solitary tract (VII, IX, X)

Inferior cerebellar peduncle

Spinal trigeminal tract (V)

Fibers of vagus nerve (X)

Rubrospinal tract

Ventral spinocerebellar tract

Anterolateral system

Fibers of hypoglossal nerve (XII)

Central tegmental tract

Medial lemniscus

Pyramid

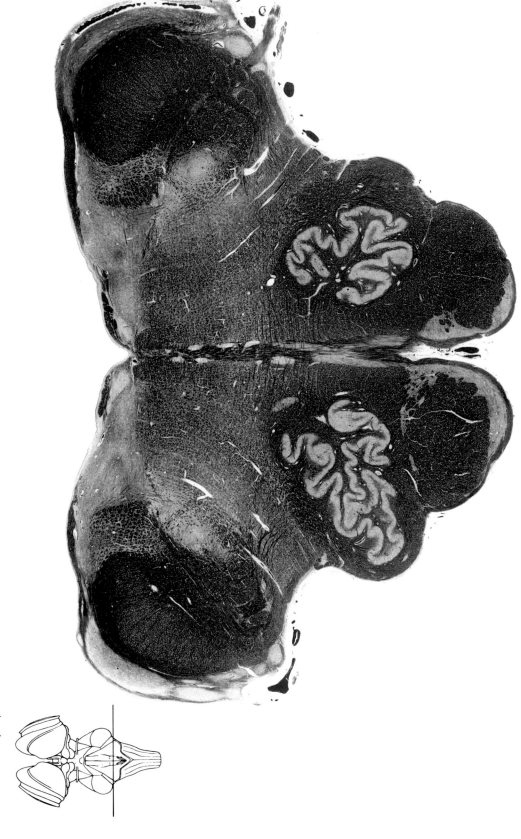

Figure II.9 Transverse section of the rostral medulla through the cochlear nuclei. (×9)

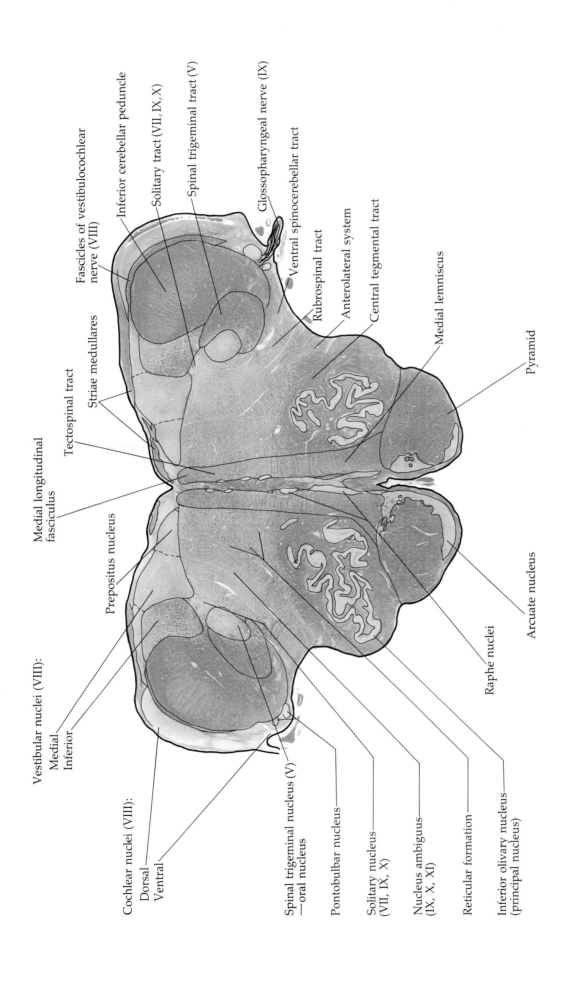

Medial longitudinal
fasciculus

Vestibular nuclei (VIII):
Medial
Inferior

Tectospinal tract

Prepositus nucleus

Striae medullares

Fascicles of vestibulocochlear
nerve (VIII)

Inferior cerebellar peduncle

Solitary tract (VII, IX, X)

Spinal trigeminal tract (V)

Glossopharyngeal nerve (IX)

Ventral spinocerebellar tract

Rubrospinal tract

Anterolateral system

Central tegmental tract

Medial lemniscus

Pyramid

Arcuate nucleus

Raphe nuclei

Inferior olivary nucleus
(principal nucleus)

Reticular formation

Nucleus ambiguus
(IX, X, XI)

Solitary nucleus
(VII, IX, X)

Pontobulbar nucleus

Spinal trigeminal nucleus (V)
—oral nucleus

Cochlear nuclei (VIII):
Dorsal
Ventral

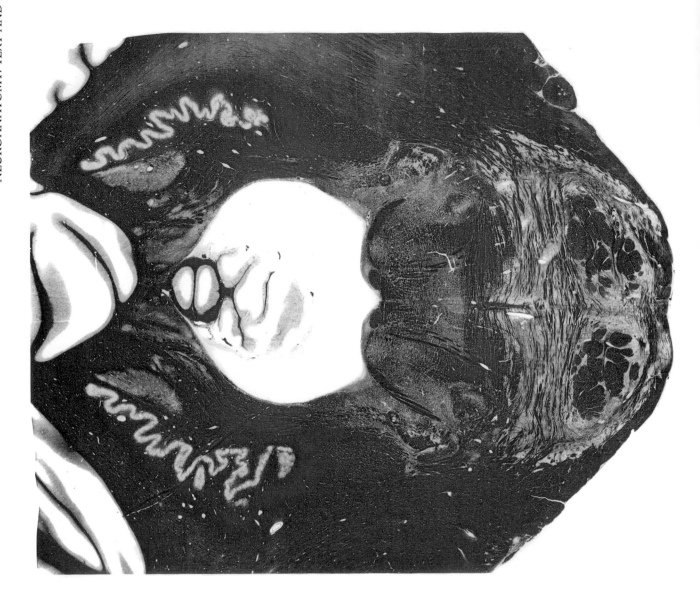

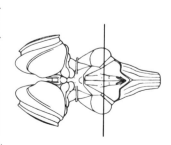

Figure II.10 Transverse section of the pons at the level of the genu of the facial nerve and the deep cerebellar nuclei. (×4.3)

Deep cerebellar nuclei:
Dentate
Interposed nuclei [Emboliform
Globose
Fastigial
Nodulus of cerebellum
Vestibular nuclei (VIII):
Superior
Lateral
Abducens nucleus (VI)
Spinal trigeminal nucleus (V)
—oral nucleus
Facial nucleus (VII)
Reticular formation
Superior olivary complex
Pontine nuclei

Medial longitudinal fasciculus
Dorsal longitudinal fasciculus
Juxtarestiform body
Cerebellar peduncles:
Superior
Inferior
Middle
Facial nerve (VII):
Genu
Fascicles
Tectospinal tract
Spinal trigeminal tract (V)
Fascicles of abducens nerve (VI)
Central tegmental tract
Ventral spinocerebellar tract
Lateral lemniscus
Anterolateral system
Rubrospinal tract
Trigeminal lemniscus
Medial lemniscus
Trapezoid body
Pontocerebellar fibers
Corticospinal and corticobulbar tracts

IV ventricle

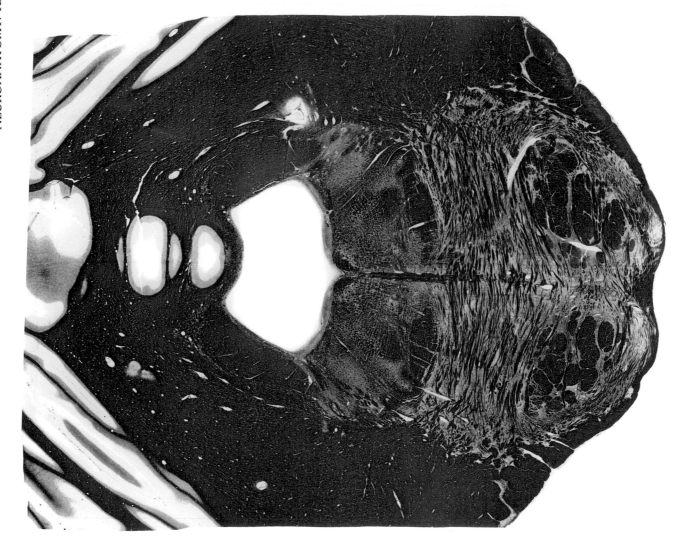

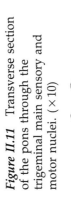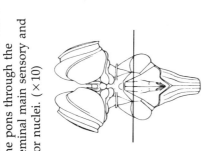

Figure II.11 Transverse section of the pons through the trigeminal main sensory and motor nuclei. (×10)

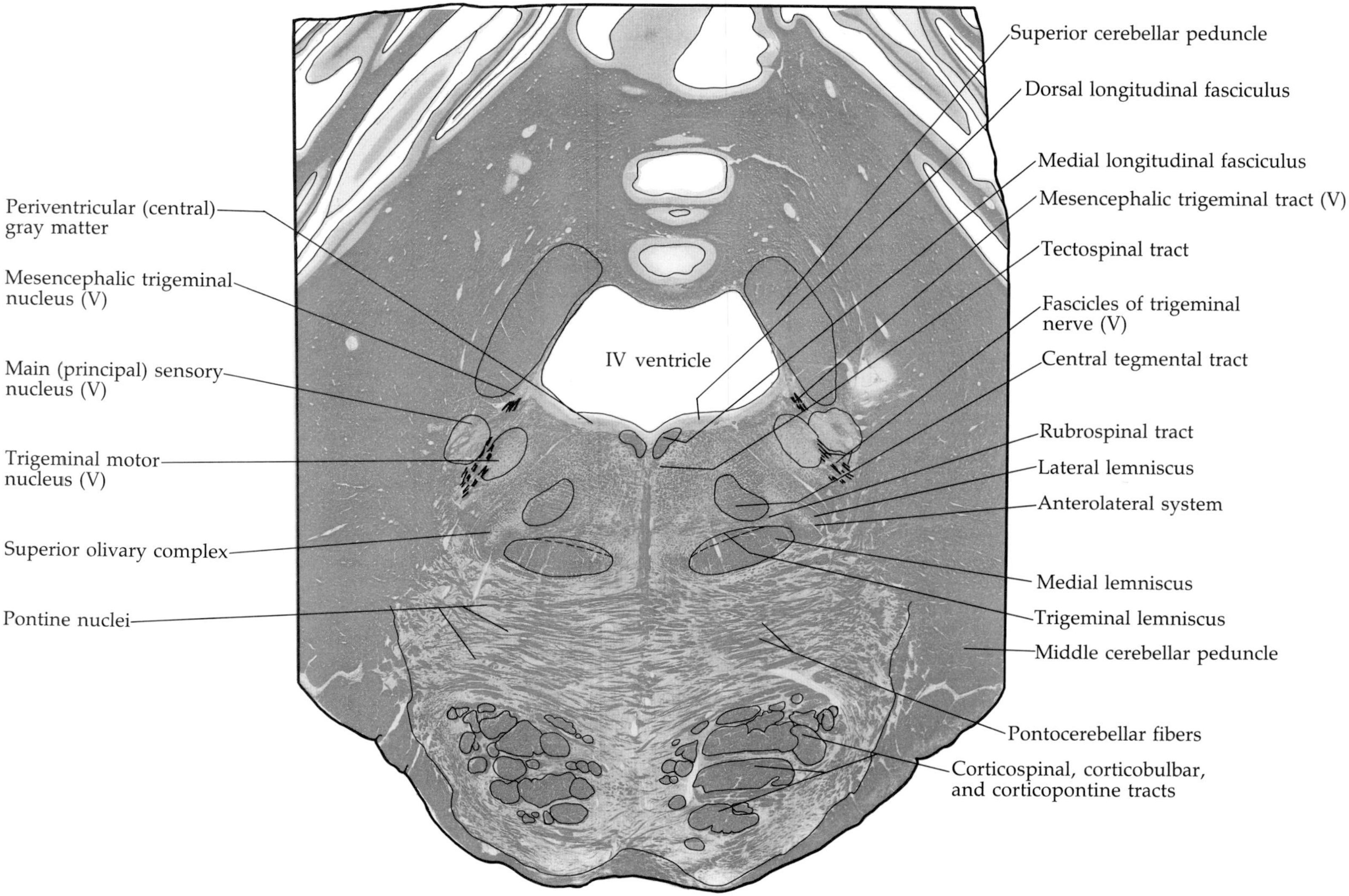

Superior cerebellar peduncle

Dorsal longitudinal fasciculus

Medial longitudinal fasciculus

Mesencephalic trigeminal tract (V)

Tectospinal tract

Fascicles of trigeminal nerve (V)

Central tegmental tract

Rubrospinal tract

Lateral lemniscus

Anterolateral system

Medial lemniscus

Trigeminal lemniscus

Middle cerebellar peduncle

Pontocerebellar fibers

Corticospinal, corticobulbar, and corticopontine tracts

IV ventricle

Periventricular (central) gray matter

Mesencephalic trigeminal nucleus (V)

Main (principal) sensory nucleus (V)

Trigeminal motor nucleus (V)

Superior olivary complex

Pontine nuclei

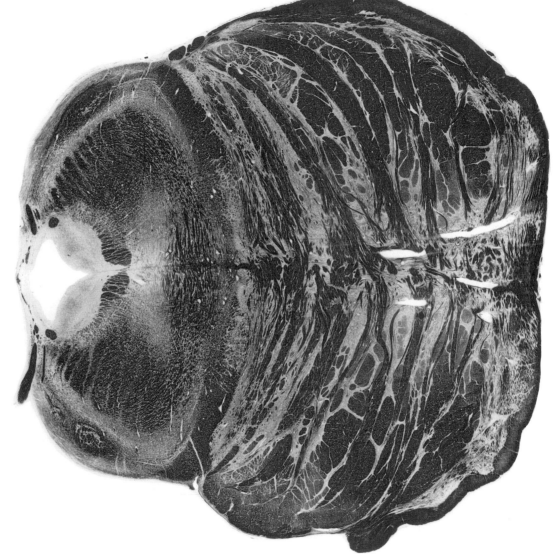

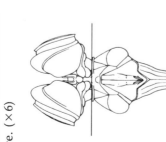

Figure II.12 Transverse section through the rostral pons (isthmus) at the level of the decussation of the trochlear nerve. (×6)

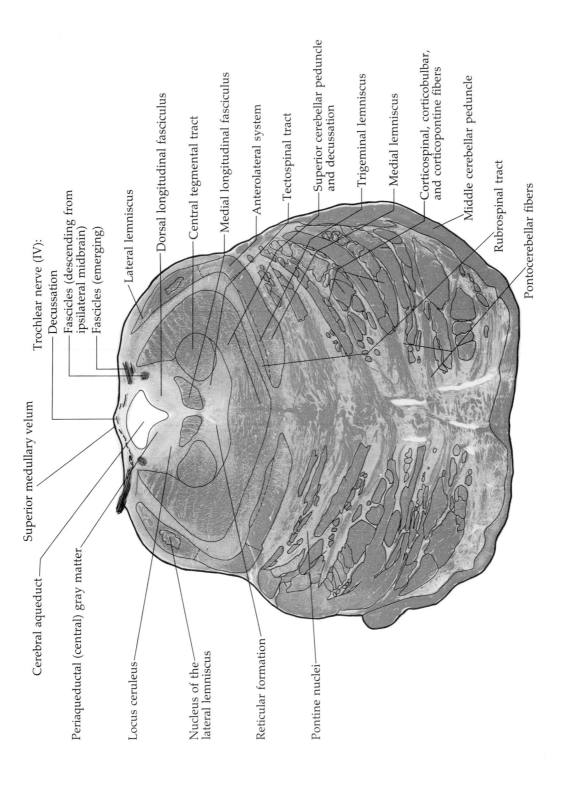

Cerebral aqueduct

Superior medullary velum

Trochlear nerve (IV):
Decussation
Fascicles (descending from ipsilateral midbrain)
Fascicles (emerging)

Lateral lemniscus

Dorsal longitudinal fasciculus

Central tegmental tract

Medial longitudinal fasciculus

Anterolateral system

Tectospinal tract

Superior cerebellar peduncle and decussation

Trigeminal lemniscus

Medial lemniscus

Corticospinal, corticobulbar, and corticopontine fibers

Middle cerebellar peduncle

Rubrospinal tract

Pontocerebellar fibers

Periaqueductal (central) gray matter

Locus ceruleus

Nucleus of the lateral lemniscus

Reticular formation

Pontine nuclei

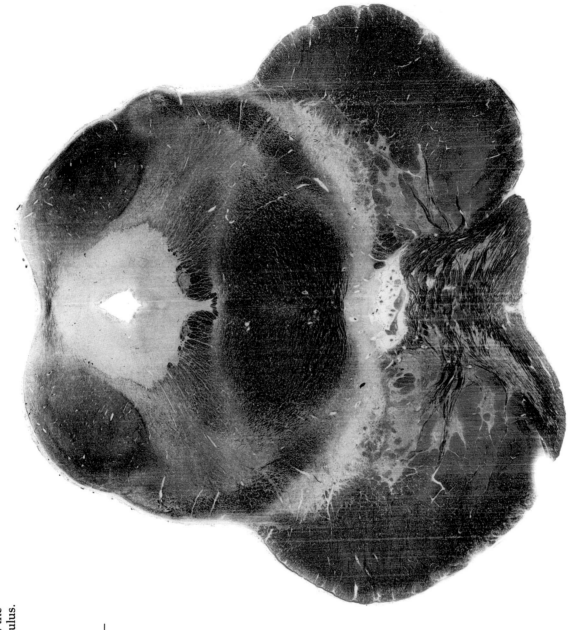

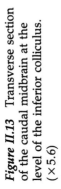

Figure II.13 Transverse section of the caudal midbrain at the level of the inferior colliculus. (×5.6)

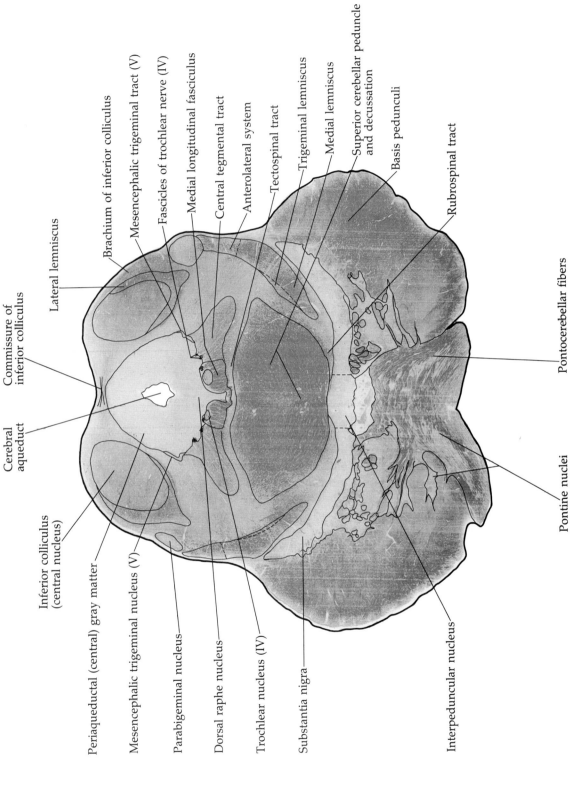

Lateral lemniscus

Commissure of
inferior colliculus

Cerebral
aqueduct

Inferior colliculus
(central nucleus)

Periaqueductal (central) gray matter

Mesencephalic trigeminal nucleus (V)

Parabigeminal nucleus

Dorsal raphe nucleus

Trochlear nucleus (IV)

Substantia nigra

Interpeduncular nucleus

Brachium of inferior colliculus

Mesencephalic trigeminal tract (V)

Fascicles of trochlear nerve (IV)

Medial longitudinal fasciculus

Central tegmental tract

Anterolateral system

Tectospinal tract

Trigeminal lemniscus

Medial lemniscus

Superior cerebellar peduncle
and decussation

Basis pedunculi

Rubrospinal tract

Pontocerebellar fibers

Pontine nuclei

Figure II.14 Transverse section of the rostral midbrain at the level of the superior colliculus. (×5.0)

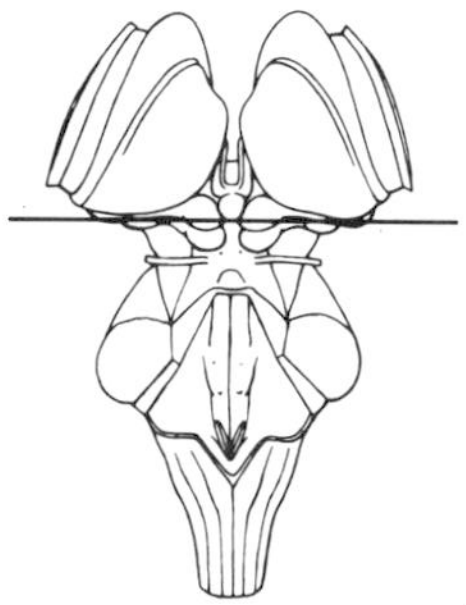

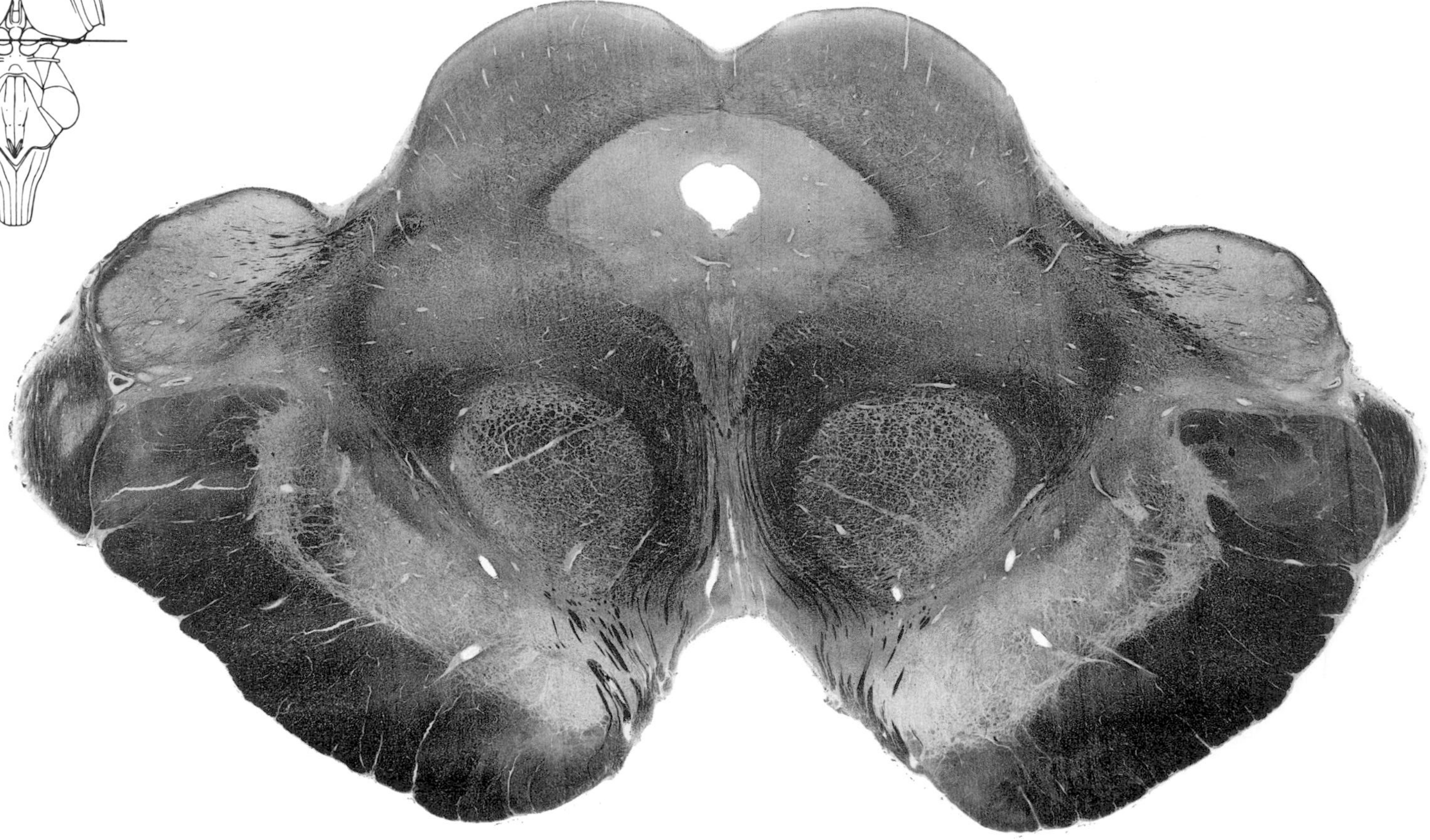

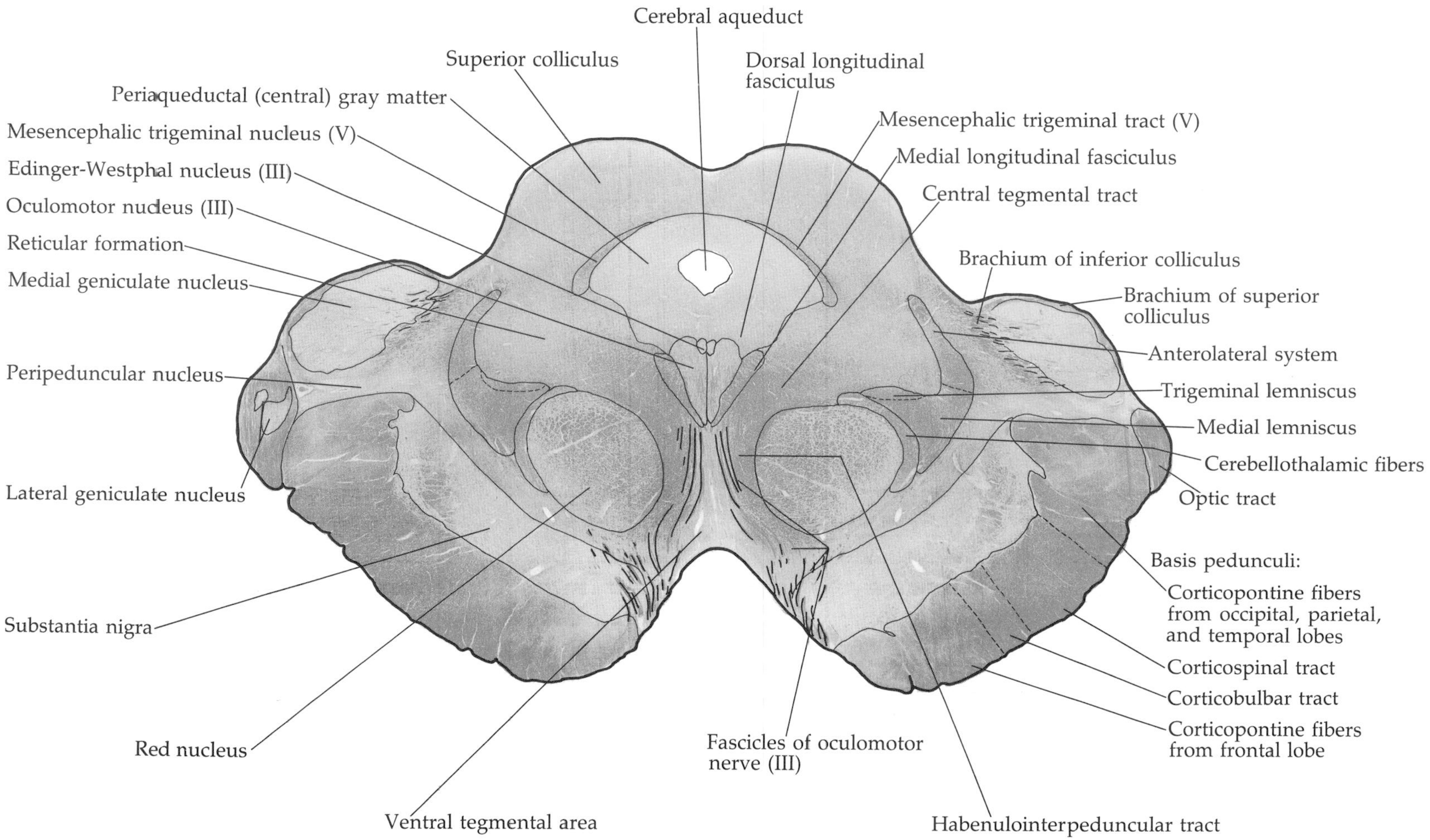

Cerebral aqueduct

Dorsal longitudinal fasciculus

Mesencephalic trigeminal tract (V)

Medial longitudinal fasciculus

Central tegmental tract

Brachium of inferior colliculus

Brachium of superior colliculus

Anterolateral system

Trigeminal lemniscus

Medial lemniscus

Cerebellothalamic fibers

Optic tract

Basis pedunculi:

Corticopontine fibers from occipital, parietal, and temporal lobes

Corticospinal tract

Corticobulbar tract

Corticopontine fibers from frontal lobe

Habenulointerpeduncular tract

Fascicles of oculomotor nerve (III)

Ventral tegmental area

Red nucleus

Substantia nigra

Lateral geniculate nucleus

Peripeduncular nucleus

Medial geniculate nucleus

Reticular formation

Oculomotor nudeus (III)

Edinger-Westphal nucleus (III)

Mesencephalic trigeminal nucleus (V)

Periaqueductal (central) gray matter

Superior colliculus

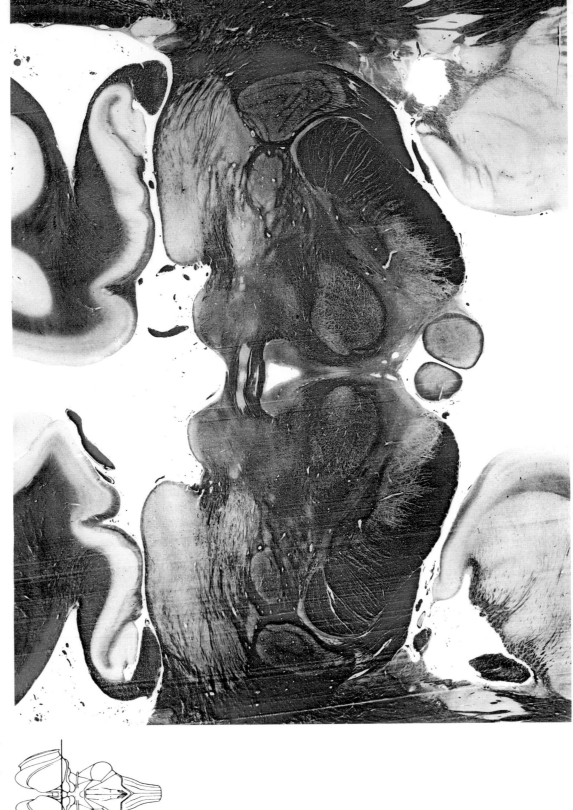

Figure II.15   Transverse section of the juncture of the midbrain and diencephalon. (×3.3)

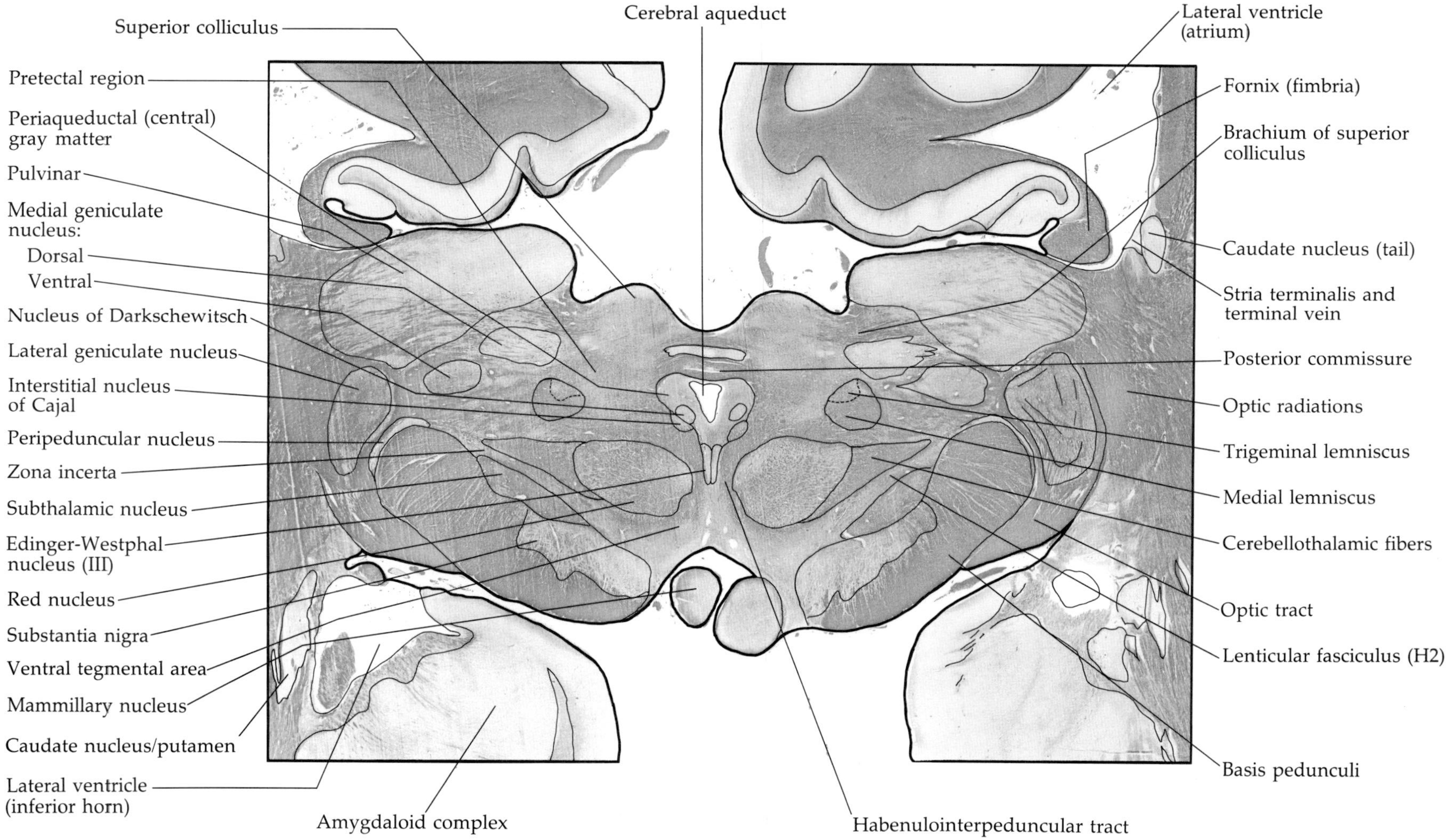

Lateral ventricle (atrium)

Fornix (fimbria)

Brachium of superior colliculus

Caudate nucleus (tail)

Stria terminalis and terminal vein

Posterior commissure

Optic radiations

Trigeminal lemniscus

Medial lemniscus

Cerebellothalamic fibers

Optic tract

Lenticular fasciculus (H2)

Basis pedunculi

Cerebral aqueduct

Habenulointerpeduncular tract

Amygdaloid complex

Superior colliculus

Pretectal region

Periaqueductal (central) gray matter

Pulvinar

Medial geniculate nucleus:
Dorsal
Ventral

Nucleus of Darkschewitsch

Lateral geniculate nucleus

Interstitial nucleus of Cajal

Peripeduncular nucleus

Zona incerta

Subthalamic nucleus

Edinger-Westphal nucleus (III)

Red nucleus

Substantia nigra

Ventral tegmental area

Mammillary nucleus

Caudate nucleus/putamen

Lateral ventricle (inferior horn)

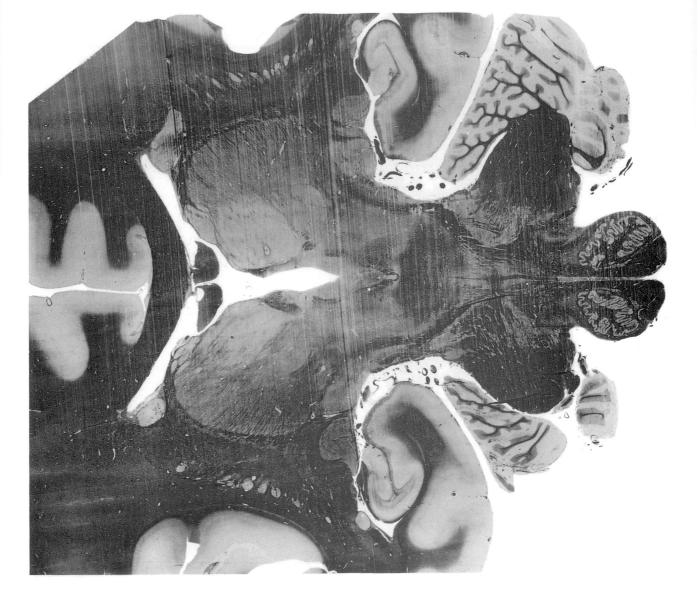

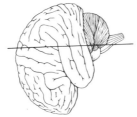

Figure II.16 Coronal section of the diencephalon and cerebral hemisphere through the posterior limb of the internal capsule and the medial and lateral geniculate nuclei. The midbrain and pontine tegmentum, lateral cerebellum, and the ventral medulla are also shown (×2.1)

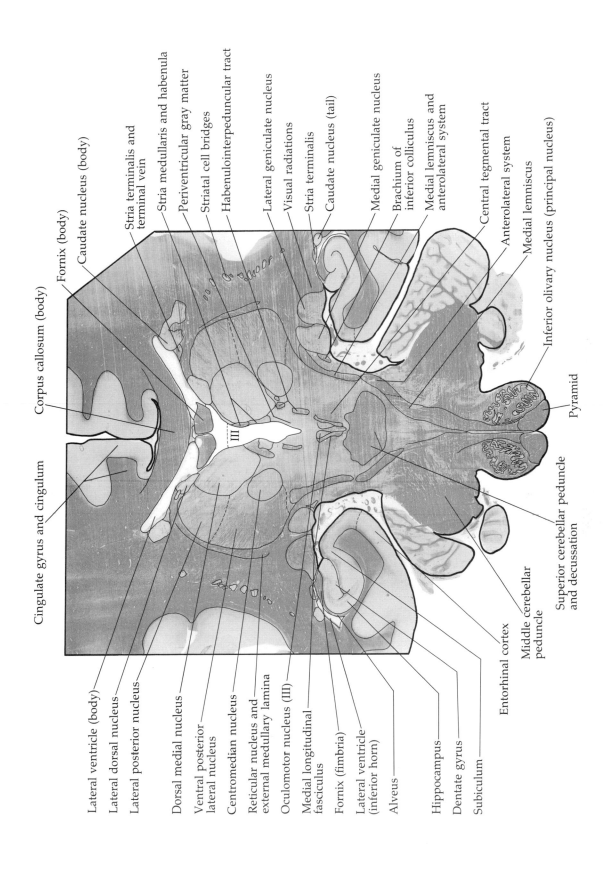

Cingulate gyrus and cingulum

Corpus callosum (body)

Fornix (body)

Caudate nucleus (body)

Stria terminalis and terminal vein

Stria medullaris and habenula

Periventricular gray matter

Striatal cell bridges

Habenulointerpeduncular tract

Lateral geniculate nucleus

Visual radiations

Stria terminalis

Caudate nucleus (tail)

Medial geniculate nucleus

Brachium of inferior colliculus

Medial lemniscus and anterolateral system

Central tegmental tract

Anterolateral system

Medial lemniscus

Inferior olivary nucleus (principal nucleus)

Pyramid

Lateral ventricle (body)

Lateral dorsal nucleus

Lateral posterior nucleus

Dorsal medial nucleus

Ventral posterior lateral nucleus

Centromedian nucleus

Reticular nucleus and external medullary lamina

Oculomotor nucleus (III)

Medial longitudinal fasciculus

Fornix (fimbria)

Lateral ventricle (inferior horn)

Alveus

Hippocampus

Dentate gyrus

Subiculum

Entorhinal cortex

Middle cerebellar peduncle

Superior cerebellar peduncle and decussation

III

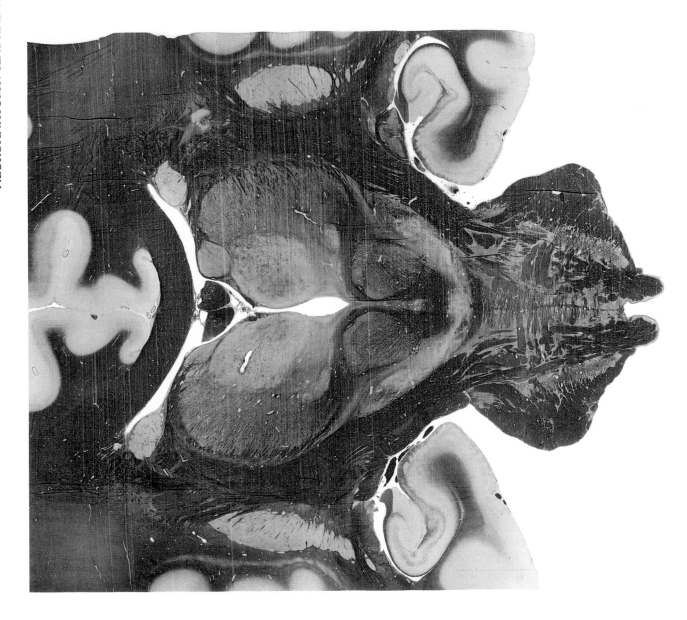

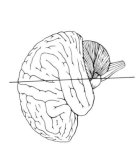

Figure II.17 Coronal section of the diencephalon and cerebral hemisphere through the posterior limb of the internal capsule and ventral posterior nucleus. The midbrain tegmentum and base of the pons are also shown. (×2.3)

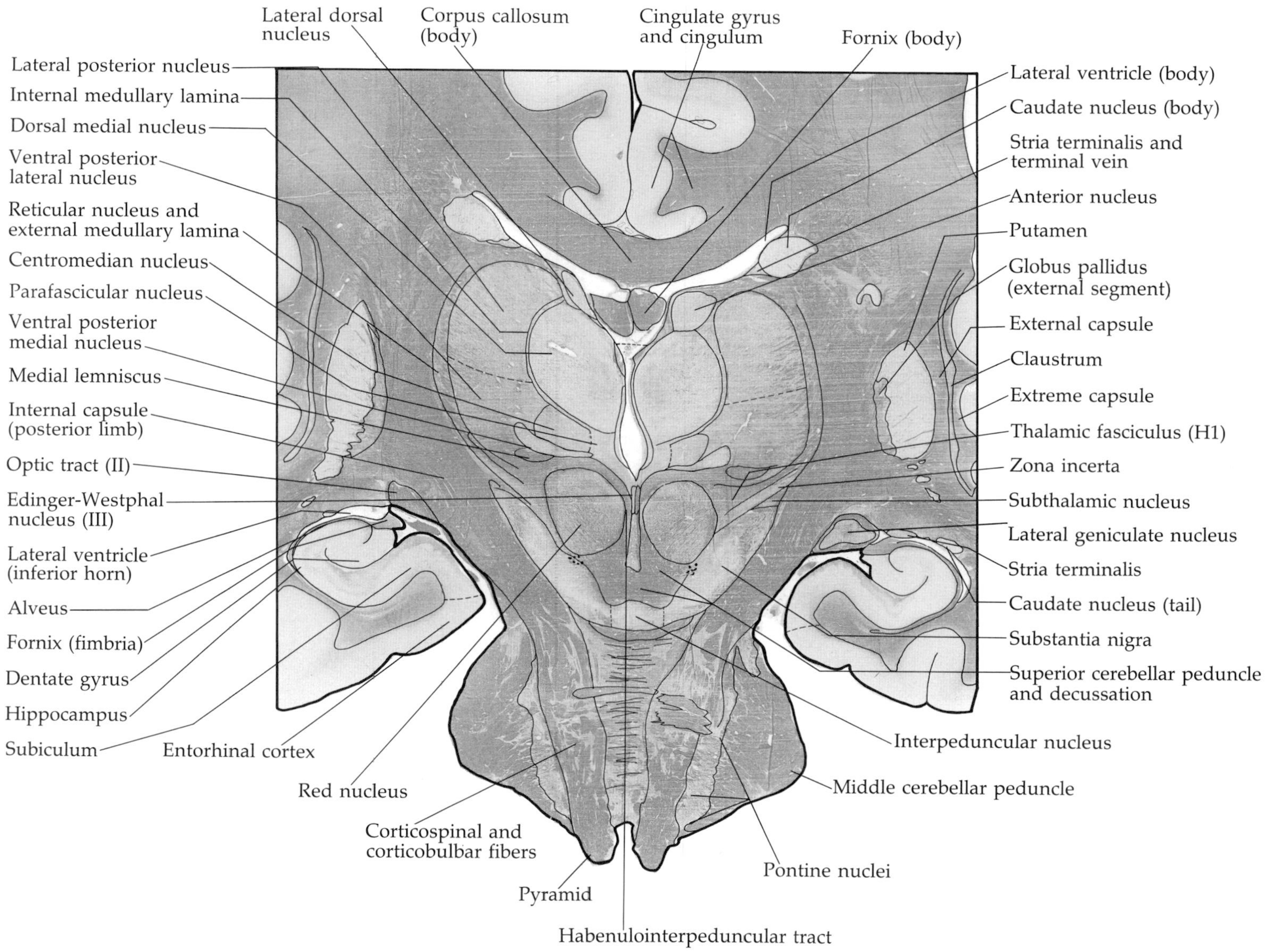

Lateral dorsal nucleus

Corpus callosum (body)

Cingulate gyrus and cingulum

Fornix (body)

Lateral ventricle (body)

Caudate nucleus (body)

Stria terminalis and terminal vein

Anterior nucleus

Putamen

Globus pallidus (external segment)

External capsule

Claustrum

Extreme capsule

Thalamic fasciculus (H1)

Zona incerta

Subthalamic nucleus

Lateral geniculate nucleus

Stria terminalis

Caudate nucleus (tail)

Substantia nigra

Superior cerebellar peduncle and decussation

Interpeduncular nucleus

Middle cerebellar peduncle

Pontine nuclei

Habenulointerpeduncular tract

Pyramid

Corticospinal and corticobulbar fibers

Red nucleus

Entorhinal cortex

Subiculum

Hippocampus

Dentate gyrus

Fornix (fimbria)

Alveus

Lateral ventricle (inferior horn)

Edinger-Westphal nucleus (III)

Optic tract (II)

Internal capsule (posterior limb)

Medial lemniscus

Ventral posterior medial nucleus

Parafascicular nucleus

Centromedian nucleus

Reticular nucleus and external medullary lamina

Ventral posterior lateral nucleus

Dorsal medial nucleus

Internal medullary lamina

Lateral posterior nucleus

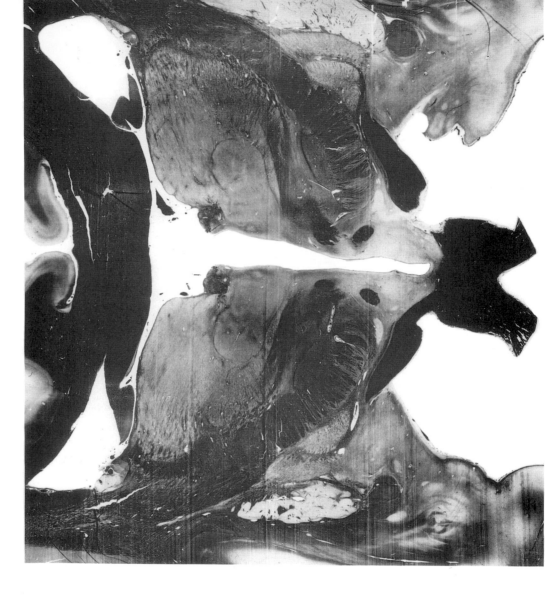

Figure II.18 Oblique section of the cerebral hemisphere and diencephalon through the optic chiasm and tracts. (×2.4)

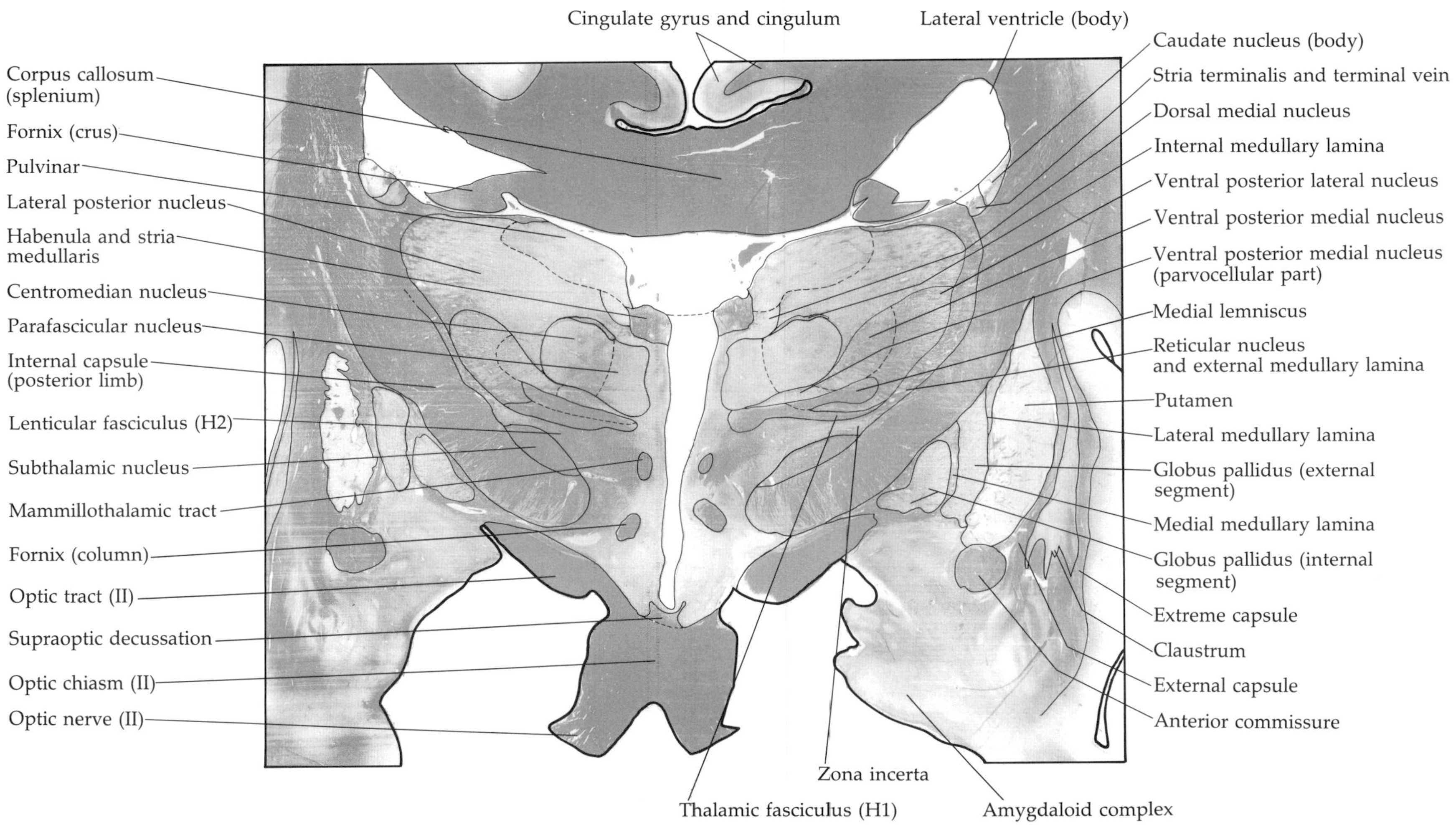

Cingulate gyrus and cingulum

Lateral ventricle (body)

Caudate nucleus (body)
Stria terminalis and terminal vein
Dorsal medial nucleus
Internal medullary lamina
Ventral posterior lateral nucleus
Ventral posterior medial nucleus
Ventral posterior medial nucleus (parvocellular part)
Medial lemniscus
Reticular nucleus and external medullary lamina
Putamen
Lateral medullary lamina
Globus pallidus (external segment)
Medial medullary lamina
Globus pallidus (internal segment)
Extreme capsule
Claustrum
External capsule
Anterior commissure

Amygdaloid complex

Zona incerta

Thalamic fasciculus (H1)

Corpus callosum (splenium)
Fornix (crus)
Pulvinar
Lateral posterior nucleus
Habenula and stria medullaris
Centromedian nucleus
Parafascicular nucleus
Internal capsule (posterior limb)
Lenticular fasciculus (H2)
Subthalamic nucleus
Mammillothalamic tract
Fornix (column)
Optic tract (II)
Supraoptic decussation
Optic chiasm (II)
Optic nerve (II)

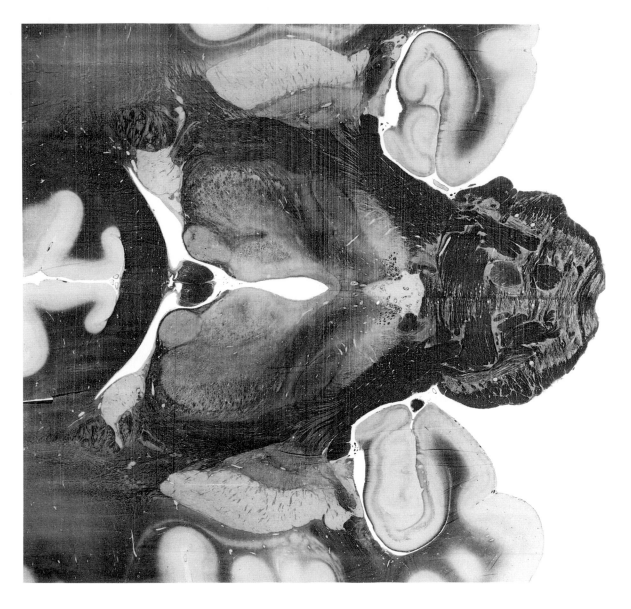

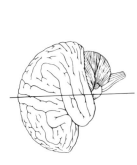

Figure II.19 Coronal section of the diencephalon and cerebral hemisphere through the posterior limb of the internal capsule and anterior thalamic nuclei. The ventral midbrain and ventral pons are also shown. (×2.2)

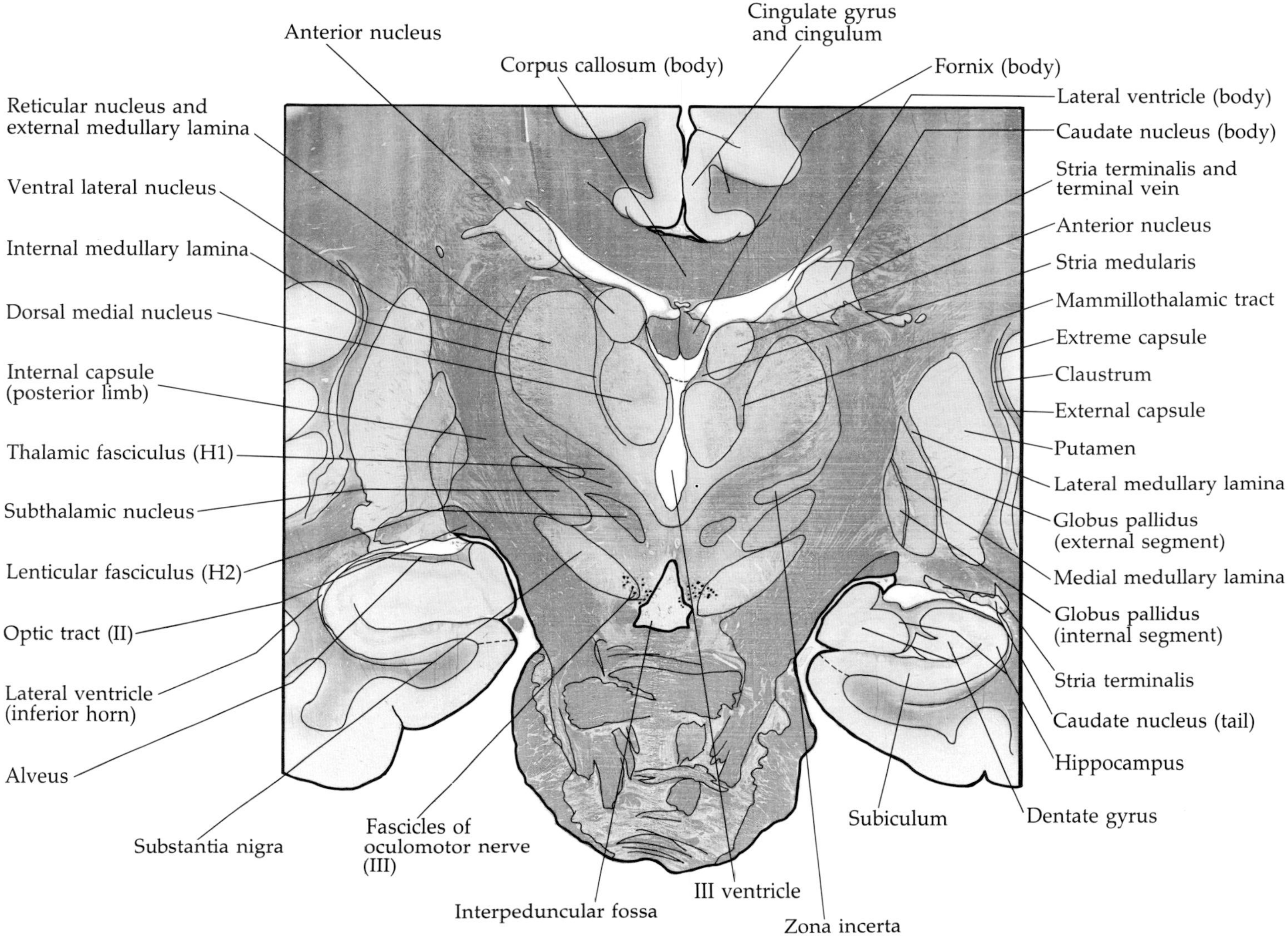

Anterior nucleus

Cingulate gyrus
and cingulum

Corpus callosum (body)

Reticular nucleus and
external medullary lamina

Ventral lateral nucleus

Internal medullary lamina

Dorsal medial nucleus

Internal capsule
(posterior limb)

Thalamic fasciculus (H1)

Subthalamic nucleus

Lenticular fasciculus (H2)

Optic tract (II)

Lateral ventricle
(inferior horn)

Alveus

Substantia nigra

Fornix (body)

Lateral ventricle (body)

Caudate nucleus (body)

Stria terminalis and
terminal vein

Anterior nucleus

Stria medularis

Mammillothalamic tract

Extreme capsule

Claustrum

External capsule

Putamen

Lateral medullary lamina

Globus pallidus
(external segment)

Medial medullary lamina

Globus pallidus
(internal segment)

Stria terminalis

Caudate nucleus (tail)

Hippocampus

Dentate gyrus

Subiculum

Zona incerta

III ventricle

Interpeduncular fossa

Fascicles of
oculomotor nerve
(III)

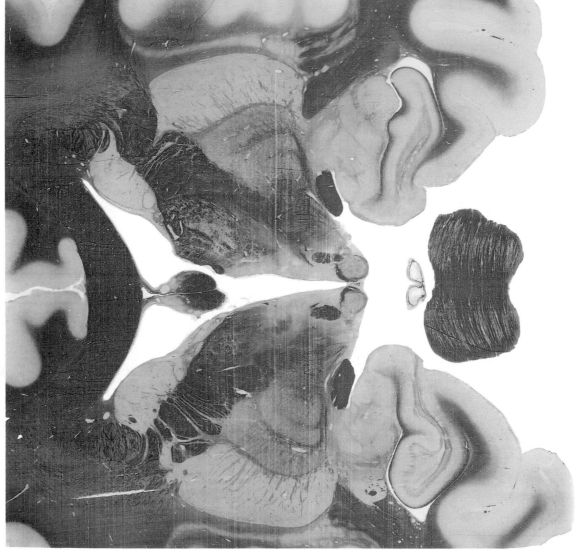

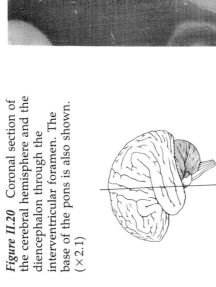

Figure II.20 Coronal section of the cerebral hemisphere and the diencephalon through the interventricular foramen. The base of the pons is also shown. (×2.1)

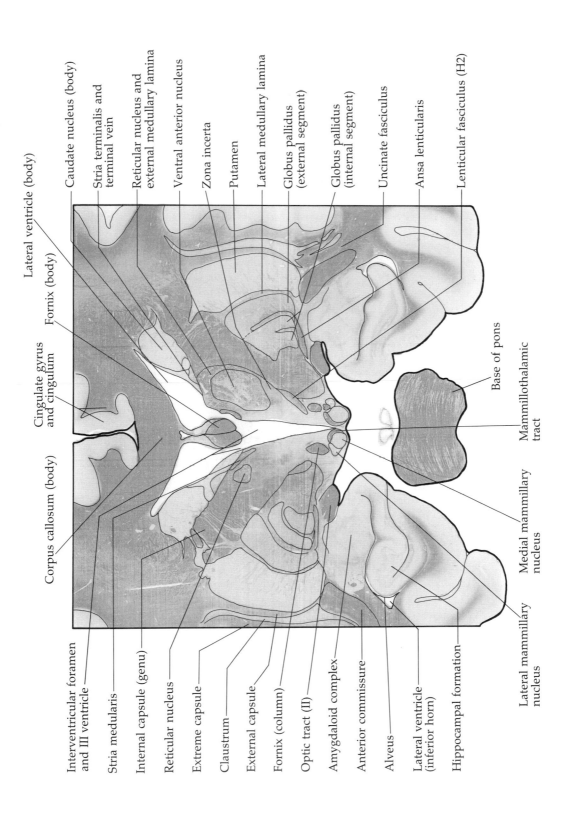

Lateral ventricle (body)

Caudate nucleus (body)

Stria terminalis and terminal vein

Reticular nucleus and external medullary lamina

Ventral anterior nucleus

Zona incerta

Putamen

Lateral medullary lamina

Globus pallidus (external segment)

Globus pallidus (internal segment)

Uncinate fasciculus

Ansa lenticularis

Lenticular fasciculus (H2)

Fornix (body)

Cingulate gyrus and cingulum

Corpus callosum (body)

Base of pons

Mammillothalamic tract

Medial mammillary nucleus

Lateral mammillary nucleus

Interventricular foramen and III ventricle

Stria medularis

Internal capsule (genu)

Reticular nucleus

Extreme capsule

Claustrum

External capsule

Fornix (column)

Optic tract (II)

Amygdaloid complex

Anterior commissure

Alveus

Lateral ventricle (inferior horn)

Hippocampal formation

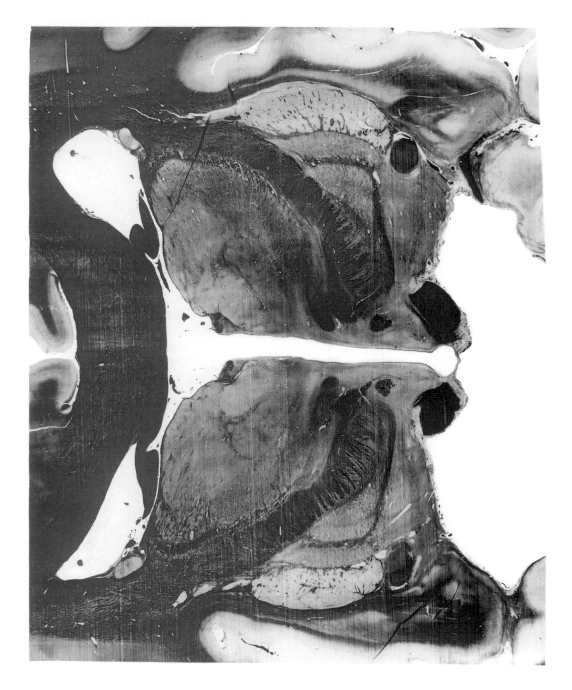

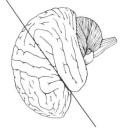

Figure II.21 Oblique section of the cerebral hemisphere and diencephalon through the ansa lenticularis and optic tract. (×2.4)

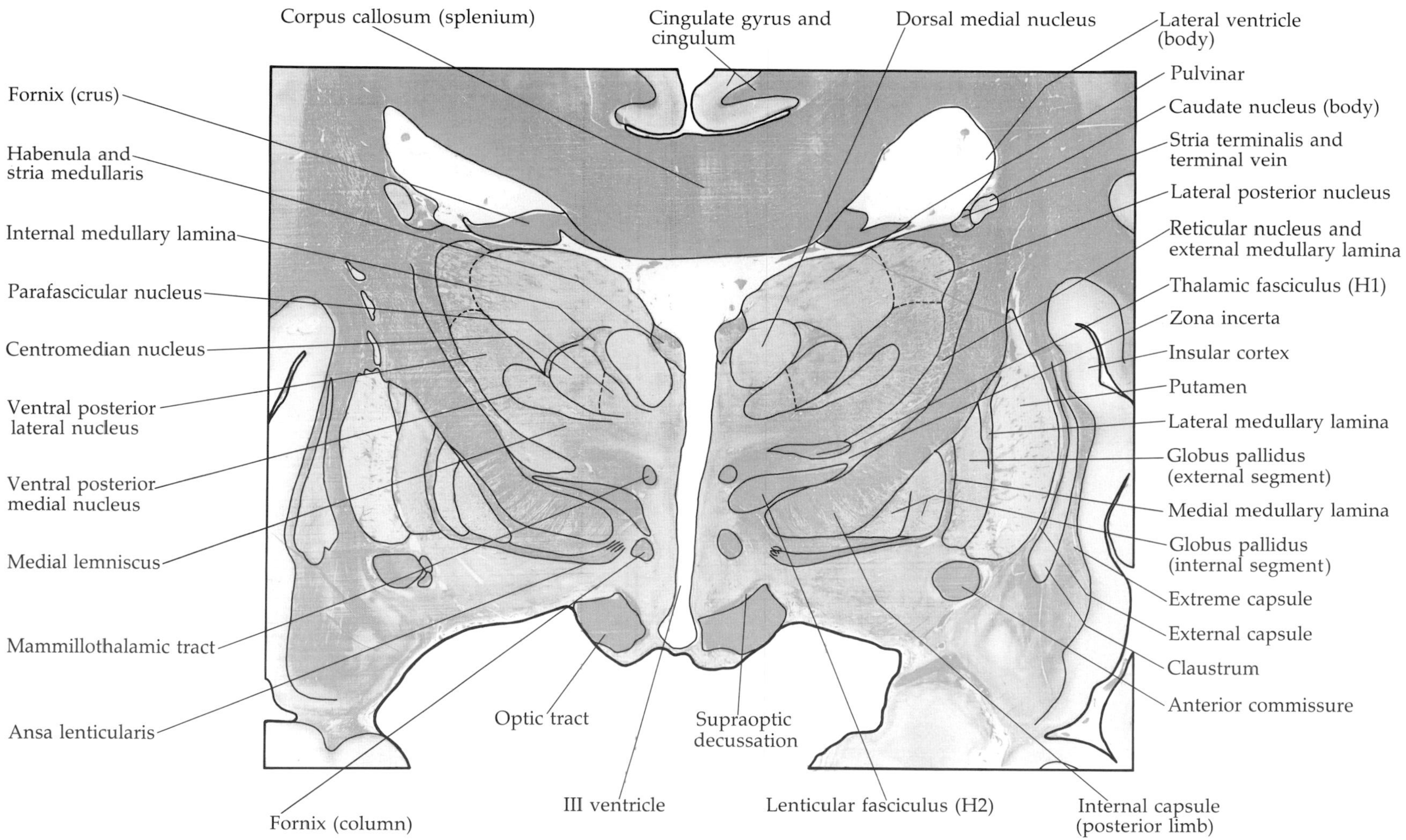

Corpus callosum (splenium)

Cingulate gyrus and cingulum

Dorsal medial nucleus

Lateral ventricle (body)

Pulvinar

Caudate nucleus (body)

Stria terminalis and terminal vein

Lateral posterior nucleus

Reticular nucleus and external medullary lamina

Thalamic fasciculus (H1)

Zona incerta

Insular cortex

Putamen

Lateral medullary lamina

Globus pallidus (external segment)

Medial medullary lamina

Globus pallidus (internal segment)

Extreme capsule

External capsule

Claustrum

Anterior commissure

Internal capsule (posterior limb)

Fornix (crus)

Habenula and stria medullaris

Internal medullary lamina

Parafascicular nucleus

Centromedian nucleus

Ventral posterior lateral nucleus

Ventral posterior medial nucleus

Medial lemniscus

Mammillothalamic tract

Ansa lenticularis

Lenticular fasciculus (H2)

Supraoptic decussation

Optic tract

III ventricle

Fornix (column)

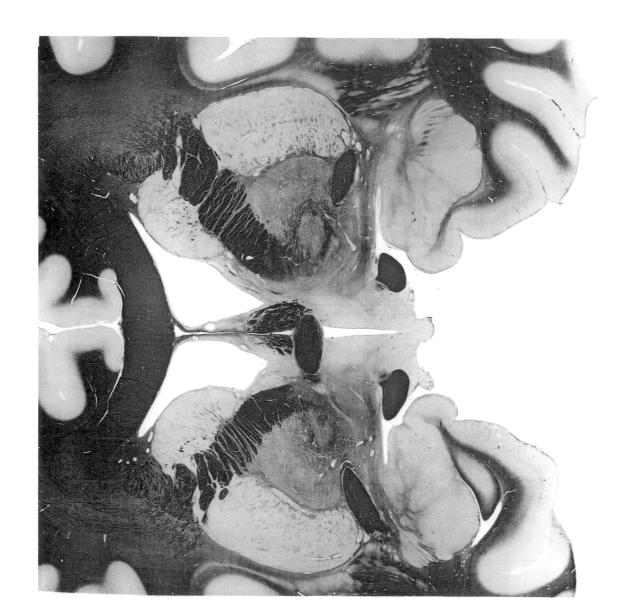

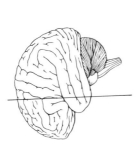

Figure II.22 Coronal section of the cerebral hemisphere through the anterior limb of the internal capsule, columns of the fornix, and amygdaloid complex. (×2.2)

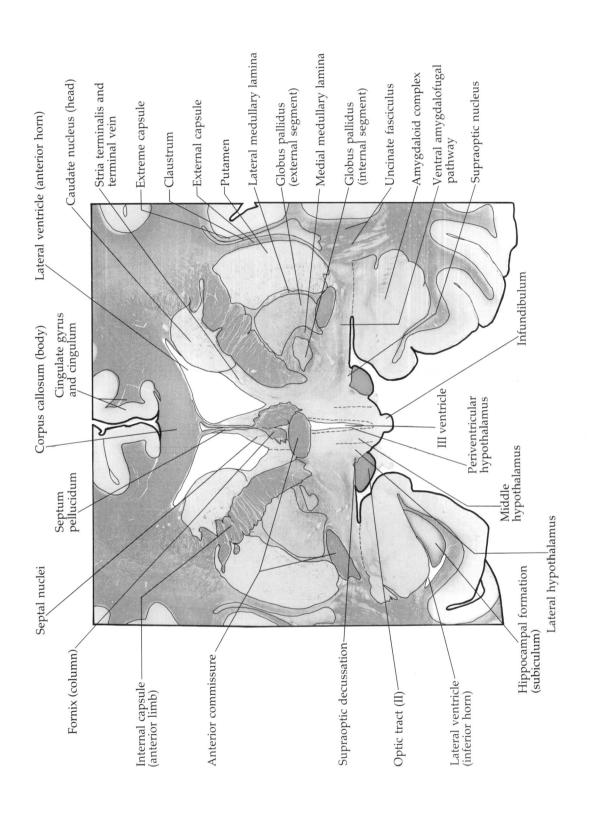

Septal nuclei

Corpus callosum (body)

Cingulate gyrus and cingulum

Septum pellucidum

Fornix (column)

Internal capsule (anterior limb)

Anterior commissure

Supraoptic decussation

Optic tract (II)

Lateral ventricle (inferior horn)

Hippocampal formation (subiculum)

Lateral hypothalamus

Lateral ventricle (anterior horn)

Caudate nucleus (head)

Stria terminalis and terminal vein

Extreme capsule

Claustrum

External capsule

Putamen

Lateral medullary lamina

Globus pallidus (external segment)

Medial medullary lamina

Globus pallidus (internal segment)

Uncinate fasciculus

Amygdaloid complex

Ventral amygdalofugal pathway

Supraoptic nucleus

Infundibulum

III ventricle

Periventricular hypothalamus

Middle hypothalamus

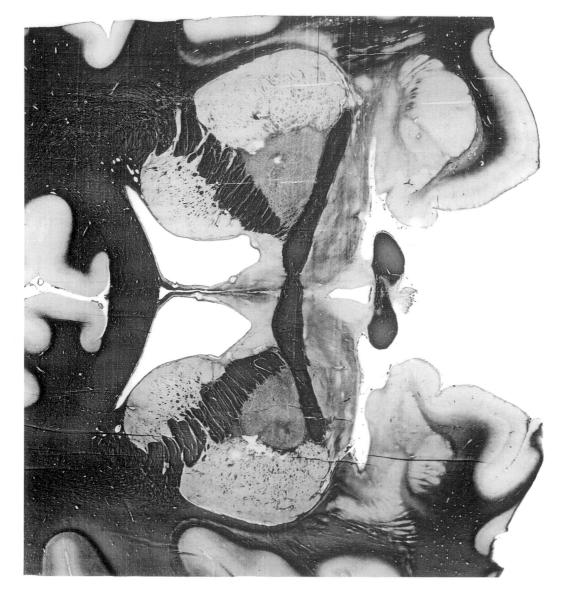

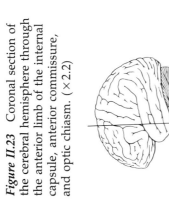

Figure II.23 Coronal section of the cerebral hemisphere through the anterior limb of the internal capsule, anterior commissure, and optic chiasm. (×2.2)

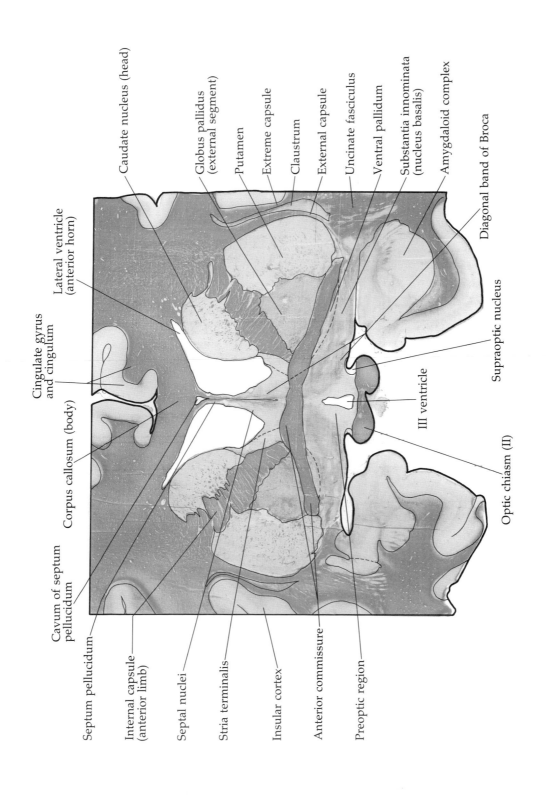

Caudate nucleus (head)

Globus pallidus
(external segment)

Putamen

Extreme capsule

Claustrum

External capsule

Uncinate fasciculus

Ventral pallidum

Substantia innominata
(nucleus basalis)

Amygdaloid complex

Diagonal band of Broca

Supraoptic nucleus

III ventricle

Optic chiasm (II)

Lateral ventricle
(anterior horn)

Cingulate gyrus
and cingulum

Cavum of septum
pellucidum

Corpus callosum (body)

Septum pellucidum

Internal capsule
(anterior limb)

Septal nuclei

Stria terminalis

Insular cortex

Anterior commissure

Preoptic region

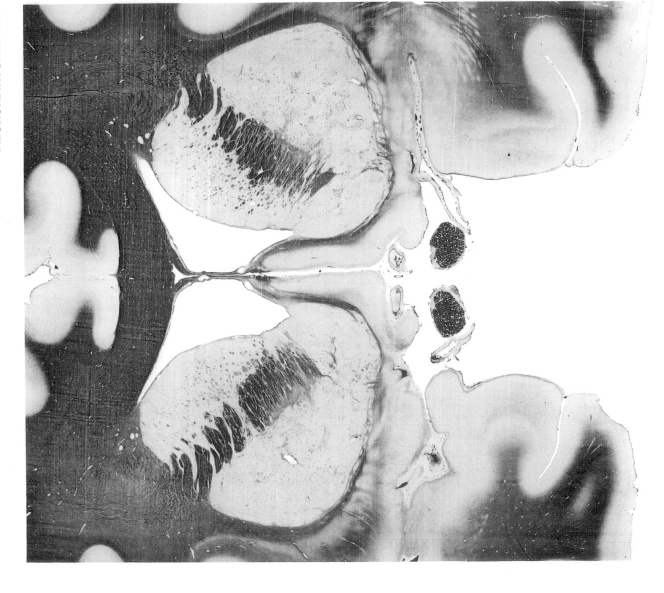

Figure II.24 Coronal section of the cerebral hemisphere through the anterior limb of the internal capsule and the head of caudate nucleus. (×2.4)

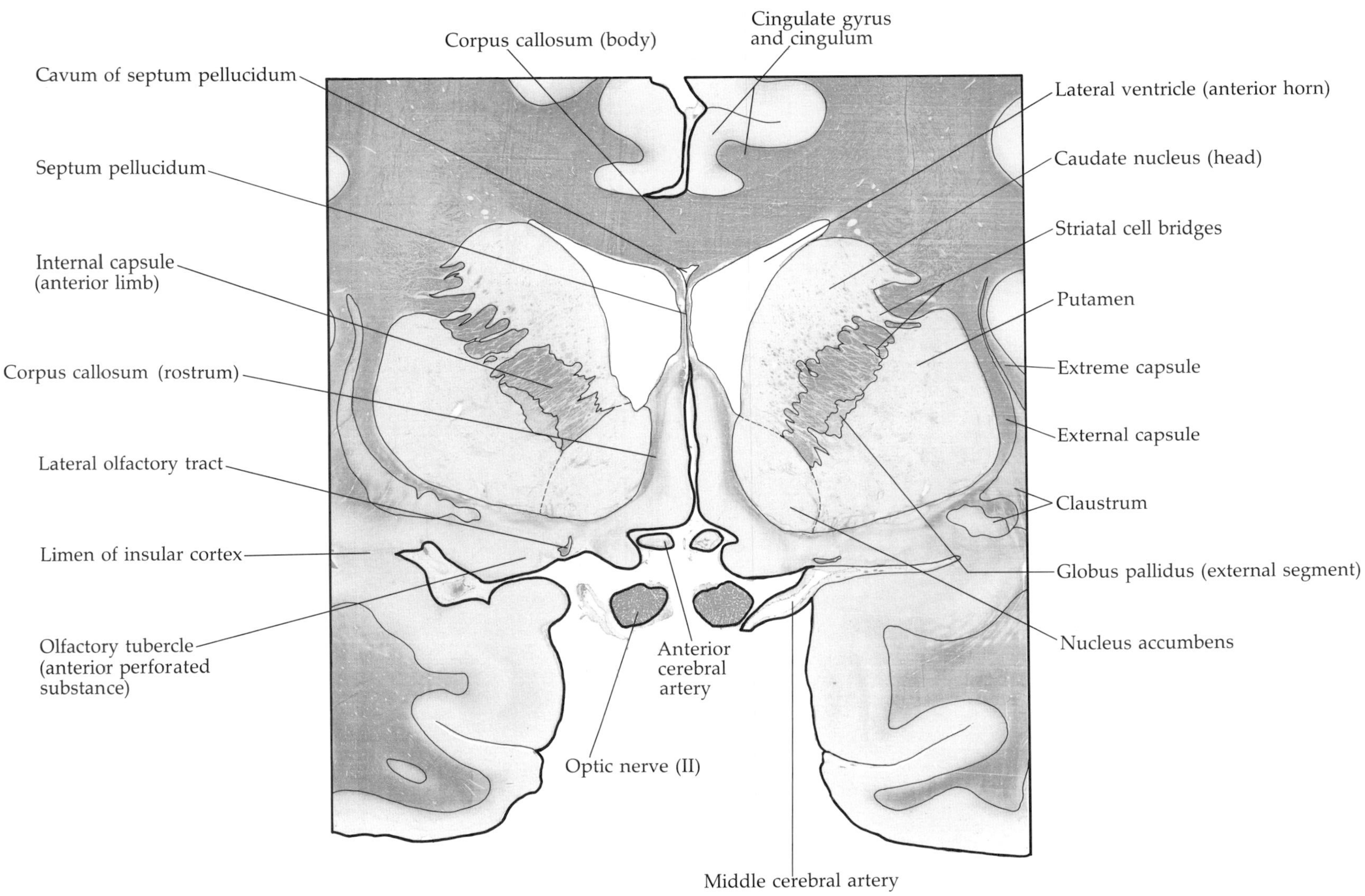

Cingulate gyrus
and cingulum

Corpus callosum (body)

Cavum of septum pellucidum

Septum pellucidum

Internal capsule
(anterior limb)

Corpus callosum (rostrum)

Lateral olfactory tract

Limen of insular cortex

Olfactory tubercle
(anterior perforated
substance)

Optic nerve (II)

Anterior
cerebral
artery

Middle cerebral artery

Lateral ventricle (anterior horn)

Caudate nucleus (head)

Striatal cell bridges

Putamen

Extreme capsule

External capsule

Claustrum

Globus pallidus (external segment)

Nucleus accumbens

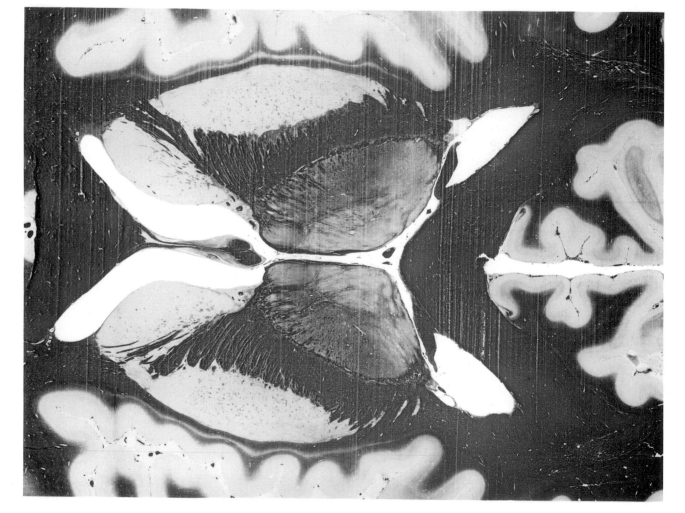

Figure II.25 Horizontal section of the cerebral hemisphere and diencephalon through the anterior thalamic nuclei. (×1.9)

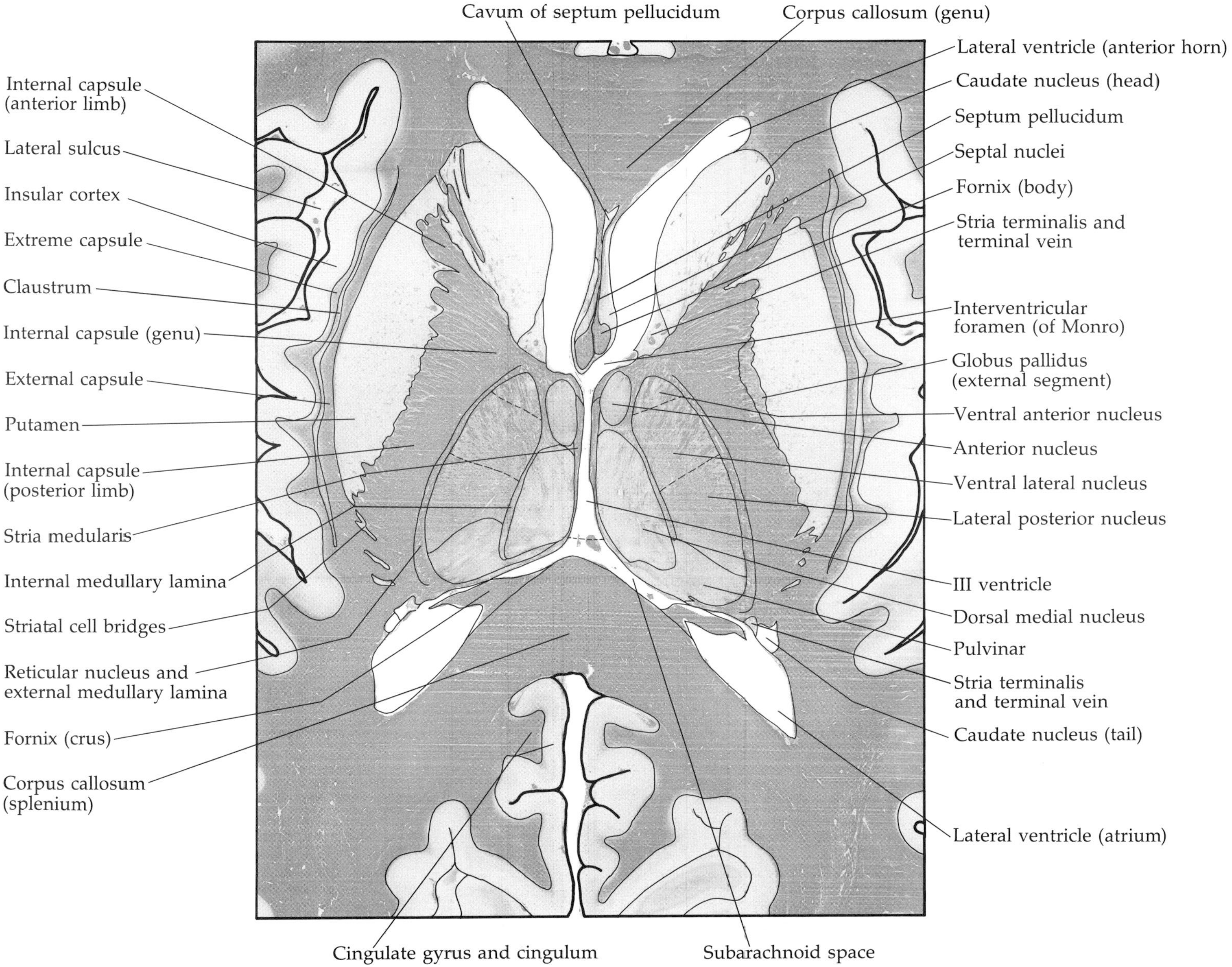

Corpus callosum (genu)

Cavum of septum pellucidum

Lateral ventricle (anterior horn)

Caudate nucleus (head)

Septum pellucidum

Septal nuclei

Fornix (body)

Stria terminalis and terminal vein

Interventricular foramen (of Monro)

Globus pallidus (external segment)

Ventral anterior nucleus

Anterior nucleus

Ventral lateral nucleus

Lateral posterior nucleus

III ventricle

Dorsal medial nucleus

Pulvinar

Stria terminalis and terminal vein

Caudate nucleus (tail)

Lateral ventricle (atrium)

Subarachnoid space

Cingulate gyrus and cingulum

Internal capsule (anterior limb)

Lateral sulcus

Insular cortex

Extreme capsule

Claustrum

Internal capsule (genu)

External capsule

Putamen

Internal capsule (posterior limb)

Stria medularis

Internal medullary lamina

Striatal cell bridges

Reticular nucleus and external medullary lamina

Fornix (crus)

Corpus callosum (splenium)

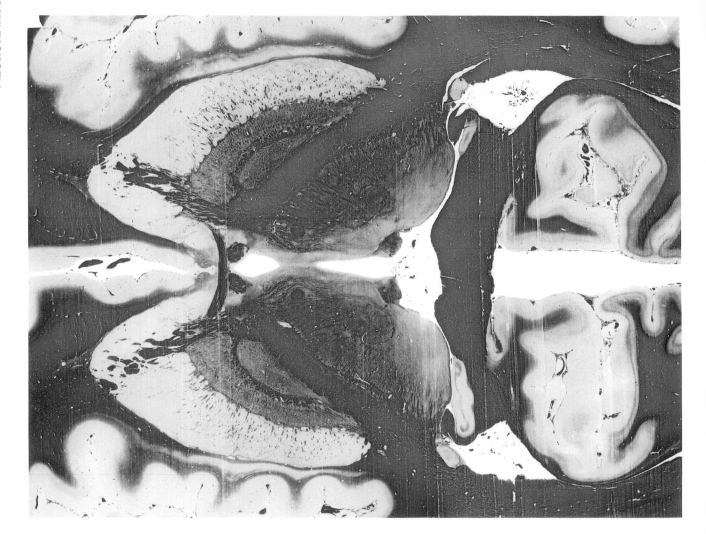

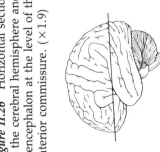

Figure II.26 Horizontal section of the cerebral hemisphere and diencephalon at the level of the anterior commissure. (×1.9)

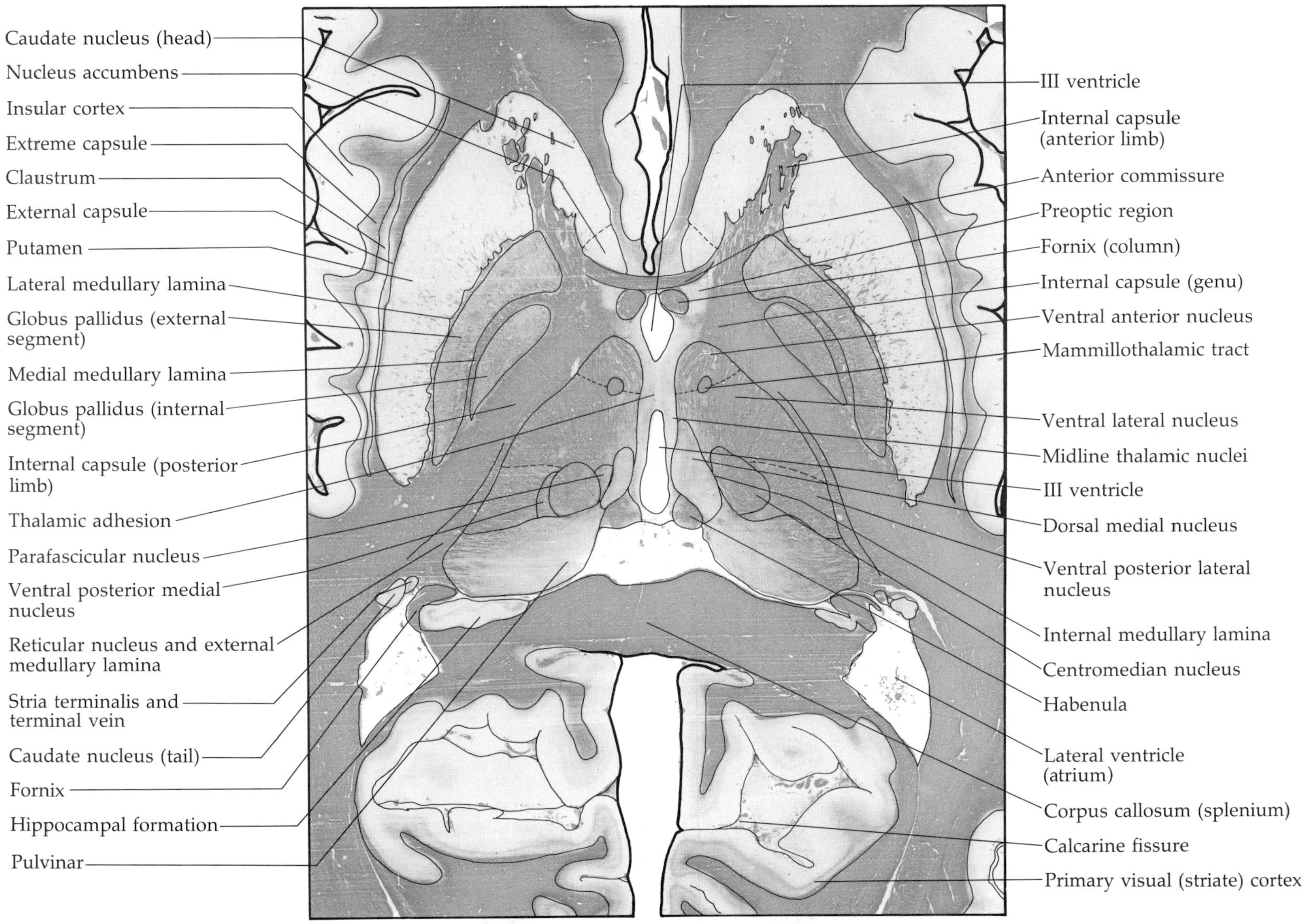

Caudate nucleus (head)

Nucleus accumbens

Insular cortex

Extreme capsule

Claustrum

External capsule

Putamen

Lateral medullary lamina

Globus pallidus (external segment)

Medial medullary lamina

Globus pallidus (internal segment)

Internal capsule (posterior limb)

Thalamic adhesion

Parafascicular nucleus

Ventral posterior medial nucleus

Reticular nucleus and external medullary lamina

Stria terminalis and terminal vein

Caudate nucleus (tail)

Fornix

Hippocampal formation

Pulvinar

III ventricle

Internal capsule (anterior limb)

Anterior commissure

Preoptic region

Fornix (column)

Internal capsule (genu)

Ventral anterior nucleus

Mammillothalamic tract

Ventral lateral nucleus

Midline thalamic nuclei

III ventricle

Dorsal medial nucleus

Ventral posterior lateral nucleus

Internal medullary lamina

Centromedian nucleus

Habenula

Lateral ventricle (atrium)

Corpus callosum (splenium)

Calcarine fissure

Primary visual (striate) cortex

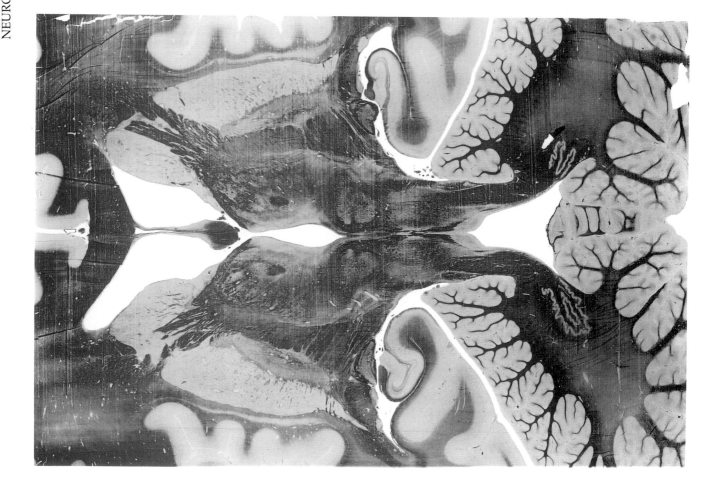

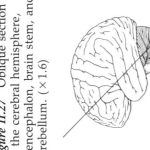

Figure II.27 Oblique section of the cerebral hemisphere, diencephalon, brain stem, and cerebellum. (×1.6)

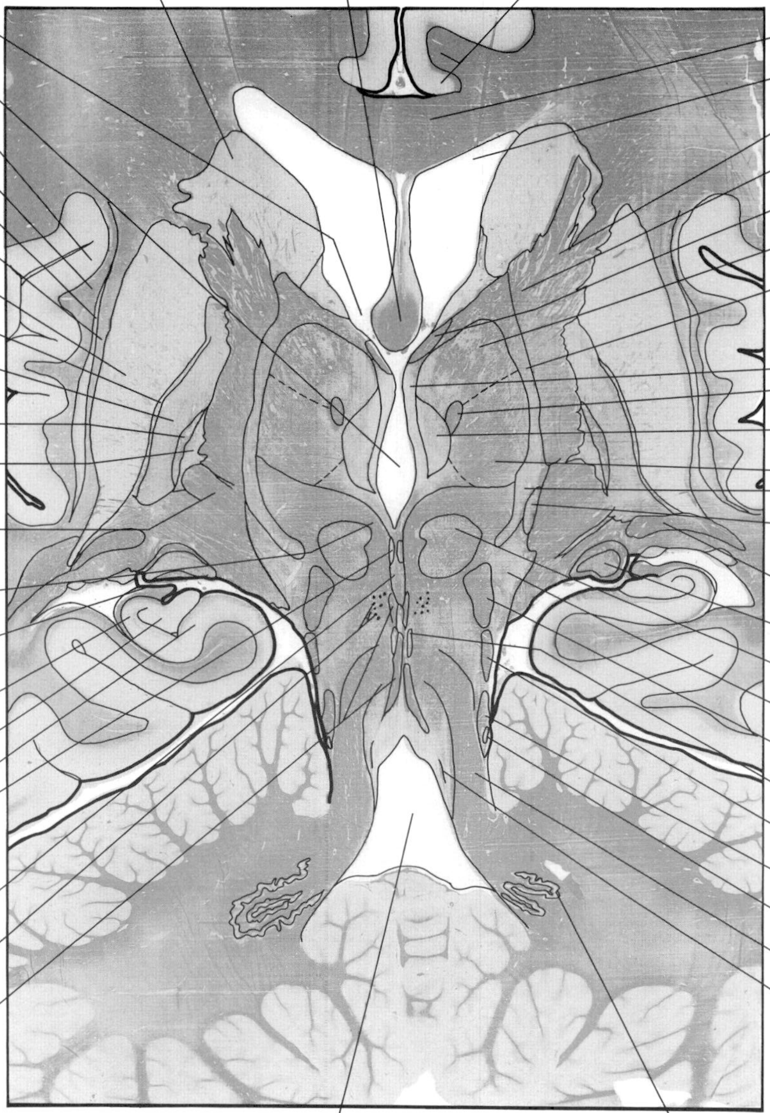

Cingulate gyrus and cingulum

Caudate nucleus (head) Fornix (body)

Interventricular foramen (of Monro)
III ventricle
Insular cortex
Extreme capsule
Claustrum
External capsule
Putamen
Lateral medullary lamina
Globus pallidus (external segment)
Medial medullary lamina
Globus pallidus (internal segment)
Internal capsule (posterior limb)
Habenulointerpeduncular tract
Fornix (fimbria)
Hippocampus
Dentate gyrus
Subiculum
Edinger-Westphal nucleus (III)
Oculomotor nucleus (III)
Fascicles of oculomotor nerve (III)
Medial longitudinal fasciculus

Corpus callosum (genu)
Lateral ventricle (anterior horn)
Internal capsule (anterior limb)
Internal capsule (genu)
Stria medullaris
Ventral anterior nucleus
Reticular nucleus and external medullary lamina
Midline thalamic nuclei
Mammillothalamic tract
Dorsal medial nucleus
Ventral lateral nucleus
Zona incerta
Subthalamic nucleus
Visual radiations
Lateral geniculate nucleus
Red nucleus
Substantia nigra
Medial lemniscus
Trochlear nucleus (IV)
Brachium of inferior colliculus
Lateral lemniscus
Nucleus of lateral lemniscus
Superior cerebellar peduncle
Mesencephalic trigeminal nucleus and tract (V)

Dentate nucleus

IV ventricle

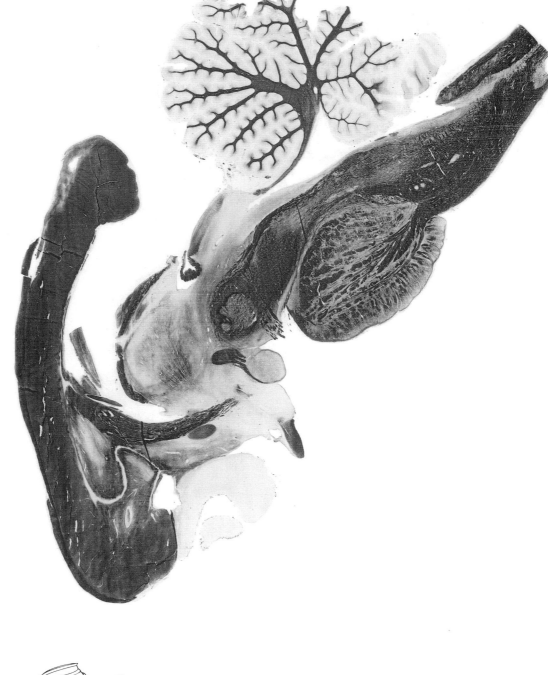

Figure II.28 Sagittal section of the cerebral hemisphere, diencephalon, brain stem, and cerebellum close to the midline. (×1.9)

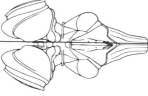

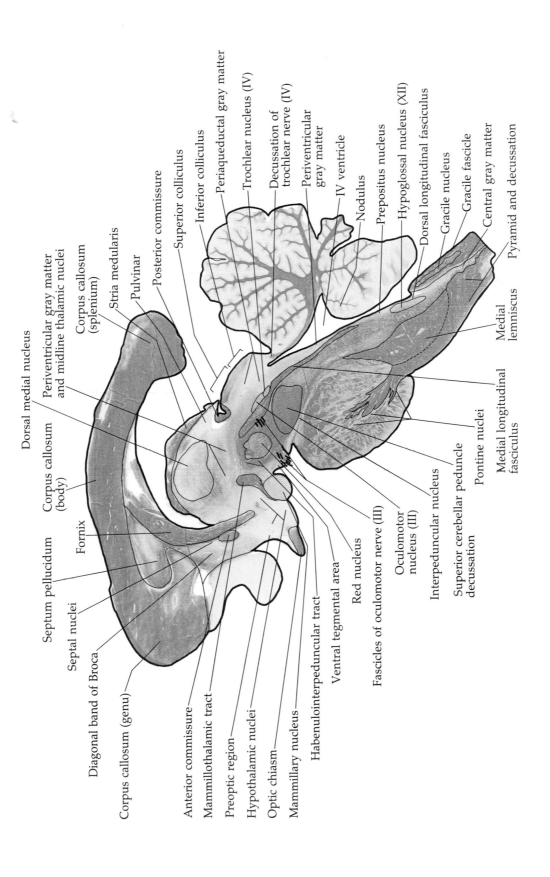

Dorsal medial nucleus

Periventricular gray matter
and midline thalamic nuclei

Corpus callosum
(body)

Corpus callosum
(splenium)

Stria medularis

Pulvinar

Posterior commissure

Superior colliculus

Inferior colliculus

Periaqueductal gray matter

Trochlear nucleus (IV)

Decussation of
trochlear nerve (IV)

Periventricular
gray matter

IV ventricle

Nodulus

Prepositus nucleus

Hypoglossal nucleus (XII)

Dorsal longitudinal fasciculus

Gracile nucleus

Gracile fascicle

Central gray matter

Pyramid and decussation

Medial
lemniscus

Septum pellucidum

Septal nuclei

Diagonal band of Broca

Corpus callosum (genu)

Anterior commissure

Mammillothalamic tract

Preoptic region

Hypothalamic nuclei

Optic chiasm

Mammillary nucleus

Habenulointerpeduncular tract

Ventral tegmental area

Red nucleus

Fascicles of oculomotor nerve (III)

Oculomotor
nucleus (III)

Interpeduncular nucleus

Superior cerebellar peduncle
decussation

Pontine nuclei

Medial longitudinal
fasciculus

Fornix

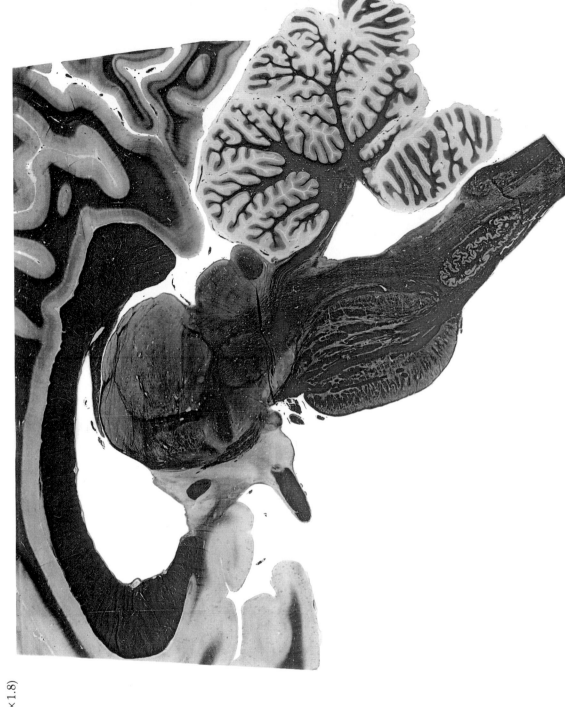

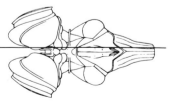

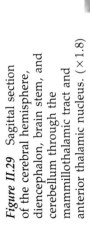

Figure II.29 Sagittal section of the cerebral hemisphere, diencephalon, brain stem, and cerebellum through the mammillothalamic tract and anterior thalamic nucleus. (×1.8)

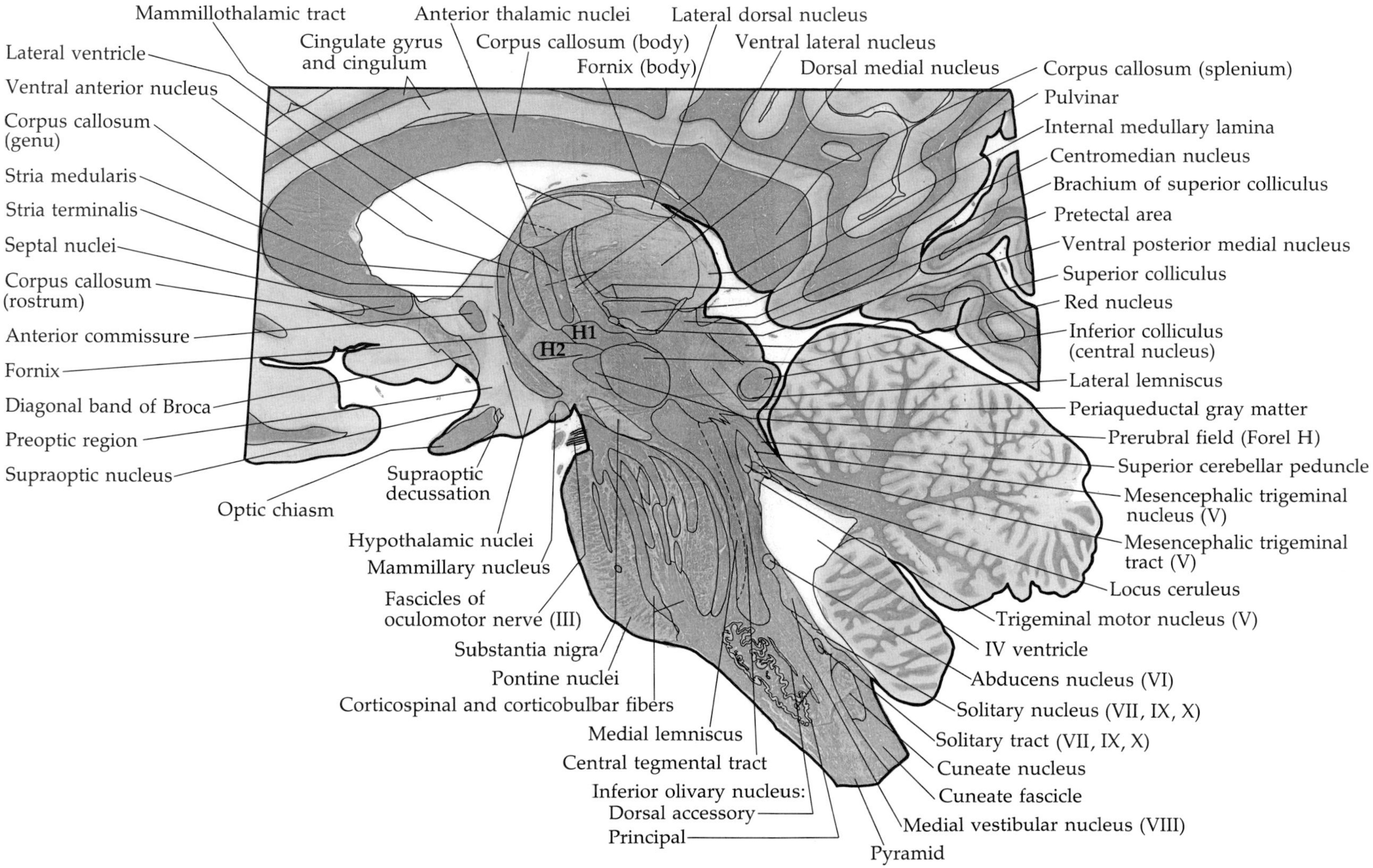

Lateral dorsal nucleus

Mammillothalamic tract

Anterior thalamic nuclei

Ventral lateral nucleus

Cingulate gyrus
and cingulum

Corpus callosum (body)

Dorsal medial nucleus

Fornix (body)

Corpus callosum (splenium)

Pulvinar

Internal medullary lamina

Centromedian nucleus

Brachium of superior colliculus

Pretectal area

Ventral posterior medial nucleus

Superior colliculus

Red nucleus

Inferior colliculus
(central nucleus)

Lateral lemniscus

Periaqueductal gray matter

Prerubral field (Forel H)

Superior cerebellar peduncle

Mesencephalic trigeminal
nucleus (V)

Mesencephalic trigeminal
tract (V)

Locus ceruleus

Trigeminal motor nucleus (V)

IV ventricle

Abducens nucleus (VI)

Solitary nucleus (VII, IX, X)

Solitary tract (VII, IX, X)

Cuneate nucleus

Cuneate fascicle

Medial vestibular nucleus (VIII)

Pyramid

Principal

Inferior olivary nucleus:
Dorsal accessory

Central tegmental tract

Medial lemniscus

Corticospinal and corticobulbar fibers

Pontine nuclei

Substantia nigra

Fascicles of
oculomotor nerve (III)

Mammillary nucleus

Hypothalamic nuclei

Optic chiasm

Supraoptic
decussation

H1

H2

Lateral ventricle

Ventral anterior nucleus

Corpus callosum
(genu)

Stria medularis

Stria terminalis

Septal nuclei

Corpus callosum
(rostrum)

Anterior commissure

Fornix

Diagonal band of Broca

Preoptic region

Supraoptic nucleus

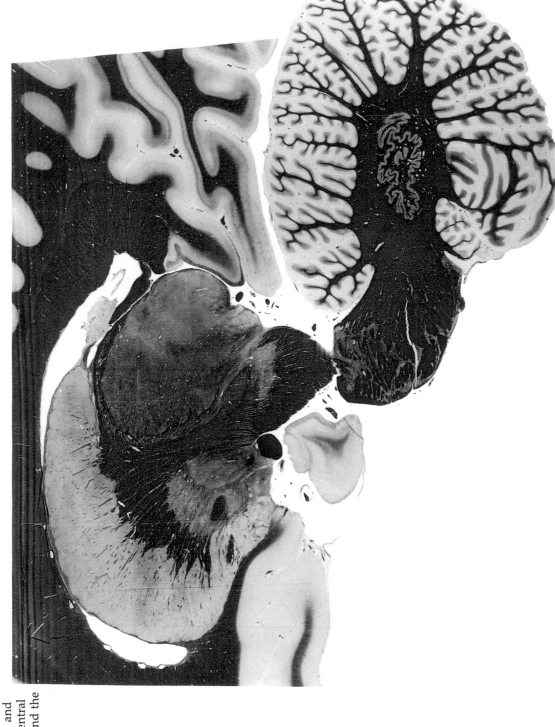

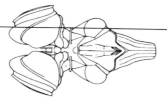

Figure II.30 Sagittal section of the cerebral hemisphere, diencephalon, brain stem, and cerebellum through the ventral posterior lateral nucleus and the dentate nucleus. (×1.9)

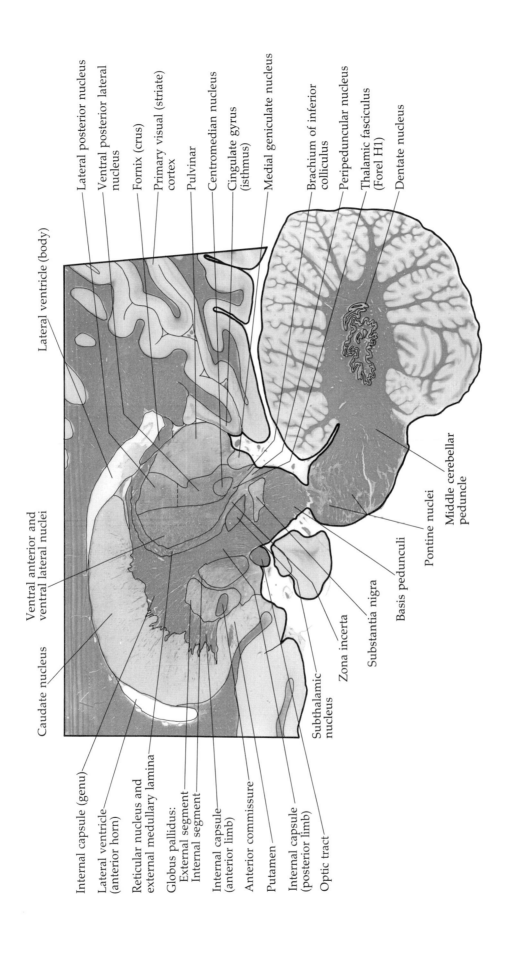

Lateral posterior nucleus

Ventral posterior lateral nucleus

Fornix (crus)

Primary visual (striate) cortex

Pulvinar

Centromedian nucleus

Cingulate gyrus (isthmus)

Medial geniculate nucleus

Brachium of inferior colliculus

Peripeduncular nucleus

Thalamic fasciculus (Forel H1)

Dentate nucleus

Lateral ventricle (body)

Ventral anterior and ventral lateral nuclei

Caudate nucleus

Internal capsule (genu)

Lateral ventricle (anterior horn)

Reticular nucleus and external medullary lamina

Globus pallidus:
External segment
Internal segment

Internal capsule (anterior limb)

Anterior commissure

Putamen

Internal capsule (posterior limb)

Optic tract

Subthalamic nucleus

Zona incerta

Substantia nigra

Basis pedunculi

Pontine nuclei

Middle cerebellar peduncle

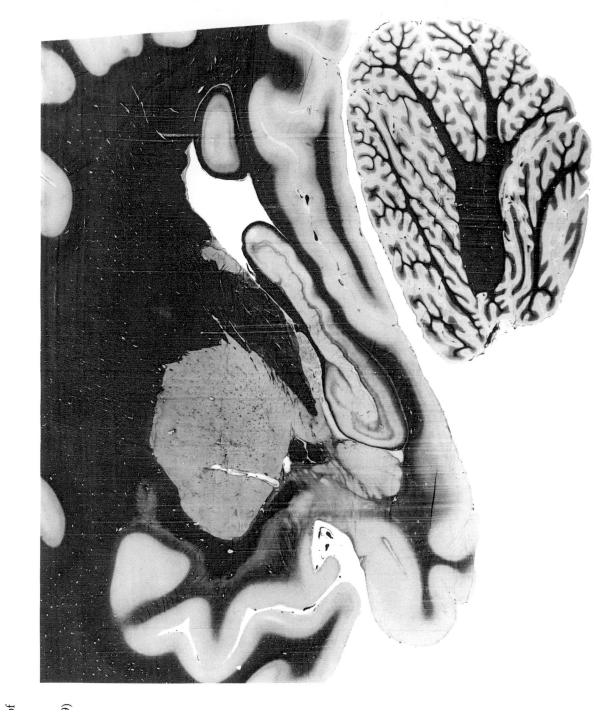

Figure II.31 Sagittal section of the cerebral hemisphere and cerebellum through the amygdaloid complex and hippocampal formation. (×1.9)

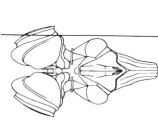

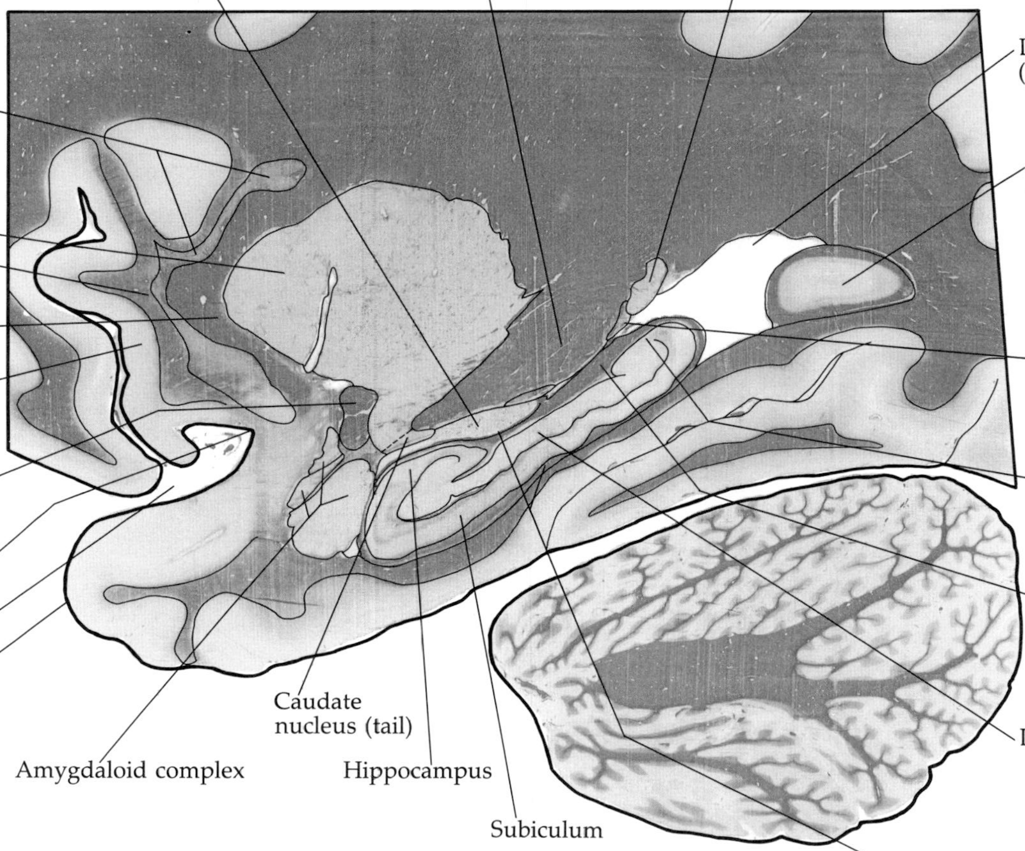

Caudate nucleus (tail)

Lateral ventricle (posterior horn)

Primary visual (striate) cortex

Stria terminalis

Hippocampus

Fornix (fimbria)

Dentate gyrus

Internal capsule (retrolenticular and sublenticular portions)

Alveus

Lateral ventricle (inferior horn)

Caudate nucleus (tail)

Hippocampus

Subiculum

Amygdaloid complex

Claustrum

Putamen

Extreme capsule

External capsule

Insular cortex

Anterior commissure

Limen of insular cortex

Lateral sulcus

Temporal pole

References

Andy, O. J., and Stephan, H. 1968. The septum of the human brain. J. Comp. Neurol. 133:383–410.

Bruce, A. 1901. A Topographical Atlas of the Spinal Cord. London: Williams and Norgate.

Carpenter, M. B., and Sutin, J. 1983. Human Neuroanatomy. Baltimore: Williams & Wilkins.

Crosby, E. C., Humphrey, T., and Lauer, E. W. 1962. Correlative Anatomy of the Nervous System. New York: Macmillan.

DeArmond, S. J., Fusco, M. M., and Dewey, M. M. 1976. Structure of the Human Brain. New York: Oxford University Press.

Haines, D. 1983. Neuroanatomy: An Atlas of Structures, Sections, and Systems. Baltimore: Urban & Schwarzenberg.

Nathan, P. W., and Smith, M. C. 1955. Long descending tracts in man. I. Review of present knowledge. Brain 78:248–303.

Olszewski, J., and Baxter, D. (eds.). 1982. Cytoarchitecture of the Human Brain Stem. Vol. I: Head, Neck, Upper Extremities. Basel: S. Karger.

Riley, H. A. 1943. An Atlas of the Basal Ganglia, Brain Stem and Spinal Cord. Baltimore: Williams & Wilkins.

Schaltenbrand, G., and Wahren, W. 1977. Atlas for Stereotaxy of the Human Brain. Chicago: Georg Thieme.

Williams, P. L., and Warwick, R. 1975. Functional Neuroanatomy of Man. Philadelphia: Saunders.

Index